MELATONIN

MIRACLE
MOLECULE

BEYOND SLEEP:

FIGHT INFECTIONS, DEGENERATIVE NEUROLOGIC DISEASE, DEPRESSION, AUTO-IMMUNITY, AGING, HEART DISEASE & CANCEER.

JOHN LIEURANCE, ND DC

Medical Disclaimer

This book details the author's personal experiences with and opinions about Melatonin.

The author and publisher are providing this book and its contents on an "as is" basis and make no representations or warranties of any kind with respect to this book or its contents. The author and publisher disclaim all such representations and warranties, including for example warranties of merchantability and healthcare for a particular purpose. In addition, the author and publisher do not represent or warrant that the information accessible via this book is accurate, complete, or current.

The statements made about products and services have not been evaluated by the U.S. Food and Drug Administration. They are not intended to diagnose, treat, cure, or prevent any condition or disease. Please consult with your own physician or healthcare specialist regarding the suggestions and recommendations made in this book.

Except as specifically stated in this book, neither the author or publisher, nor any authors, contributors, or other representatives will be liable for damages arising out of or in connection with the use of this book. This is a comprehensive limitation of liability that applies to all damages of any kind, including (without limitation) compensatory; direct, indirect, or consequential damages; loss of data, income, or profit; loss of or damage to property and claims of third parties.

You understand that this book is not intended as a substitute for consultation with a licensed healthcare practitioner, such as your physician. Before you begin any healthcare program, or change your lifestyle in any way, you will consult your physician or another licensed healthcare practitioner to ensure that you are in good health and that the examples contained in this book will not harm you.

This book provides content related to health issues. As such, use of this book implies your acceptance of this disclaimer.

DEDICATIONS

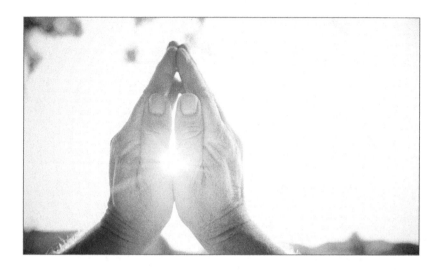

First and foremost, I would like to dedicate this book to my mother Pamela for always supporting and believing in me. I'm happy to say that she has been benefiting greatly from high-dose melatonin as well.

I'd also like to dedicate this book to Dr. Russell Reiter who has spent most of his career working to understand and share the secrets of melatonin and its functions, with the desire to showcase its potential role in our healthcare system. Also, Dr. Frank Shallenberger because without his suggestion that I personally start taking high doses of melatonin this book may have never been born.

I would further like to acknowledge Dr. Shallenberger for his tireless efforts over the years to highlight many powerful and natural strategies such as ozone and high-dose melatonin, professor Venkataramanujam Srinivasan for a lifelong dedication to conducting research unveiling the secrets of melatonin, colleagues such as Dr. Patrick Gentempo and his wife Lauri, Dr. Joe Mercola & Dr. Daniel Pompa. Also, my staff including Sarah Carnigie, Candace Johnson, Irene Melendez, Dr. Daniel Kirschner, and all the other people that have been on my journey to share melatonin's story.

Lastly, to all of the people that have trusted me and started their own journey using melatonin to improve their lives.

CONTENTS

Dedications .... *v*

1. Intro to the Miracle Molecule 1

2. Melatonin & Mental Emotional Stress 13

3. How Melatonin Supports the Mitochondria 29

4. Melatonin & Neurological Health 41

5. Melatonin & Immune System 51

6. Melatonin & Infections 77

7. Melatonin & Autoimmune Diseases 89

8. Melatonin & Cardiovascular 99

9. Melatonin & Sex Hormones 109

10. Melatonin & Degenerative Neurologic Disease 117

11. Melatonin & Gut 145

12. Melatonin for Jet Lag & Disrupted Sleep-Wake Cycle in Shift Workers ... 159

13. Melatonin & Skin 175

14. Melatonin, EMF & Melatonin Disruptors 193

15. Melatonin for Children 213

16. Melatonin for Diabetes 223

17. Cannabis & Sleep, Melatonin's Pot Connection 237

18. Melatonin for the Management of Liver Disorders 255

19. Melatonin & Cancer 279

20. Pineal Gland 305

21. Supra-Physiological Dosing 313

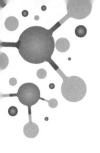

INTRO TO THE MIRACLE MOLECULE

Melatonin, commonly called the sleep hormone or the hormone of darkness, holds enormous importance which the public is in the dark about! Melatonin works for sleep; however, in this book you will find it works around the clock protecting you. Many doctors poorly understand melatonin and the public is told false and misleading information such as that it's dangerous to take too much or that the body will become reliant on melatonin, and you will stop making your own. I have interviewed the top scientists in the world, and I've read through almost all the research and have found that not only is melatonin safe in much higher doses than what is typically recommended, but it can be lifesaving and work on your health at a cellular level like no other substance can do. I have come to understand that this hormone has many medicinal properties outside of just assisting restorative sleep. As scientists dig deeper, they are finding new uses for melatonin in the treatment and prevention of many diseases. This has caused researchers and doctors to sitting up and taking notice of melatonin.

It's not surprising to me that this miracle molecule has been ignored by modern medicine. Big Pharma has tried extremely hard to reproduce a molecule that is structurally close to melatonin in an effort to have a molecule they can patent; however, they have not been successful. When you change this molecule even slightly it doesn't offer up the magic that natural melatonin does.

We live in a world where cures are not what Big Pharma is putting their research dollars into, nor are budgets allocated to "un patent-able" molecules like melatonin. What they prefer is a long-term dosing schedule that keeps the dollars rolling in, stock price up, and the shareholders happy. If you're looking for a miraculous compound that can heal, cure, and prevent disease, you found it with melatonin.

Big Pharma owns the media now and COVID censorship is at its worst in the USA. Even with recent research showing melatonin can be lifesaving for those infected with COVID-19, it has been silenced. I have even been silenced by the FDA and FTC. I have shared a plethora of scientific data on my MitoZen.com site related to melatonin and its relationship to viral infection and COVID-19, with subsequent explanations on the mechanisms and links to leading hospitals who are administering doses in the hundreds of milligrams. I was asked to take it all down. Denying the public this crucial information is so they can keep the public attention on vaccines touted to be the answer to this pandemic.

Please know, the vaccines can do nothing to keep you from becoming ill with COVID—only prevent the severe and critical stages of the disease. This severe stage is rare and is typically found in aged demographics and individuals with poor health. Chapter 6 covers how melatonin can protect you from these effects and many other serious and lethal infections such as EBOLA and COVID.

Melatonin may be a better answer than vaccines, with zero risks. However, this would never see the light of day due to the current medical system, which is sadly based on money and politics. It's up to YOU to look outside of mainstream media and demand answers, understand risks associated with vaccines, as well as judge alternative options, and the potential safety and efficacy based on years of research. This book aims to unravel the hidden benefits of melatonin and shed some light on its potential to be what I call the "miracle molecule" versus a mere sleep hormone.

In this book, I will dig into all the research and provide my own insights surrounding the use of high-dose melatonin with my own patients. But first, let me begin with what sparked my interest in melatonin and its benefits.

My first encounter with high dose melatonin

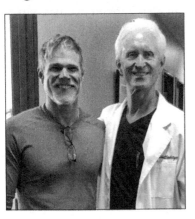

I was first introduced to using higher than normal doses of melatonin when I attended a large presentation in Fort Lauderdale in 2017. A presenter was discussing using melatonin in extremely high doses.

The doctor sitting next to me said that this was one of the most exciting clinical pearls he had learned in recent times, and he had begun using high doses of melatonin for his patients in his own clinic. This got my attention!

Shortly after, I was doing an internship with Dr. Frank Sha llenberger in Reno Nevada, and I was shocked to see Dr. Sha llenberger utilizing hundreds of milligrams of melatonin for his cancer patients as well as for many of his neurologic cases such as Alzheimer's, Parkinson's, and TBI or traumatic brain injuries.[1] [2] [3]

I myself suffered a brain injury from chronic Lyme disease and mold illness and had arranged to be a patient with Dr. Shallenberger while I was there interning.

I was having problems with finding correct words in speech, difficulty with memory, and concentration. Dr. Sha llenberger prescribed 200 mg of melatonin taken orally at bedtime. He even suggested if I could tolerate it, to take 200 mg each day for my condition. Wow, wouldn't I sleep all day? Maybe not, we will get into this later.

This is where my journey began into the miraculous benefits of melatonin!

The more I started to dig into melatonin research, the more excited I became, not just for myself, but for my patients as well.

Melatonin works at the deepest cellular level, which involves the cell's ability to make "clean" and efficient energy. Melatonin is almost like a quarterback of the cell. And we all know what happens when someone has a great quarterback like with Tampa Bay in 2021. Or what occurs when the quarterback gets sacked, and the play goes dead!

If you don't understand football, then understand that the game begins and ends with this position, but let' get back to the game of biology. This game is played inside our cells with many individual players - and melatonin's critical position as a quarterback! When we speak about the chemistry that's occurring in every cell of your body, we need to consider the burning of glucose as energy in the presence of oxygen. This process is the heart of the energy of life within your body and each cell.

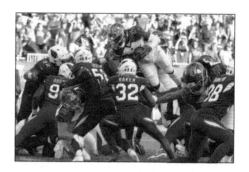

We're going to be taking a deep dive into this process and how melatonin is vitally important to keep this process or "game" organized and clean, just like a quarterback in football calling the shots.[4]

When one starts to ponder and consider the amazing benefits shown in research that has been conducted over the last several decades, it is difficult to wrap one's head around why melatonin is not used more commonly for a multitude of conditions. Due to melatonin's ability to regulate your body and cells at such a deep level, it is an important molecule to consider with many different diseases that are rooted in chronic inflammation. Most diseases are rooted in inflammation which is itself rooted in dirty and inefficient energy production at a cellular level. In this book you will discover that poor cellular energy leads to a build-up of toxins, thus allowing infections to run wild.

When researchers first started to study this miracle molecule, I had a difficult time determining the benefits that melatonin provides to all animals including humans. In fact, when scientists first started studying melatonin, they didn't find any health benefits. Not surprising since melatonin is primarily involved with stress protection and when giving melatonin to animal models in a normal environment (stress-free) they saw no benefit. In other words, they

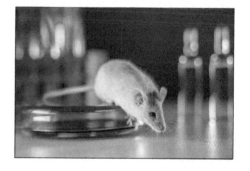

gave melatonin to mice that were living at the Ritz Carlton (stress-free) and they did not see a significant difference in the melatonin group versus the placebo group. Again, this is mainly due to melatonin's ability to protect the body at a cellular level from stress.

It was not until they started to stress the animals in the study that melatonin's miracle healing abilities began to shine. What they did is place them in tiny tubes with just little pin holes for several hours a day to simulate a stressful situation for these animals. Then when they looked at the melatonin group, they saw significant improvements. The melatonin group had less weight loss, lived significantly longer, and avoided diseases when compared to the animals that had no melatonin.

If you're looking to slow aging, improve brain function, or maybe you're suffering from a disease that's rooted in a lack of efficient energy production at a cellular level which is resulting in excess inflammation then this book is for you, as we'll take a close look at how melatonin can quench this inflammation or "cytokine storm".

The lack of adequate secretion of melatonin can affect these cellular processes and increase the risk of several disorders including infections like Lyme, influenza, and COVID-19, as well as cancer, and autoimmune diseases.[5][6][7][8]

Later, we will discuss melatonin supplements and how you can use them to restore optimum health by protecting your body against oxidation and inflammation at the cellular level.

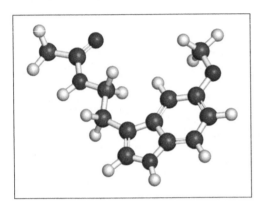

What is melatonin?

Generally, melatonin is referred to as the "hormone of darkness" and is naturally produced in our body. This hormone is stored in our pineal gland during the daytime and then released by the gland as the night approaches or when the body is exposed to darkness.[9] [10] [11] Besides the pineal gland, melatonin is also secreted by our mitochondria in all cells throughout the body.

Furthermore, melatonin is also produced in your gut for protection purposes, and to help stimulate microbiome health. Some amount of melatonin is also produced within eye fluids, called intraocular fluid.

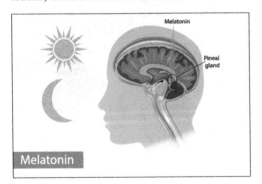

Melatonin is basically a methoxyindole compound, which, under normal environmental conditions, follows an endogenous rhythm of secretion. This means the secretion of melatonin is regulated by the endogenous or internal rhythm set by your body's own biological clock or the circadian rhythm.

The endogenous rhythm of melatonin secretion is attuned to the cycle of bright light during daytime and darkness in the evening and night. The intensity of light your body is exposed to is able to synchronize or suppress melatonin production.

That's not all.

There are various factors at play when it comes to the amount and timing of melatonin secretion.

The suprachiasmatic nuclei in the brain play a vital role in determining the amount of melatonin secreted in your body at different times of the day. Moreover, the production of melatonin also adjusts to the length of the night or darkness to be more in phase with the seasons.

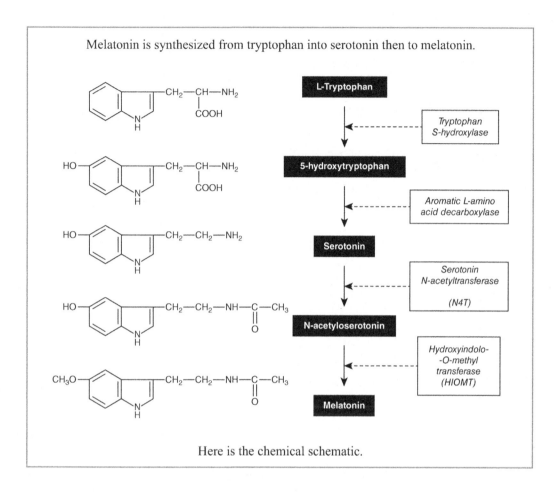

Here is the chemical schematic.

What is considered the primary function of melatonin?

The primary physiological function of melatonin for the sleep-wake cycle is to convey information about your exposure to light and darkness to all organs, especially the brain. The information conveyed by melatonin can then be used by the organs for the organization of different functions that respond to the changes in photoperiod, such as seasonal rhythms.

In addition, daily melatonin secretion serves as a robust biochemical mechanism signaling nighttime. This mechanism can

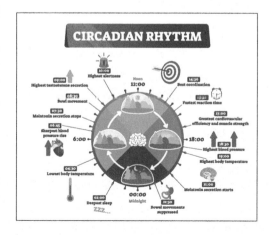

be used by the tissues and organs for the organization and regulation of the circadian rhythm.

Melatonin can further stabilize and strengthen the coupling of circadian rhythms with the sleep-wake rhythms and the body's core temperature. The circadian organization controls such things as antioxidant and immune defenses, glucose regulation, and hemostasis - which also depend on the biochemical signals carried by melatonin.

Melatonin has generated a great deal of interest as a therapeutic modality for various diseases, particularly diseases related to poor sleep. You would be shocked to find out how many diseases are correlated with poor sleep. This miracle molecule possesses antioxidant, anti-inflammatory, endothelial-protective, and anticoagulant properties.

This is just a glimpse of what melatonin can do. We will learn a lot more about the functions and benefits of melatonin as we move through the next chapters of this book.

The pineal gland is the primary seat of the production of melatonin. We discuss the pineal gland in the chapter on pineal in great depth.

History of pineal science?

The first evidence that the Pineal gland produced a biologically active hormone, now famously known as melatonin, was revealed by the medicinal potential of the pineal tissue extracts obtained from bovine sources. It was found that this extract of the pineal gland could modify melatonin pigmentation in frogs by regulating melanin aggregation.

Melatonin got its name due to its particular property to regulate melanin aggregation, thus prompting the researchers to name it melatonin. These findings later led to the attempts to use melatonin for treating vitiligo, which proved to be effective. We will dive deep into this in chapter 13. This research also led to the incidental discovery of the sleep-promoting effects of melatonin.[12][13][14][15]

The secretion, release, and storage of melatonin

Melatonin is the primary hormone secreted in the pineal gland. It is synthesized in response to darkness giving it the name, "the hormone of darkness".[16]

Melatonin is produced from a hormone called serotonin. Serotonin is a neurotransmitter derived from the amino acid called tryptophan through a chain of enzymatic reactions. Serotonin is acetylated in the pineal gland and later, methylated to produce melatonin.

The last two steps in this pathway involve the conversion of serotonin to NAS (N-acetylserotonin) catalyzed by another enzyme called AANAT (arylalkylamine N acetyltransferase). This is followed by the conversion of NAS to melatonin. This process is further catalyzed by the enzyme HIOMT (hydroxyl-indole-O-methyltransferase).[17][18]

You might be wondering how the whole process begins? It so happens that the pineal gland receives signals from some fibers called the postganglionic fibers, thus leading to the production and release of serotonin. The same process also results in an increased production of cyclic AMP, thereby activating AANAT, which is critical to the secretion of melatonin.

Melatonin is secreted by the pineal gland and released into the bloodstream through which it can penetrate all tissues. The pineal gland is stimulated to secrete melatonin primarily in the presence of darkness, whereas exposure to bright light can inhibit these mechanisms thereby reducing melatonin production.[19][20]

The mechanisms behind the unique pattern of melatonin secretion during the darkness cycle can be attributed to the activities of NAT, a rate-limiting enzyme that is lower during daylight and tends to peak during the dark phase. So, when the NAT levels are higher, which is when you are exposed to darkness, the melatonin levels would peak and vice versa.

However, the activities of another enzyme called methyltransferase involved in the conversion of serotonin to melatonin does not show this form of regulation linked to the pattern of light exposure. Darkness is the primary criterion needed for melatonin secretion; there are also a few other factors linked to methyltransferase that could determine the amount of melatonin secreted in the body.

Understanding the role of the blood-brain barrier in melatonin production

Interestingly, the pineal gland, despite being part of the brain during its embryological stage (while it is still being formed in the fetus), is situated outside the blood-brain barrier. As a result, it loses its direct connection with the brain or the central nervous system.

This explains why the pineal gland must rely on the stimulation by sympathetic nerves and serotonin for regulating melatonin production.

The ability of the pineal gland to escape the restrictions imposed by the blood-brain barrier also accounts for its capacity to have a larger uptake of tryptophan, allowing for an increased melatonin production in response to darkness.

The freedom to escape the blood-brain barrier offers relative protection to melatonin against premature enzymatic degradation leading to a 10 to 20-fold rise in melatonin levels.

We will discuss the exact role of the blood-brain barrier as we move to future chapters.

Right now, as we are discussing the various processes involved in melatonin secretion, it is essential to understand that the production of this hormone is somewhat independent of the blood-brain barrier, thanks to its unique location.[21]

How is melatonin secretion regulated?

The daily rhythmic production of melatonin in the pineal gland is driven by the circadian clock. This 'clock', in turn, is regulated by a region in the brain called the suprachiasmatic nuclei that express a series of clock genes, which tend to oscillate continuously throughout the day.

This oscillation is synchronized with the solar day and night through light rays falling onto the retina. The suprachiasmatic nuclei are linked to the pineal gland via a complex pathway. The pathway passes through different areas in the brain in the spinal cord, ultimately reaching the pineal gland.

During the daytime, the suprachiasmatic nuclei block melatonin secretion by sending inhibitory signals to the pineal gland. However, at night, the suprachiasmatic nuclei are not as active. So obviously, the inhibition induced during the daytime is withdrawn, following which the melatonin production is resumed with a greater force by the pineal gland.

From this, it is clear that light is the most important regulator for melatonin production. First, it can reset a specific part of the brain - the suprachiasmatic nuclei - and control the timing of melatonin secretion. Second, exposure of the body to light, or to be precise the LACK of light during the biological night-time reduces melatonin secretion.[22]

Safety profile and administration of melatonin for sleep

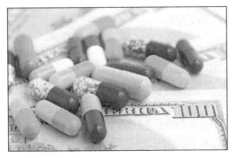

If you google Melatonin multiple sites including WebMD state reported side effects including dizziness, headache, nausea, or agitation can occur. However, these were based on a study where these side effects happened just as much in the placebo group. This creates confusion for the public and does not accurately reflect the real potential side effects of melatonin. Could this be our beloved Big Pharma putting out false information to discourage melatonin use?[23]

With regard to the administration of melatonin in the form of a supplement for sleep aid, the time of administration might be as important as the actual dosage in determining its effectiveness to support sleep. For example, research studies have found that when melatonin is administered at bedtime, it may not be effective unless high doses are used. On the other hand, when smaller doses of melatonin are administered about 2 to 4 hours before bedtime, it tends to be more effective in reducing sleep latency.

But what is sleep latency? It is the period that we usually spend waiting to fall asleep after going to bed. Higher sleep latency is common in patients who suffer from severe mental stress, depression, or pain disorders like arthritis.

The use of melatonin during early evening hours, even in low doses, could help reduce the latency period and allow you to fall asleep shortly after your head hits the pillow. That is the beauty of melatonin! It all depends on when you use it, and how well you integrate it with your body's internal circadian rhythm. [24][25][26]

Obviously, if you were using a product like Sandman with 200 mg of melatonin this would be considered a high dose, and the application time would not be a factor. Yet, if you're using smaller dosing for sleep you might consider taking your melatonin earlier.

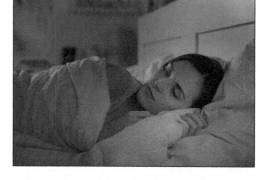

The safety profile of melatonin therapy is quite reassuring and much superior to the commonly used sleep-inducing agents, including sedatives. For example, unlike benzodiazepines and Zolpidem, melatonin therapy is not known to cause dependence and withdrawal symptoms.

There have been studies done where dosages reaching the equivalent of 150,000 mg in a 150 lb. human had no toxic effect.[27][28][29][30]

What is the difference between the pharmacological and physiological effects of melatonin?

The difference between the physiological effects produced by melatonin secreted in the body vs the pharmacological effects created by exogenous melatonin needs to be understood clearly.

A "physiological" dose refers to the plasma level of the same magnitude as that produced during the nocturnal peak. A pharmacological dose, on the other hand, usually provides supra-physiological, or higher than the normal, physiological levels of melatonin. When a lower dose of melatonin is used, a narrow hormonal signal is created that may not mimic the expected effects of endogenous secretion.

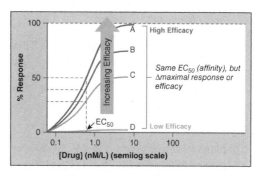

This is the reason why most experts recommend using supra-physiological doses of melatonin, to create signals that could bring about the expected improvements in sleep and other health-related parameters.[31][32]

Conclusion

Melatonin is such an important hormone, perhaps the most important one we make. Its therapeutic value reaches into almost every disease known to us and we will be diving into many of them in this book. We will get into the substantial body of research done over the years which has expanded our understanding of this amazing molecule and demystified the potential benefits of this hormone.

Melatonin is indeed the miracle molecule and is made in every cell of your body and in the miracle gland, the pineal. It is time we dig deeper into all aspects of this hormone and learn how it can help us be more resilient to stress, stay healthier, live longer, and enjoy more vitality.

Reference

1. Tordjman, S., Chokron, S., Delorme, R., Charrier, A., Bellissant, E., Jaafari, N., & Fougerou, C. (2017). Melatonin: Pharmacology, Functions and Therapeutic Benefits. *Current neuropharmacology*, *15*(3), 434–443. https://doi.org/10.2174/1570159X14666161228122115

2. MELATONIN: Overview, Uses, Side Effects, Precautions, Interactions, Dosing and Reviews (webmd.com)

3. Kostoglou-Athanassiou I. (2013). Therapeutic applications of melatonin. *Therapeutic advances in endocrinology and metabolism*, *4*(1), 13–24. https://doi.org/10.1177/2042018813476084

4. Savage RA, Zafar N, Yohannan S, et al. Melatonin. [Updated 2021 Aug 15]. In: StatPearls [Internet]. Treasure Island (FL): StatPearls Publishing; 2021 Jan-. Available from: https://www.ncbi.nlm.nih.gov/books/NBK534823/

5. Lin, G. J., Huang, S. H., Chen, S. J., Wang, C. H., Chang, D. M., & Sytwu, H. K. (2013). Modulation by melatonin of the pathogenesis of inflammatory autoimmune diseases. *International journal of molecular sciences*, *14*(6), 11742–11766. https://doi.org/10.3390/ijms140611742

6. Arushanian EB. [MELATONIN TREATMENT OF AUTOIMMUNE AND ALLERGIC PATHOLOGY]. Eksp Klin Farmakol. 2015;78(8):29-34. Russian. PMID: 26591580.

7. Cutando A, López-Valverde A, Arias-Santiago S, DE Vicente J, DE Diego RG. Role of melatonin in cancer treatment. Anticancer Res. 2012 Jul;32(7):2747-53. PMID: 22753734.

8. Wang, Y., Wang, P., Zheng, X., & Du, X. (2018). Therapeutic strategies of melatonin in cancer patients: a systematic review and meta-analysis. *OncoTargets and therapy*, *11*, 7895–7908. https://doi.org/10.2147/OTT.S174100

9. Costello, R. B., Lentino, C. V., Boyd, C. C., O'Connell, M. L., Crawford, C. C., Sprengel, M. L., & Deuster, P. A. (2014). The effectiveness of melatonin for promoting healthy sleep: a rapid evidence assessment of the literature. *Nutrition journal*, *13*, 106. https://doi.org/10.1186/1475-2891-13-106

10. Xie Z, Chen F, Li WA, Geng X, Li C, Meng X, Feng Y, Liu W, Yu F. A review of sleep disorders and melatonin. Neurol Res. 2017 Jun;39(6):559-565. doi: 10.1080/01616412.2017.1315864. Epub 2017 May 1. PMID: 28460563.

11. Ferracioli-Oda E, Qawasmi A, Bloch MH. Meta-analysis: melatonin for the treatment of primary sleep disorders. PLoS One. 2013 May 17;8(5):e63773. doi: 10.1371/journal. pone.0063773. PMID: 23691095; PMCID: PMC3656905.

12. Paus, Ralf & Bomirski, A. (1989). Hypothesis: Possible Role for the Melatonin Receptor in Vitiligo: Discussion Paper. Journal of the Royal Society of Medicine. 82. 539-41. 10.1177/014107688908200911.

13. Lerner A, Case J, Heinselman R, (1959) Structure of Melatonin, Journal of American Chemical Society. 81. 6084-6085

14. Pandi-Perumal SR, Zisapel N, Srinivasan V, Cardinali DP. Melatonin and sleep in aging population. Exp Gerontol. 2005 Dec;40(12):911-25. doi: 10.1016/j.exger.2005.08.009. Epub 2005 Sep 23. PMID: 16183237.

15. ON THE EFFECTS OF MELATONIN ON SLEEP AND BEHAVIOR IN MAN (inist.fr)

16. Luboshizsky R, Lavie P. Sleep-inducing effects of exogenous melatonin administration. Sleep Med Rev. 1998 Aug;2(3):191-202. doi: 10.1016/s1087-0792(98)90021-1. PMID: 15310501.

17. Pandi-Perumal SR, Zisapel N, Srinivasan V, Cardinali DP. Melatonin and sleep in aging population. Exp Gerontol. 2005 Dec;40(12):911-25. doi: 10.1016/j.exger.2005.08.009. Epub 2005 Sep 23. PMID: 16183237.

18. The Pineal Gland and Melatonin (colostate.edu)

19. Luboshizsky R, Lavie P. Sleep-inducing effects of exogenous melatonin administration. Sleep Med Rev. 1998 Aug;2(3):191-202. doi: 10.1016/s1087-0792(98)90021-1. PMID: 15310501.

20. Hardeland R. Chronobiology of Melatonin beyond the Feedback to the Suprachiasmatic Nucleus-Consequences to Melatonin Dysfunction. Int J Mol Sci. 2013 Mar 12;14(3):5817-41. doi: 10.3390/ijms14035817. PMID: 23481642; PMCID: PMC3634486.

21. WURTMAN RJ, AXELROD J, POTTER LT. THE UPTAKE OF H3-MELATONIN IN ENDOCRINE AND NERVOUS TISSUES AND THE EFFECTS OF CONSTANT LIGHT EXPOSURE. J Pharmacol Exp Ther. 1964 Mar;143:314-8. PMID: 14161142.

22. Melatonin - an overview | ScienceDirect Topics

23. Andersen LP, Gögenur I, Rosenberg J, Reiter RJ. The Safety of Melatonin in Humans. Clin Drug Investig. 2016 Mar;36(3):169-75. doi: 10.1007/s40261-015-0368-5. PMID: 26692007.

24. Luboshizsky R, Lavie P. Sleep-inducing effects of exogenous melatonin administration. Sleep Med Rev. 1998 Aug;2(3):191-202. doi: 10.1016/s1087-0792(98)90021-1. PMID: 15310501.

25. Cramer H, Rudolph J, Consbruch U, Kendel K. On the effects of melatonin on sleep and behavior in man. Adv Biochem Psychopharmacol. 1974;11(0):187-91. PMID: 4367644.

26. Zhdanova IV, Wurtman RJ, Morabito C, Piotrovska VR, Lynch HJ. Effects of low oral doses of melatonin, given 2-4 hours before habitual bedtime, on sleep in normal young humans. Sleep. 1996 Jun;19(5):423-31. doi: 10.1093/sleep/19.5.423. PMID: 8843534.

27. Hardeland R, Poeggeler B, Srinivasan V, Trakht I, Pandi-Perumal SR, Cardinali DP. Melatonergic drugs in clinical practice. Arzneimittelforschung. 2008;58(1):1-10. doi: 10.1055/s-0031-1296459. PMID: 18368944.

28. Maestroni GJ, Cardinali DP, Esquifino AI, Pandi-Perumal SR. Does melatonin play a disease-promoting role in rheumatoid arthritis? J Neuroimmunol. 2005 Jan;158(1-2):106-11. doi: 10.1016/j.jneuroim.2004.08.015. PMID: 15589043.

29. Pandi-Perumal SR, Srinivasan V, Maestroni GJ, Cardinali DP, Poeggeler B, Hardeland R. Melatonin: Nature's most versatile biological signal? FEBS J. 2006 Jul;273(13):2813-38. doi: 10.1111/j.1742-4658.2006.05322.x. PMID: 16817850.

30. Masters, A., Pandi-Perumal, S. R., Seixas, A., Girardin, J. L., & McFarlane, S. I. (2014). Melatonin, the Hormone of Darkness: From Sleep Promotion to Ebola Treatment. *Brain disorders & therapy*, 4(1), 1000151. https://doi.org/10.4172/2168-975X.1000151

31. Claustrat B. (2014) Melatonin: An Introduction to Its Physiological and Pharmacological Effects in Humans. In: Srinivasan V., Brzezinski A., Oter S., Shillcutt S. (eds) Melatonin and Melatonergic Drugs in Clinical Practice. Springer, New Delhi. https://doi.org/10.1007/978-81-322-0825-9_14

32. Masters, A., Pandi-Perumal, S. R., Seixas, A., Girardin, J. L., & McFarlane, S. I. (2014). Melatonin, the Hormone of Darkness: From Sleep Promotion to Ebola Treatment. *Brain disorders & therapy*, 4(1), 1000151. https://doi.org/10.4172/2168-975X.1000151

33. Masters, A., Pandi-Perumal, S. R., Seixas, A., Girardin, J. L., & McFarlane, S. I. (2014). Melatonin, the Hormone of Darkness: From Sleep Promotion to Ebola Treatment. *Brain disorders & therapy*, 4(1), 1000151. https://doi.org/10.4172/2168-975X.1000151

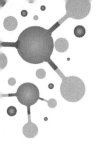

2

MELATONIN & MENTAL EMOTIONAL STRESS

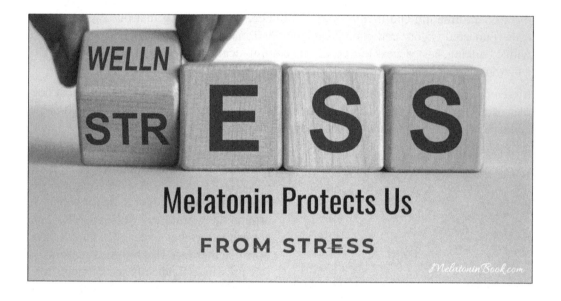

When I was extremely sick with Lyme EBV and mold illness—yes, I had all those at one time—I had severe anxiety and depression. Because I didn't find a doctor that properly worked me up with the right lab work, I was just told my problem was in my head and that it was emotionally based. I spent years meditating for hours a day to try to work through this and it had limited effects. It was not until I began to clear these stressors that I really found relief to my mental emotional afflictions. If I only knew about melatonin back then. Melatonin would have provided support against the toxic infection stress my body and brain was suffering from.

Stress presents itself in many ways within our bodies. There are various forms of stress such as physical stress, chemical stress, infections, mental and emotional stress, psycho-social stress, and electromagnetic stress (EMF). Yet a common downstream effect from all of these varying stressors is how it affects us on a cellular level.[1][2][3][4]

All of these stressors oftentimes lead to increased inflammation, oxidation, and cytokines (as described in another chapter), and they can further lead to a negative cycle of mental and emotional problems. Nevertheless, this is where melatonin comes in! The beneficial actions melatonin offers eases anxiety directly, as well as helping to act as a buffer for almost all the stressors in our world. In my case, I benefited from the support to the immune system, the detoxification, and the buffering effect from exposure to toxins. Read my history as a child in chapter 15 and learn how I was exposed to toxins early on in life. We live in a very toxic world today and EVERY one of us needs to consider that they are polluted and needs to have a regular plan to detox. Melatonin can play a role here, but binder and cell membrane support are also important. We get more into this in Chapter 3,4 & 10.

In our modern, technologically advanced, and industrialized world toxins and stress have become synonymous with life. For instance, humans now endure a constant bombardment of information and media. And while there is no denying that our capacity to be ever-connected via our cell phones brings with it many advantages such as social media, online banking, easy access to emails, and communication with loved ones at the click of a button- the 24/7 endless supply of stimuli can be extremely stressful.

Moreover, as humans, we often try to shift blame, and a hectic lifestyle is the most popular excuse. However, the uncertainties and stressors surrounding life are unavoidable, and instead of trying to fight this fact, learning how to better cope would serve as a more proactive solution.

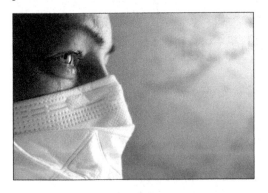

As I sit here today penning this book, COVID-19 seems to have highlighted just how detrimental stress can be for people all around the world. And while COVID-19 is a transient global event, it's important to note that there are also routine stressors like job pressure, finance-based anxiety, relationship hardships, and many other things which we tend to worry about on a daily basis. Nowadays, it's becoming painfully clear that nobody is able to completely escape stress. Even those who are aware of all the health implications that can ensue after prolonged periods of fight or flight such as our healthcare providers, psychiatrists, yoga instructors, and meditation teachers are susceptible to stress. Moreover, with our current fast-paced and busy societies, there appears to be little escape from the potentially devastating and life-taking impacts of stress.[5][6]

All this makes it painstakingly clear that the solution no longer lies in striving to avoid stress. In fact, I'm about to suggest quite the opposite! The real key lies in providing adaptive support, so that not only can we tolerate more stress, but we can benefit from stress.

Hormesis is a term used to describe the beneficial reaction your body responds with from a stressful event. Hormetic stress can be described as a form of stress that given in the right dosage—not too much and not too little—can give you a net gain in health. Examples of hormetic stressors can be fasting, cold and heat stress, physical stress like exercise, and even infections.

Melatonin is like the electromagnetic field of the earth. Just like the electromagnetic field is produced by an internal force due to the metals putting off the energy that extends beyond the surface and protects life on our planet from the harmful UV rays from our sun, melatonin also is made within each cell of your body and works to protect your cells from stress. Throughout this book you will find out how melatonin can protect you from things like cancer, metabolic diseases like diabetes, all infections including COVID and Ebola, heart disease, digestive disease, sexual dysfunction, mood disorders, neurological diseases like Parkinson's, Alzheimer's, and cognitive decline. It can even extend life too!

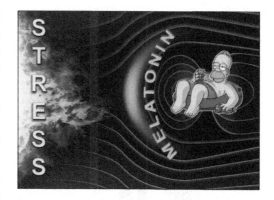

If you look at the graph on hormesis, you can see there is a certain level of stress that you can receive, and as long as you don't accede to this, your body responds to this stress with an action that actually strengthens rather than weakens the body.

For example, if you do too much exercise you will exceed the stress your body can deal with, and therefore you might get sick or feel worn out for a few days until the body can recover from the stressful injury incurred by overtraining. In our clinic, we do ozone therapy, and ozone is the most oxidative substance on the planet. Meaning it is a huge stressor to our body. Why then would I want to run this as an IV to a sick individual? It's all about hormesis. Ozone is a stressor, however, in

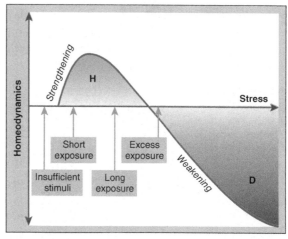

the right dose, it can be a way to activate the endogenous antioxidant systems in the body. In other words, the high levels of oxidation delivered from brief periods of infusion, when exposed to your blood cells can activate enzymes and oxidize the lipids in your blood. Those oxidized lipids then become signaling factors that tell the body to do some work to be better prepared for oxidation next time. Even the most core part of your cells—the mitochondria, are told to recycle the poor functioning mitochondria, and build new strong ones, in a process called mitochondrial biogenesis.

I use ozone as an example of hormetic stress because it's the best medical hermetic therapy I know of and it is used very often in my practice. What's important to know with IV ozone is that you need to be able to tolerate the dosage of ozone. This depends on your antioxidant capacity.

Melatonin is the primary antioxidant for all your cells and is involved in the beneficial effects received by IV ozone. Supplementing with melatonin can allow you to better adapt to stress and enable you to receive larger amounts and stay within the hermetic curve. This means you may stand a better chance of benefitting from stressors, versus becoming worn down, leading to disease and aging.

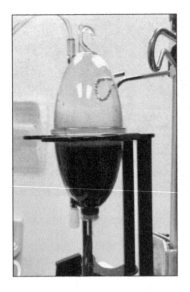

It makes good sense to minimize the negative impacts stress can have on your health by leveraging the use of "stress protecting" supplements, such as melatonin. I'm also a proponent of many other stress-reducing activities such as exercise, breathing, and meditation for stress reduction. However, sleep is at the top of my list which is another factor that melatonin can help with. Yet the numerous advantages of melatonin go far beyond sleep, as you will discover in this book.

Stress has indeed become synonymous with our life. The irony that medical professionals including psychiatrists who emphasize avoiding stress are not able to escape its impact speaks volumes. In this chapter, we will be considering stress as the accumulation of all the activities over the day such as overworking both physical and mentally, exercise, toxic exposures such as pesticides and mold, poor nutrition, lack of sleep, infections both acute and chronic, and electromagnetic stress from cell phones and Wi-Fi.

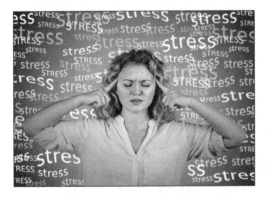

Mental-emotional stress and anxiety disorders have become the most common of mental illnesses, affecting nearly 40 million adults per year in the US alone.[7]

While the list of factors that can contribute to your mental and emotional stress is endless, the anxiety-driven feeling is not. Stress can be buffered, consequently diminishing the impact on your mental and physical health.

It is amazing that a molecule that is not only produced in the brain but like I've mentioned before, produced in every cell in your body, can be so intrinsic to our mental, emotional, and overall well-being.

Throughout this chapter we're going to dive a little deeper into various aspects of melatonin, and how it works similar to the electromagnetic field protecting the earth. It protects and lessens the effects of stress and allows the body to handle different stressors in a more optimized manner. Plus, by using melatonin we can further benefit from greater forms of hormesis.

Melatonin for mental-emotional stress

Besides improved sleep, which has a balancing effect on the brain, the autonomics play a large role in supporting proper mental emotional stress responses. Sympathetic dominance is common where we get stuck in a fight or flight response, and it can also cause confusion and depression. Consider how powerfully melatonin supports the parasympathetic side keeping the sympathetics calmed down. In a minute we will dive into heart rate variability (HRV) and how it can be a measure into your sympathetic system - and how melatonin can support this.

First let's look at the sleep side of this equation and then dive into HRV. Sleep disorders like insomnia are intricately linked to stress, anxiety, and depression. The more nights you spend feeling restless without any sleep, the more stressed you're going to be during the daytime.[8][9]

In fact, it works both ways.

I like to use the analogy of a revolving door. For instance, most of us are more than familiar with the consequences of a bad night's sleep. We end up in a bad mood the following day, tired, with low energy, and most likely running into further problems. Humorously enough, it's these same anxieties that are capable of leaving you without being able to sleep the following night. As you can see, it becomes somewhat of a perpetual cycle. Part of this is related to a stress hormone called cortisol which we will talk about later in this chapter.[10]

It's comparable to a case of what came first - the chicken or the egg? I guess it really doesn't matter because using melatonin could offer a way to tackle both sides of that revolving door; And by this, I mean, the stress on one end and the sleeplessness on the other.

Moreover, research studies have suggested that sleep aids like melatonin could reduce stress while also improving your cognitive function and boosting overall mood.[11][12]

Melatonin is effective for managing mild day-to-day stress that we all experience as well as severe mental stress that can lead to complications like depression and generalized anxiety. This is primarily due to the mechanism of action melatonin provides towards regulating the circadian rhythm, promoting sleep quality, and easing negative emotions.[13]

Melatonin works to support your autonomic nervous system and particularly the parasympathetic system. By doing this, melatonin works to improve something called heart rate variability or HRV.

HRV is a sign of health and the body's adaptation to stress. It's a great metric to track if you're trying to figure out if you are working out too hard for example. It goes up when you're healthy and it's lowered due to less variability when you're poorly adapting, or the stress is too high.

Consider that the HRV is controlled through 2 opposite sides of your autonomic nervous system, the sympathetic (or fight or flight) and your parasympathetic or resting and digesting

side. One side is telling your heart when to contract and the other when to relax, thus when one side is overactive you get lower variability.

Can you guess which side is overactive typically? If you guessed the sympathetic you are correct. It's the "stress" side of your nervous system, so it's obviously the part of our nervous system that gets lots of activation, therefore it becomes stronger. To counteract this, we need to work on things that support the parasympathetic system, like deep breathing, my personal favorite - meditation, laughing, and doing things you love.[14]

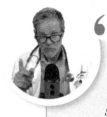

" *"Melatonin is protective in CNS on several different levels: It reduces free radical burden, improves endothelial dysfunction, reduces inflammation and shifts the balance between the sympathetic and parasympathetic system in favor of the parasympathetic system."*

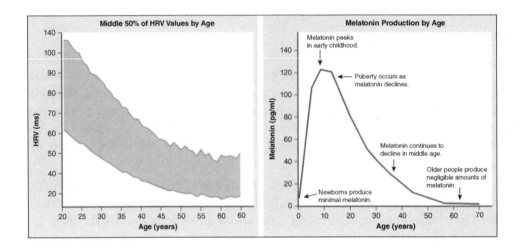

Moreover, there are receptors in the brain called G-protein melatonin receptors. The two called MT1 and MT2 work with the brain, and melatonin affects the brain through the activation of these receptors. Let's circle back to HRV and consider the graph of how this becomes more problematic as we get older.

The graph highlights a direct relationship of a reduction in stress-enduring capacity as we age. But what's interesting is that this graph when compared to the melatonin levels chart bears many similarities.

Is it the relationship melatonin has with HRV that reflects this? With the science pointing toward that being true, supplementing with melatonin when one is under stress makes more sense now than ever before.

The aforementioned is exactly what we're going to dive deeper into throughout the next section.

How does melatonin work to reduce mental stress?

Stress and getting the correct amount of sleep are two opposing forces.

REM Sleep is the primary phase of sleep that allows our subconscious mind to work out all the challenges that it met throughout the day. I think of it as a computer that must go through a defrag for it to function optimally. Think about how conflicted we get throughout the day due to the multitude of situations and experiences that arise, such as someone cutting us off on the road or the way your siblings and parents interacted with you. We all know that over time, things tend to calm down from an emotional standpoint and this is what primarily happens during our REM sleep.

Incidentally, alcohol and high THC (Tetrahydrocannabinol) levels can further inhibit REM sleep thereby creating a devastating effect on our emotional well-being. THC is nothing more than a compound secreted by the cannabis plant. Cannabis has been shown to be hugely beneficial when administered in the right dosages. The right type of full-spectrum hemp product with a small amount of THC can work wonders for sleep cycle health. We recommend the brand NeuroDiol found at Mitozen.com as it has been shown clinically to improve sleep dramatically.

Furthermore, there is something called a C1 receptor that a small amount of THC activates, which is the brake system that many of us need, especially after the age of 40. Most of the research has shown that extremely high levels of CBD are necessary to induce quality REM sleep. Personally, I've found success with suppositories in the hundred and 125 to 300 mg range to be quite effective, as well as oral tinctures using higher milligram dosages.

Taking melatonin in conjunction with the right type of full-spectrum CBD health product can be a great way to improve sleep. Another compound to look at is glutathione as it is one of the more successful sleep-promoting substances, along with uridine.[15]

Another curious thing to note when it comes to melatonin and sleep is that while your REM sleep can be adversely affected by alcohol or narcotics, melatonin has shown to buffer the negative effects, therefore, allowing for a more peaceful night's sleep.[16][17]

Sleep, melatonin, and mechanism of action

The effect of melatonin on your mental health is not limited to how it promotes sleep quality. It can also take care of the after-effects of insufficient sleep and allow you to avoid additional stressors that could worsen your emotional well-being.

Melatonin, being a sleep hormone, helps to maintain your body's circadian rhythm and enables you to get a sound sleep every night, thereby protecting you against the consequences of insomnia.

Conversely, the indirect benefits of sleep improvement brought about by melatonin can go a long way towards preventing stress, as well as the factors that cause it.

This brings us to understanding the first mechanism of action to which melatonin contributes that can help you avoid stress and anxiety. It basically works by improving your sleep pattern.[18]

Yet, that's not all.

The stress-relieving action of melatonin is not limited to the improvement of sleep. It also helps to regulate the production and release of stress hormones like cortisol, and feel-good hormones like dopamine and serotonin, to help you better absorb the impact of unpleasant stress on your mental health.

The complex interplay between melatonin and mood-regulating hormones

Your mood, whether happy, sad, or anxious, depends on the complex interplay between the levels of different hormones in the body. Other than melatonin, hormones like dopamine, serotonin, and cortisol are also responsible for mood regulation.

Among these, cortisol is largely responsible for increasing mental stress and anxiety. Moreover, the production and release of melatonin and cortisol in the nervous system are interdependent.

Since melatonin secretion is light-sensitive, it reacts to morning light, which is how the brain is signaled to slow down or pull back on melatonin secretion and release.

At the same time, the morning light also signals your brain to produce more cortisol, which is your "awake" hormone. The increased production of cortisol in the early morning hours is what nudges us to wake up. During the daytime, the release of cortisol continues to increase and reaches its peak, thus allowing us to feel more alert.[19]

This is how melatonin and cortisol work in opposite ways, yet at the same time symbiotically, to manage our sleep-wake cycle. When melatonin secretion is high, the cortisol levels reduce and vice versa.

When the secretion of either of these hormones is out of balance, your ability to sleep at night or stay awake throughout the day becomes affected.

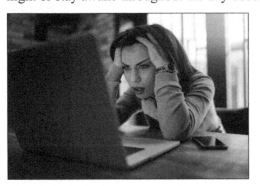

Increased cortisol production reduces melatonin secretion, and this is the reason why your stressful day can subsequently lead to a poor night's sleep.

On top of this possible dysregulation, you throw in the constant text messages, Instagram posting, returning emails, TV watching, and any other form of screen staring, which are known to emit tons of blue and green light, and the mystery behind the suppression of melatonin starts to become more apparent. When you are in a distressed state, you're not in the best mindset to make positive changes in your life, which then leads to further mental-emotional stress. This prevents you from falling asleep thereby, once again, contributing to your stress and anxiety. This is one reason why it's important to ensure your body has a higher level of melatonin to counter these fast-paced changes and adapt to the new age that we live in now.[20][21]

Nevertheless, the effects of cortisol are not limited to improving your wakefulness and poor sleep. Chronically high cortisol levels are also linked to a higher risk of cardiovascular disease, psychological disorders, anxiety disorders, depression, postpartum depression, post-traumatic stress syndrome (PTSD), OCD, and many other psychological disorders.[22][23]

Any form of stressor including toxic, chemical, emotional, and psychological stressors can cause your cortisol levels to rise. Furthermore, all of these stressors can lead to inflammation in the body, as well as an activation of the sympathetic nervous system. This ultimately triggers higher cortisol levels, insufficient sleep, and depressed melatonin production and release. Diseases such as diabetes, sleep apnea, chronic infections, cancers, allergies, and autoimmune disorders are all linked to elevated levels of cortisol. This is why regulating cortisol production is important when trying to minimize the impact of stressors on your physical and mental health. Besides getting a deeply restorative night's sleep, melatonin can buffer the negative effects of chronic inflammation, cancer, immune dysregulation such as autoimmune disease and allergies, as well as acute and chronic infections. Again, this is why we refer to melatonin as being the "quarterback". Meaning that there's one player that can have a widespread effect on the game.

The increased secretion of cortisol could be addressed by supplementation of melatonin. The interdependency between the secretion of melatonin and cortisol allows for the regulation of the levels of cortisol in the nervous system. An increased melatonin level would subsequently signal the brain to reduce cortisol production.[24][25]

Dopamine, serotonin, and melatonin

Now, let's take a quick look at the other two hormones that play a role in determining your moods and mental health.

These are dopamine and serotonin.

While cortisol is largely considered a stress hormone, dopamine and serotonin are commonly referred to as the feel-good hormones, which ultimately means these hormones play an important role in mood regulation. Just like cortisol, the secretion of dopamine and serotonin is also linked to the levels of melatonin in the nervous system. The higher secretion of melatonin at night is essential for inducing deep sleep, which, in turn, can improve the production of serotonin and dopamine. The increased levels of these two feel-good hormones induce a sense of relaxation, thereby reducing anxiety.

But how do melatonin levels affect the balance of feel-good hormones in the brain?

Serotonin is a neurotransmitter, the deficiency of which is associated with a higher risk of depression. A research study revealed that mice exhibited more fears when serotonin receptors were deleted.

Another experiment compared the levels of serotonin of healthy individuals with those in patients with panic disorders using a PET scan. This study showed that patients who experienced panic attacks had about two-thirds of the regular serotonin level of 1A receptors in certain parts of the brain including midbrain raphe, anterior cingulate, and posterior cingulate.[26]

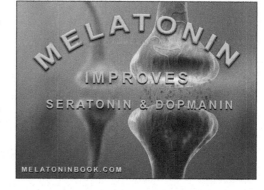

This indicates how depleted serotonin levels are intricately linked to negative emotions like fear and anxiety.

Similarly, dopamine is another neurotransmitter commonly associated with social anxiety and reward-motivated behavior. A research study found that patients with generalized social phobia have a lower dopamine level compared to healthy subjects.[27] While on the other hand, higher dopamine levels are linked to improved mental health, higher self-confidence, and reduced risk of depression and anxiety.

This suggests that a higher secretion of dopamine and serotonin could help to improve mood and avoid anxiety.

There is evidence to prove that melatonin, when injected in rats, can help to control anxiety allowing them to spend a longer time in the plus-size maze. It's also believed to work by improving the quality and duration of sleep, thereby allowing you to feel more refreshed and energetic during the daytime. Getting adequate amounts of sleep at night ultimately improves brain functions and enables higher secretion of dopamine and serotonin, thus relieving anxiety.[28]

This is how the anxiety-relieving effect of melatonin is linked to its capacity to improve the secretion of dopamine and serotonin.

The complex interplay between melatonin and stress hormones, like cortisol and feel-good hormones such as dopamine and serotonin, may help you avoid anxiety. It might also improve your self-confidence and enhance your cognitive and creative skills.[29]

The discovery of the anxiolytic properties of melatonin

One of the primary and beneficial effects of melatonin is its potential to help protect us from the impact of poor mental health.[30]

When scientists first started researching this miracle molecule, they had a difficult time determining the benefits that melatonin could provide to all animals, including humans. They did not notice a significant difference when melatonin was given in a conventional environment.

Initially, they gave melatonin to mice that were not under stress to assess if it could improve their health status. However, they didn't notice any significant improvement in the mice that were administered melatonin.

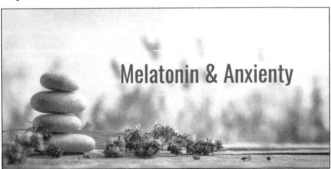

The lack of noticeable improvement was mainly due to the protective effect of melatonin on the body at a cellular level, which is particularly notable during stress.

It wasn't until the researchers started to stress the animals in the study by placing them in tiny tubes with little holes for several hours a day, that the protective effects of melatonin became obvious. The simulation of a stressful situation induced these animals to activate the protective effects of melatonin, from which a subsequent improvement was observed in their health status.[31][32]

What does the research say about the anxiolytic properties of melatonin?

Several research studies have confirmed the anxiety-relieving properties of melatonin, which have further shown to be effective for improving mental health.

Let's take a brief look at what the research has to say about the anxiolytic action of melatonin.

Animal studies

One animal study conducted in 2017 revealed that melatonin can increase the levels of GABA (gamma-aminobutyric acid) in specific parts of the brain. A higher GABA level may induce a calming effect on the mind and body, ultimately relieving symptoms of anxiety.

In fact, some medications commonly recommended for treating anxiety, including benzo-diazepines, also function by increasing GABA levels.[33]

Human studies

Studies have linked the use of melatonin supplementation to relief from presurgical anxiety. It's common for patients to feel anxious before a planned surgical procedure. Moreover, the clinical trials conducted to assess the effect of melatonin administration in surgical patients revealed that it can positively reduce the anxiety that patients usually experience before surgery.

The anxiety-relieving effect was significantly higher compared to the patients who were given a placebo. These studies have indicated the wider application of the anxiolytic properties of melatonin across different use cases.

Also, medications such as benzodiazepines are commonly used to reduce anxiety in pre-surgical patients. In an analysis of clinical studies conducted in 2015, it was found that the anxiolytic effect of melatonin was comparable to benzodiazepines such as midazolam when given before a surgical procedure.

Most of the research studies conducted have revealed that melatonin works better than placebo, and as effectively as midazolam for lessening anxiety when given to pre-surgical patients.[34]

In another study, the use of melatonin was evaluated in patients who had undergone a major procedure to open up blood vessels within the heart. This study showed that the anxiolytic effect of melatonin was superior to that of oxazepam.[35][36]

Conclusion

In addition to supporting our brain and brain chemistry through quality sleep, melatonin supports our cells and energy supply. It's becoming ever clearer that melatonin, the quarterback, has the potential to be of great assistance in the management of mental and emotional stress, both directly and indirectly. With melatonin's ability to improve sleep and regulate the secretion of cortisol, dopamine, and serotonin it can be highly effective in reducing these afflictions and improving your mental-emotional wellbeing.

Other important avenues to consider:

- Meditation.
- Breathing Exercises- Look into Wim Hof breathing or other techniques.
- The use of glutathione as an additional antioxidant to buffer stress, as well as improve sleep quality.
- Get tested for toxins such as heavy metals and or pesticides.
- Get tested for chronic infections such as viral bacterial, fungal, and intestinal parasites.
- Test food allergies such as gluten, dairy, night shades.
- Try a ketogenic diet to improve brain power which supports stress resilience.
- Try Mito Fast or other fasting programs to support your mitochondria.
- Try NAD+ supplementation. (precursors such as NR and NMN are also good).
- Full-spectrum CBD can also be leveraged for sleep and stress management.
- Magnolia bark extract can help anxiety and sleep.
- Ketamine assisted psychotherapy.
- Sometimes, chronic infections in the sinuses can cause a lot of s stress symptoms as well. If you feel like this might possibly be affecting your stress levels, consider a 30-day nasal cleanse, and if you're able to test the microbial health of your sinuses it's highly recommended. Systemic infections with viruses such as Lyme disease and mold illness can cause a lot of chronic mental-emotional stress as well. Although melatonin could be extremely helpful in most of these cases if this is the underlying root cause one needs to make sure they get the appropriate testing and diagnosis so that they could better understand the correct treatment.

I would suggest melatonin would be a great adjunct to any plan to support becoming healthier and feeling better mentally and emotionally. Consider some testing to see if there are stressors that have gone undiagnosed such as toxicity, infections, sinus health, food sensitivities and gut health.

Reference

1. Hirotsu, C., Tufik, S., & Andersen, M. L. (2015). Interactions between sleep, stress, and metabolism: From physiological to pathological conditions. *Sleep science (Sao Paulo, Brazil)*, *8*(3), 143–152. https://doi.org/10.1016/j.slsci.2015.09.002

2. Mahdavi, S. M., Sahraei, H., Yaghmaei, P., & Tavakoli, H. (2014). Effects of electromagnetic radiation exposure on stress-related behaviors and stress hormones in male wistar rats. *Biomolecules & therapeutics*, *22*(6), 570–576. https://doi.org/10.4062/biomolther.2014.054

3. Kim, E. J., & Dimsdale, J. E. (2007). The effect of psychosocial stress on sleep: a review of polysomnographic evidence. *Behavioral sleep medicine*, *5*(4), 256–278. https://doi.org/10.1080/15402000701557383

4. Lichtveld K, Thomas K, Tulve NS. Chemical and non-chemical stressors affecting childhood obesity: a systematic scoping review. J Expo Sci Environ Epidemiol. 2018 Jan;28(1):1-12. doi: 10.1038/jes.2017.18. Epub 2017 Sep 27. PMID: 28952603; PMCID: PMC6097845.

5. Wilkins K. Work stress among health care providers. Health Rep. 2007 Nov;18(4):33-6. PMID: 18074995.

6. Boo YL, Liam CCK, Lim SY, Look ML, Tan MH, Ching SM, Wan JL, Chin PW, Hoo FK. Stress and burnout syndrome in health-care providers treating dengue infection: A cross-sectional study. Med J Malaysia. 2018 Dec;73(6):371-375. PMID: 30647206.

7. Facts & Statistics | Anxiety and Depression Association of America, ADAA

8. Kalmbach DA, Anderson JR, Drake CL. The impact of stress on sleep: Pathogenic sleep reactivity as a vulnerability to insomnia and circadian disorders. J Sleep Res. 2018 Dec;27(6):e12710. doi: 10.1111/jsr.12710. Epub 2018 May 24. PMID: 29797753; PMCID: PMC7045300.

9. Sanford LD, Suchecki D, Meerlo P. Stress, arousal, and sleep. Curr Top Behav Neurosci. 2015;25:379-410. doi: 10.1007/7854_2014_314. PMID: 24852799.

10. Hirotsu, C., Tufik, S., & Andersen, M. L. (2015). Interactions between sleep, stress, and metabolism: From physiological to pathological conditions. *Sleep science (Sao Paulo, Brazil)*, *8*(3), 143–152. https://doi.org/10.1016/j.slsci.2015.09.002

11. Jean-Louis G, von Gizycki H, Zizi F. Melatonin effects on sleep, mood, and cognition in elderly with mild cognitive impairment. J Pineal Res. 1998 Oct;25(3):177-83. doi: 10.1111/j.1600-079x.1998.tb00557.x. PMID: 9745987.

12. Riemersma-van der Lek RF, Swaab DF, Twisk J, Hol EM, Hoogendijk WJ, Van Someren EJ. Effect of bright light and melatonin on cognitive and noncognitive function in elderly residents of group care facilities: a randomized controlled trial. JAMA. 2008 Jun 11;299(22):2642-55. doi: 10.1001/jama.299.22.2642. PMID: 18544724.

13. Zisapel N. (2018). New perspectives on the role of melatonin in human sleep, circadian rhythms and their regulation. *British journal of pharmacology*, *175*(16), 3190–3199. https://doi.org/10.1111/bph.14116

14. Pechanova, O., Paulis, L., & Simko, F. (2014). Peripheral and central effects of melatonin on blood pressure regulation. *International journal of molecular sciences*, *15*(10), 17920–17937. https://doi.org/10.3390/ijms151017920

15. Angarita, G. A., Emadi, N., Hodges, S., & Morgan, P. T. (2016). Sleep abnormalities associated with alcohol, cannabis, cocaine, and opiate use: a comprehensive review. *Addiction science & clinical practice*, *11*(1), 9. https://doi.org/10.1186/s13722-016-0056-7

16. Gendy, M., Lagzdins, D., Schaman, J., & Le Foll, B. (2020). Melatonin for Treatment-Seeking Alcohol Use Disorder patients with sleeping problems: A randomized clinical pilot trial. *Scientific reports*, *10*(1), 8739. https://doi.org/10.1038/s41598-020-65166-y

17. Onaolapo, O. J., & Onaolapo, A. Y. (2018). Melatonin in drug addiction and addiction management: Exploring an evolving multidimensional relationship. *World journal of psychiatry*, *8*(2), 64–74. https://doi.org/10.5498/wjp.v8.i2.64

18. Valdez P. (2019). Circadian Rhythms in Attention. *The Yale journal of biology and medicine*, *92*(1), 81–92.

19. Melatonin and Cortisol - Thriven Functional Medicine Clinic

20. Erbay, L. G., & Kartalci, S. (2015). Neurosteroid Levels in Patients with Obsessive-Compulsive Disorder. *Psychiatry investigation*, *12*(4), 538–544. https://doi.org/10.4306/pi.2015.12.4.538

21. Evans, L. M., Myers, M. M., & Monk, C. (2008). Pregnant women's cortisol is elevated with anxiety and depression - but only when comorbid. *Archives of women's mental health*, *11*(3), 239–248. https://doi.org/10.1007/s00737-008-0019-4

22. Nandam, L. S., Brazel, M., Zhou, M., & Jhaveri, D. J. (2020). Cortisol and Major Depressive Disorder-Translating Findings From Humans to Animal Models and Back. *Frontiers in psychiatry*, *10*, 974. https://doi.org/10.3389/fpsyt.2019.00974

23. Rafael A. Caparros-Gonzalez , Borja Romero-Gonzalez , Helen Strivens-Vilchez, Raquel Gonzalez-Perez , Olga Martinez-Augustin, Maria Isabel Peralta-Ramirez; Hair cortisol levels, psychological stress and psychopathological symptoms as predictors of postpartum depression. Published: August 28, 2017 https://doi.org/10.1371/journal.pone.0182817

24. Zisapel, Nava & Tarrasch, Ricardo & Laudon, Moshe. (2005). The relationship between melatonin and cortisol rhythms: Clinical implications of melatonin therapy. Drug Development Research. 65. 119 - 125. 10.1002/ddr.20014.

25. Premkumar, M., Sable, T., Dhanwal, D., & Dewan, R. (2013). Circadian Levels of Serum Melatonin and Cortisol in relation to Changes in Mood, Sleep, and Neurocognitive Performance, Spanning a Year of Residence in Antarctica. *Neuroscience journal*, *2013*, 254090. https://doi.org/10.1155/2013/254090

26. Jean Kim, Jack Gorman, The psychobiology of anxiety, Clinical Neuroscience Research, Volume 4, Issues 5–6, 2005, Pages 335-347, ISSN 1566-2772, https://doi.org/10.1016/j.cnr.2005.03.008.

27. Schneier FR, Liebowitz MR, Abi-Dargham A, Zea-Ponce Y, Lin SH, Laruelle M. Low dopamine D(2) receptor binding potential in social phobia. Am J Psychiatry. 2000 Mar;157(3):457-9. doi: 10.1176/appi.ajp.157.3.457. PMID: 10698826.

28. Golombek DA, Martini M, Cardinali DP. Melatonin as an anxiolytic in rats: time dependence and interaction with the central GABAergic system. Eur J Pharmacol. 1993 Jun 24;237(2-3):231-6. doi: 10.1016/0014-2999(93)90273-k. PMID: 8103462.

29. Krishnakumar, D., Hamblin, M. R., & Lakshmanan, S. (2015). Meditation and Yoga can Modulate Brain Mechanisms that affect Behavior and Anxiety-A Modern Scientific Perspective. *Ancient science*, *2*(1), 13–19. https://doi.org/10.14259/as.v2i1.171

30. Yi WJ, Kim TS. Melatonin protects mice against stress-induced inflammation through enhancement of M2 macrophage polarization. Int Immunopharmacol. 2017 Jul;48:146-158. doi: 10.1016/j.intimp.2017.05.006. Epub 2017 May 12. PMID: 28505494.

31. Feng, P., Hu, Y., Vurbic, D., & Guo, Y. (2012). Maternal stress induces adult reduced REM sleep and melatonin level. *Developmental neurobiology*, *72*(5), 677–687. https://doi.org/10.1002/dneu.20961

32. Huang, Y., Xu, C., He, M., Huang, W., & Wu, K. (2020). Saliva cortisol, melatonin levels and circadian rhythm alterations in Chinese primary school children with dyslexia. *Medicine*, *99*(6), e19098. https://doi.org/10.1097/MD.0000000000019098

33. Zhang, L., Guo, H. L., Zhang, H. Q., Xu, T. Q., He, B., Wang, Z. H., Yang, Y. P., Tang, X. D., Zhang, P., & Liu, F. E. (2017). Melatonin prevents sleep deprivation-associated anxiety-like behavior in rats: role of oxidative stress and balance between GABAergic and glutamatergic transmission. *American journal of translational research*, *9*(5), 2231–2242.

34. Halladin NL, Rosenberg J, Gögenur I, Møller AM; Melatonin for pre- and postoperative anxiety in adults, Cochrane Database of Systematic Reviews, 2015; 4, 1465-1858; PB: John Wiley & Sons, Ltd DOI: 10.1002/14651858.CD009861.pub2; US: https://doi.org//10.1002/14651858.CD009861.pub2

35. Ghaeli P, Solduzian M, Vejdani S, Talasaz AH. Comparison of the Effects of Melatonin and Oxazepam on Anxiety Levels and Sleep Quality in Patients With ST-Segment-Elevation Myocardial Infarction Following Primary Percutaneous Coronary Intervention: A Randomized Clinical Trial. Ann Pharmacother. 2018 Oct;52(10):949-955. doi: 10.1177/1060028018776608. Epub 2018 May 11. PMID: 29749262.

36. Laudon, M., & Frydman-Marom, A. (2014). Therapeutic effects of melatonin receptor agonists on sleep and comorbid disorders. *International journal of molecular sciences*, *15*(9), 15924–15950. Therapeutic effects of melatonin receptor agonists on sleep and comorbid disorders - PubMed (nih.gov)

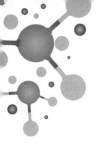

3

HOW MELATONIN SUPPORTS THE MITOCHONDRIA

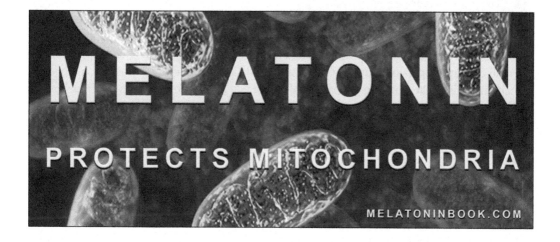

MELATONIN PROTECTS MITOCHONDRIA

MELATONINBOOK.COM

Mitochondria are the important cellular organelles that make up 1/3 of your body weight. Your mitochondria play a critical role in determining how efficiently your body's organs can work by simply producing the energy needed for their everyday function. This energy is critical for your body to deal with stressful events, which include all types of stress factors. Do you recall them? They are mental/emotional, chemical/toxic, infection, physical & EMFs.

Mitochondrial function has been linked to many diseases and it's thought that the aging process is closely related to this dysfunction that occurs over our lifetime. Meaning that, our bodies accumulate more and more stress in the form of toxins, chronic infections, nutrient depletion, poor antioxidant status, NAD+ levels, senescent cells, and physical stress.

Mitochondria play a key role in energy production. This gives them the common name of the 'powerhouses of the cell/body'.

The mitochondria ultimately make energy by converting glucose from within the cells to form energy in the form of ATP, which is in the presence of oxygen of course. This process is known and commonly referred to in health and biology circles. It's basically biology 101. This process of energy production is called the tricarboxylic acid cycle (TAC) or the Krebs cycle.[1][2][3]

Besides the pineal gland and endothelial tissues, the mitochondria in each of your cells produce melatonin.

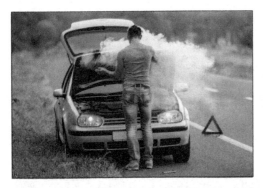

Let's dive into why melatonin is produced by your cells:

Although the pineal gland releases melatonin into the bloodstream to be used by other organs and tissues, when your mitochondria in your cells produce the melatonin, it is not secreted into the bloodstream. This precious melatonin within the cell is utilized and is extremely important. In other words, the cells selfishly hold onto this melatonin, and we will learn later that this action is critical to protect and buffer stress where we need it most. Imagine that you had a boat that had one motor. You were out at sea and your engine stopped. If you have no backup propulsion, you're dead in the water. At a cellular level, it is much the same. Except instead of that motor on the back of the boat you have thousands of little mitochondria floating around each cell working hard to make energy. Just like any engine, there needs to be a cooling system and an exhaust. These systems are critical to the mitochondria as well. The stress involved in producing energy needs to be buffered so that there is not a build-up of stress around the energy-producing entity, whether it's a boat engine or your little mitochondria's.

You may be asking; how does melatonin play this role and buffer stress at the energy-producing level of the mitochondria?

The type of stresses the mitochondria experience universally result in inflammation, thus cytokines are mental/emotional, chemical, infection, physical & EMFs. Think about a log you place on a fire, one burns for 10 hours (the one with no stress or lots of melatonin), and the other only burns for 1 hour. This is efficiency at its finest when it comes to making energy, but there is another factor which is the pollution that log puts out. The second log not only creates solely one burning hour of energy, but it puts out much more pollution or smoke. This is a similar action to what occurs in the form of oxidative stress. Since melatonin shields oxidation when you don't have enough you can't buffer it, and build-up can occur causing a further choking off of your mitochondrial and cellular functions.[4]

In a perfect scenario, when things are functioning normally this process leads to the release of 36 ATP molecules as a byproduct from the breakdown of each molecule of glucose. Remember this number, it's going to be important later.

Again, just to emphasize how important this energy is. It's used by the organs and tissues including your brain, heart, and lungs to perform critical functions. The muscles in your body also use the energy that's generated to support bodily movements.

Routine stressors affect the optimal function of the mitochondria and reduce the energy available for the cells to use, as well as increase oxidative stress in the cells. This can have a critical and devastating cascading negative effect on the functions of the cells and in turn, affect the activities of the organs, tissues, and body as a whole.

I hope you're starting to see just how important it is to address issues that encompass the energy production of mitochondria. Before we discuss how melatonin plays a role in protecting mitochondria, let us have an idea of the factors that affect energy production in mitochondria.

Factors that affect energy production in mitochondria

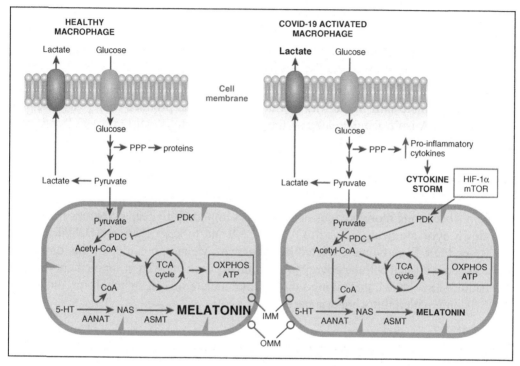

The process of energy production is severely affected in the presence of stressors because they lead to both inflammation and oxidation. These stressors often lead to excess free radicals within cells which causes oxidation. This action is also referred to as a reactive oxygen species or abbreviated as ROS. When this oxidation exceeds a certain threshold, it forces the cell to continue to make energy another way. It's still producing energy in the presence of oxygen; however, it is no longer going through the Krebs cycle.

This part of the melatonin story is fascinating, so hang on because we're going to get a little technical, but it will be well worth it for your overall understanding of this miracle molecule.

So, there's an enzyme produced in each of your mitochondria called pyruvate dehydro-genase kinase (PDK). PDK can hold phosphates derived from the energy released in the formation of ATP. It can attach a phosphate to the pyruvate dehydrogenase complex (PDC), thus disabling it. If you look at the above diagram, you'll be able to see how energy goes from glucose to pyruvate which enters into the cell and then converts it into Acetyl-CoA. This can then enter the crab cycle to make those 36 ATP. Even though we're using the image demonstrating the inflammatory storm in an infection from COVID-19 as an example, this process is affected the same way through most of the other stresses we've been discussing. So again, we go from glucose to pyruvate to Acetyl-CoA then into the Krebs cycle. This process is taken out in the face of inflammation through the PDK enzyme, where pyruvate will no longer get converted to Acetyl-CoA. This would be like the engine in your boat still running, but barely. What's also important to understand is that that same Acetyl-CoA also goes on to produce melatonin within the mitochondria. So, when the PDK enzyme gets taken out so does your cell's ability to make melatonin. Melatonin is produced in the mitochondria to protect the cell from overheating through this mechanism of energy production and trust me when I say that it's not a good situation when it gets cut off. It's like both the cooling system and the exhaust system going out on the boat engine causing it to completely choke.

What happens here is a devastating blow to the energy potential of the mitochondria. There is a complete shift in the way that the mitochondria produce energy at this point. The Acetyl-CoA isn't being created so the pyruvate has to do all the work. Pyruvate is then shuffled out of the mitochondria into the part of the cell called the cytosol, and it's there that it will be converted into ATP through a process called aerobic glycolysis. This energy system is much less efficient than Krebs cycle, hence we only get 4 ATP versus 36. That's approximately a 90% loss of the cells capacity to make energy!

I hope it's becoming more obvious now why it is important to keep cytokines from shutting down pyruvate being moved to Acetyl-CoA and to keep Pyruvate Dehydrogenase Kinase or PDK from being activated by cytokines. Melatonin can calm this down and help to restore normal cellular energy production even when taken in supplement form. In fact, studies have shown that taking supplemental melatonin can switch the production of the melatonin within mitochondria back on.

What is it that exactly regulates this PDK?

PDK is activated in the presence of pro-inflammatory substances called cytokines in cells, which ensue because of various forms of stress. Much of this is seen within the immune system at the level of the macrophage, which is one of your body's immune cells. Macrophages are released to fight infectious pathogens and they produce these pro-inflammatory cytokines, such as interleukins and human necrosis factors.

Moreover, one of the most amazing aspects of melatonin is that it will suppress PDK. Melatonin can suppress some of the production of PDK when the cell and mitochondria are under stress. This can break the cycle created by PDK allowing the production of ATPs by mitochondria to resume through Krebs cycle again back to 36 ATP versus 4.

There's another way by which melatonin helps mitochondria, and that action is linked to its anti-inflammatory potential. Let me reveal more about this as we go ahead.

How does the anti-inflammatory property of melatonin protect mitochondria?

Chronic stress oftentimes includes infections that can trigger inflammation and oxidation, leading to the immunological involvement of macrophages and neutrophils on a chronic level. This action makes your immune system weaker. The defense mechanisms stimulated by the immune cells in the event of infections may also lead to the destruction of cells, along with the mitochondria, which will result in the creation of debris from dead cells and cellular parts. These particles simply float around and lead to immunological activation.

This can stimulate the innate immune system leading to macrophages eating up the cellular debris along with their damaged mitochondria. This happens because macrophages consider the debris as antigens due to which the cycle of inflammation is triggered, releasing even more inflammatory cytokines which then activate the PDK pathway even further. It's a bit of that cycle that potentiates itself. Moreover, the inflammation caused due to macrophages can worsen the damage to healthy tissues and cells, leading to an increased risk of life-threatening consequences such as many autoimmune conditions, cancer, degenerative neurologic diseases, heart disease, etc.

The most sensitive organs toward mitochondrial function are the brain and the heart because they're the most metabolically active. It's no surprise that we see problems in those two areas in any mitochondrial challenged situation. Yet on the flip side, improving mitochondrial function can also create great improvements for those organ systems.

Melatonin can help in these endless cycles of inflammation by regulating the immune system and inhibiting excessive inflammation through the quenching of the oxidation within the mitochondria, as well as the restoration of the PDC pathway and the blocking of the PDK pathway.

Furthermore, melatonin in cells can support energy production and reduce the activities of interleukins and other inflammatory cytokines. This can help to calm the cytokine storm from most all infections, as well as minimize tissue damage which is sometimes related to autoimmune diseases such as multiple sclerosis, rheumatoid arthritis, ankylosing spondylitis, and ALS. It's my opinion that many of these autoimmune conditions have their root causes in chronic infections that are typically associated with toxicity. It's these pathways that are at the core of many of these diseases.[5]

Could melatonin really be that beneficial to this many diseases? Let's take a look at how it relates to cancer as an example.

How does melatonin influence the Warburg effect and regulate energy production in cancer cells?

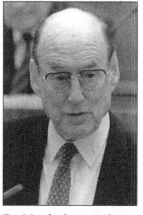

To start, let's circle back to our inefficient form of producing energy called aerobic glycolysis. This energy pathway, called the Warburg effect, has a major role in cancer cells. For this one reason melatonin has been demonstrated in literature to inhibit cancer growth. I was first introduced to the work of Otto Warburg back in the late 90s. I was working with a therapy called exercise with oxygen therapy or EWOT. The

Dr. Manfred von Ardenne

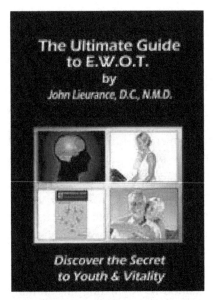

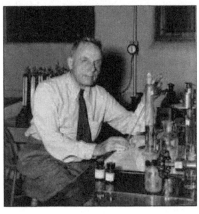

concept of exercising with oxygen was pioneered by Warburg's protégé, Dr. Van Arden.

I created the Ultimate Guide to EWOT and was promoting the use of this therapy as early as 1999.

Who was Otto Warburg?

Otto Warburg was a German scientist in the early 1990s who won the Nobel prize for discovering that oxygen and cancer can't coexist, and in the process was able to understand cancer at a much deeper level than anyone prior to him had. He was the first to observe aerobic glycolysis. This is the primary means that the mitochondria in cancer cells make energy, and as mentioned prior, is referred to as the "Warburg Effect".[6]

Warburg effect refers to a phenomenon that is observed predominantly in cancer cells. This phenomenon occurs when the cells ferment glucose to produce lactic acid during glycolysis in the presence of oxygen. It was Otto Warburg, in 1926, who postulated it as the fundamental cause of cancer.

This dysfunctional, energy-producing process that leads to the production of 4 ATP is called glycolysis. During glycolysis, 1 glucose is broken down into 2 molecules of pyruvate along with a small amount of ATP.[7] [8] As mentioned before, in a normal situation your healthy mitochondria will break down the glucose into pyruvate and then Acetyl-CoA which

subsequently goes into the Krebs cycle. At this point, the mitochondria "burn" the pyruvate molecules released from glycolysis to form much more ATP, up to 90% more!

One of the hallmarks of cancer is a change in cellular metabolism which skips the mitochondria.

CELLULAR FERMENTATION OR AEROBIC GLYCOLYSIS DIAGRAM

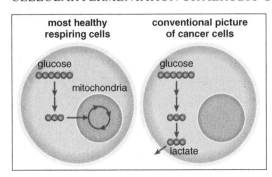

Nevertheless, in the absence of oxygen, the cells can complete only the first step, which is glycolysis, releasing only 2 molecules of ATP from each molecule of glucose. This is where in addition to that inhibition of the PDK you also have a depletion of oxygen.

Otto Warburg observed how the process of oxidative phosphorylation is altered in cancer cells. He also described how cancer cells function differently, even in the presence of oxygen. He postulated that while healthy cells can entirely "burn" the molecules of sugar, cancer cells do so only partially. They tend to overindulge in the step of glycolysis during respiration without completing the second step of oxidative phosphorylation.

Now that we've described the science of this you now know what's really happening at a cellular level to understand the difference between these two cells. [9][10][11]

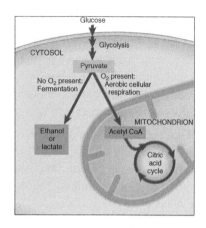

What's the downstream effect of this?

As a result, only 2 molecules of ATP are released from each glucose molecule. This reduced amount of energy is not adequate for cancer cells to survive. Without these massive amounts of glucose, cancer cells can't receive the energy needed for their survival. This is one of the reasons that avoidance of sugars in the diet and even a strict ketogenic diet can be so helpful. By starving cancer cells of glucose, you can give your cells and body the advantage, because cancerous cells rely heavily on sugars and thrive in high-sugar environments.

Furthermore, various fasting strategies are used by many alternative cancer doctors to rob cancer cells of glucose. An interesting alternative medical technique called Insulin Potentiation Therapy (IPT) has been becoming more popular. IPT is where a practitioner will give insulin to a fasting patient to put them into a severe hypoglycemic state. Then they will intravenously introduce substances that would be toxic to the cancer cells (chemo agents) along with glucose. Because the cancer cells are so hungry for this glucose, they will pull in the material from the IV very rapidly and more robustly than your normal cells. It's like the trojan horse!

A surprising increase in science was discovered back in these early days in Germany. Otto Warburg is one of my most admired scientists of that era. He was the first to observe this unusual behavior of energy-deprived cancer cells. He described how cancer cells utilize only glycolysis and oxidative phosphorylation when oxygen supply is adequate.I often wonder if we were to put Russell Reiter, MD together with Otto Warburg, MD today what would transpire?

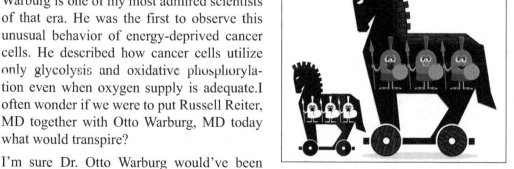

I'm sure Dr. Otto Warburg would've been a huge fan of melatonin supplementation, especially when considering the interplay between how the mitochondria become dysfunctional and how super-antioxidants like melatonin can quench some of the negative effects of this condition. Several research studies have revealed that melatonin can reverse the 'Warburg effect".[12] [13] [14]

In cancer cells, glucose is metabolized to form pyruvate, and later to lactate. Melatonin can support the conversion of pyruvate into acetyl-CoA in mitochondria. Moreover, in studies, this mechanism has shown to have the potential to reprogram the metabolism of glucose in cancer cells to that of normal cells.[15]

This means melatonin has the potential to inhibit the Warburg-dependent cancer cells by redirecting glucose oxidation to the mitochondria. It works as a glycolytic agent and inhibits cancer growth. Melatonin can compel the cancer cells to abandon partial breakdown of glucose and switch to the conventional oxidative phosphorylation or the Krebs cycle.[16][17][18][19]

While doing so, melatonin also stops and slows down the proliferative activities of cancer cells, and reduces their metastatic potential, thus forcing them to undergo apoptosis more readily. This explains how the use of melatonin has the potential to restore cellular functions and support the recovery of cancer patients.

Finally, the same effects of melatonin on cancer cells can also explain why tumors that have become resistant to chemotherapy are re-sensitized to the treatment when melatonin is administered in the form of supplements.[20][21][22][23][24][25]

Conclusion

This is probably the chapter I was most excited about writing and one of the core reasons I wanted to bring forth this book. The idea that melatonin is so intrinsically involved at the cellular level and in the most important area of the cell, the mitochondria, is not something most people or even healthcare providers are familiar with.

I mentioned the above from experience, as it is now 2021 and I've become somewhat of an advocate of melatonin, consequently teaching other doctors as well as working closely with many chronic patients. It is rare that any of them have been exposed to this information previously, and this is usually new material for them. I believe this chapter provides an argument for the supplementation of melatonin in almost all cases of the disease.

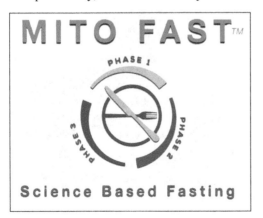

We promote MitoFast which is an anti-aging technique utilizing a 3 phase fasting strategy to improve mitochondria function along with melatonin. The MitoFast is a 3 phase fasting program where we preload with NAD+ prior to the fast then use plant polyphenols during the fasting period to support autophagy, mitophagy, and cleanup zombie-like cells called senescent cells which are extremely inflammatory.

We didn't have time to really dive into this subject, however, if this is something you're interested in you can find more information at ultimatecellularreset.com. Moreover, fasting techniques can be hugely beneficial to calm chronic inflammation and there are various ways these protocols can be executed safely. See my article on MitoFast here.

I think in today's toxic and stressful world we need to rely on more strategies than just melatonin.

Nevertheless, if you're looking to have more energy, less inflammation, less oxidative stress, better immune function, and stronger detoxification pathways, melatonin supplementation could certainly be very helpful.

We will be getting more into dosage, super physiologic melatonin dosing, routes of delivery like suppositories and liposomal in the chapters to come.

Reference

1. Reyes-Toso CF, Rebagliati IR, Ricci CR, Linares LM, Albornoz LE, Cardinali DP, Zaninovich A. Effect of melatonin treatment on oxygen consumption by rat liver mitochondria. Amino Acids. 2006 Oct;31(3):299-302. doi: 10.1007/s00726-005-0280-z. Epub 2006 Mar 24. PMID: 16554975.

2. Srinivasan, V., Spence, D. W., Pandi-Perumal, S. R., Brown, G. M., & Cardinali, D. P. (2011). Melatonin in mitochondrial dysfunction and related disorders. *International journal of Alzheimer's disease, 2011*, 326320. https://doi.org/10.4061/2011/326320

3. Erdal S. Melatonin promotes plant growth by maintaining integration and coordination between carbon and nitrogen metabolisms. Plant Cell Rep. 2019 Aug;38(8):1001-1012. doi: 10.1007/s00299-019-02423-z. Epub 2019 May 8. PMID: 31069499.

4. Owino, S., Buonfiglio, D., Tchio, C., & Tosini, G. (2019). Melatonin Signaling a Key Regulator of Glucose Homeostasis and Energy Metabolism. *Frontiers in endocrinology, 10*, 488. https://doi.org/10.3389/fendo.2019.00488

5. Sanchez-Sanchez AM, Antolin I, Puente-Moncada N, Suarez S, Gomez-Lobo M, Rodriguez C, et al. (2015) Melatonin Cytotoxicity Is Associated to Warburg Effect Inhibition in Ewing Sarcoma Cells. PLoS ONE 10(8): e0135420. https://doi.org/10.1371/journal.pone.0135420

6. Liberti, M. V., & Locasale, J. W. (2016). The Warburg Effect: How Does it Benefit Cancer Cells?. *Trends in biochemical sciences, 41*(3), 211–218. https://doi.org/10.1016/j.tibs.2015.12.001

7. Kannagi, R. Molecular mechanism for cancer-associated induction of sialyl Lewis X and sialyl Lewis A expression—The Warburg effect revisited. *Glycoconj J* **20,** 353–364 (2003). https://doi.org/10.1023/B:GLYC.0000033631.35357.41

8. Bayley, Jean-Pierrea; Devilee, Petera,b The Warburg effect in 2012, Current Opinion in Oncology: January 2012 - Volume 24 - Issue 1 - p 62-67 doi: 10.1097/CCO.0b013e32834deb9e

9. Vander Heiden MG, Cantley LC, Thompson CB. Understanding the Warburg effect: the metabolic requirements of cell proliferation. Science. 2009 May 22;324(5930):1029-33. doi: 10.1126/science.1160809. PMID: 19460998; PMCID: PMC2849637.

10. Burns JS, Manda G. Metabolic Pathways of the Warburg Effect in Health and Disease: Perspectives of Choice, Chain or Chance. Int J Mol Sci. 2017 Dec 19;18(12):2755. doi: 10.3390/ijms18122755. PMID: 29257069; PMCID: PMC5751354.

11. Burns, J. S., & Manda, G. (2017). Metabolic Pathways of the Warburg Effect in Health and Disease: Perspectives of Choice, Chain or Chance. *International journal of molecular sciences*, *18*(12), 2755. https://doi.org/10.3390/ijms18122755

12. Hevia D, Gonzalez-Menendez P, Fernandez-Fernandez M, Cueto S, Rodriguez-Gonzalez P, Garcia-Alonso JI, Mayo JC, Sainz RM. Melatonin Decreases Glucose Metabolism in Prostate Cancer Cells: A ^{13}C Stable Isotope-Resolved Metabolomic Study. *International Journal of Molecular Sciences*. 2017; 18(8):1620. https://doi.org/10.3390/ijms18081620

13. Hevia, D., Gonzalez-Menendez, P., Fernandez-Fernandez, M., Cueto, S., Rodriguez-Gonzalez, P., Garcia-Alonso, J. I., Mayo, J. C., & Sainz, R. M. (2017). Melatonin Decreases Glucose Metabolism in Prostate Cancer Cells: A ^{13}C Stable Isotope-Resolved Metabolomic Study. *International journal of molecular sciences*, *18*(8), 1620. https://doi.org/10.3390/ijms18081620

14. Sanchez-Sanchez, A. M., Antolin, I., Puente-Moncada, N., Suarez, S., Gomez-Lobo, M., Rodriguez, C., & Martin, V. (2015). Melatonin Cytotoxicity Is Associated to Warburg Effect Inhibition in Ewing Sarcoma Cells. *PloS one*, *10*(8), e0135420. https://doi.org/10.1371/journal.pone.0135420

15. Reiter, R. J., Sharma, R., & Rosales-Corral, S. (2021). Anti-Warburg Effect of Melatonin: A Proposed Mechanism to Explain its Inhibition of Multiple Diseases. *International journal of molecular sciences*, *22*(2), 764. https://doi.org/10.3390/ijms22020764

16. Reiter, R.J., Sharma, R., Ma, Q. *et al.* Melatonin inhibits Warburg-dependent cancer by redirecting glucose oxidation to the mitochondria: a mechanistic hypothesis. *Cell. Mol. Life Sci.* **77,** 2527–2542 (2020). https://doi.org/10.1007/s00018-019-03438-1

17. Liberti, M. V., & Locasale, J. W. (2016). The Warburg Effect: How Does it Benefit Cancer Cells?. *Trends in biochemical sciences*, *41*(3), 211–218. https://doi.org/10.1016/j.tibs.2015.12.001

18. Liberti, M. V., & Locasale, J. W. (2016). The Warburg Effect: How Does it Benefit Cancer Cells?. *Trends in biochemical sciences*, *41*(3), 211–218. https://doi.org/10.1016/j.tibs.2015.12.001

19. Warburg Effect (cellsignal.com)

20. Venkatesh K.V., Darunte L., Bhat P.J. (2013) Warburg Effect. In: Dubitzky W., Wolkenhauer O., Cho KH., Yokota H. (eds) Encyclopedia of Systems Biology. Springer, New York, NY. https://doi.org/10.1007/978-1-4419-9863-7_703

21. Tan, D. X., Manchester, L. C., Qin, L., & Reiter, R. J. (2016). Melatonin: A Mitochondrial Targeting Molecule Involving Mitochondrial Protection and Dynamics. *International journal of molecular sciences*, *17*(12), 2124. https://doi.org/10.3390/ijms17122124

22. Sharafati-Chaleshtori, R., Shirzad, H., Rafieian-Kopaei, M., & Soltani, A. (2017). Melatonin and human mitochondrial diseases. *Journal of research in medical sciences : the official journal of Isfahan University of Medical Sciences*, *22*, 2. https://doi.org/10.4103/1735-1995.199092

23. Leon J, Acuña-Castroviejo D, Sainz RM, Mayo JC, Tan DX, Reiter RJ. Melatonin and mito-chondrial function. Life Sci. 2004 Jul 2;75(7):765-90. doi: 10.1016/j.lfs.2004.03.003. PMID: 15183071.

24. Tan, D.-X. and Reiter, R.J. 2019. Mitochondria: the birth place, battle ground and the site of melatonin metabolism in cells. *Melatonin Research*. 2, 1 (Feb. 2019), 44-66. DOI:https://doi.org/https://doi.org/10.32794/mr11250011.

25. León J, Acuña-Castroviejo D, Escames G, Tan DX, Reiter RJ. Melatonin mitigates mitochon-drial malfunction. J Pineal Res. 2005 Jan;38(1):1-9. doi: 10.1111/j.1600-079X.2004.00181.x. PMID: 15617531.

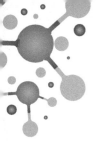

4

MELATONIN & NEUROLOGICAL HEALTH

Blood Brain-Barrier, Glymphatics & mTOR

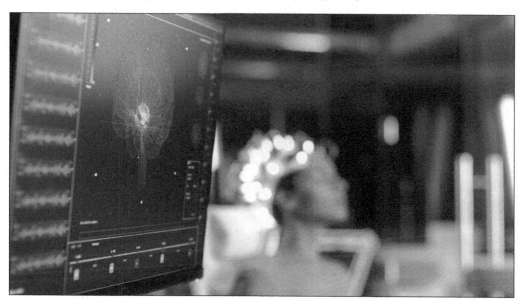

More important than nutrition is your sleep! Sleep and melatonin do more than just allow you to have good sleep, but this process as well as the miracle molecule itself does more for your brain than you could ever imagine.

Over the last 26 years, being a Naturopath and Functional Neurologist, I have taken a lot of time to research this topic to help my patients have a better brain. It is a common theme for most patients that don't get proper sleep to also have poor neurology and brain health. Besides not feeling fresh in the morning, inadequate sleep and poor melatonin levels can be detrimental to your brain, therefore enjoyment of life.

If you don't sleep, the repair activities do not happen the way they should. This can accelerate the process of aging. This is also one of the reasons why neurological diseases have become so rampant. Lack of sleep and lack of proper healing! These factors are at the root of most age-related diseases.

In this chapter, I will be getting into some ideas on how poor sleep can lead to toxic build-up in the brain, ultimately causing a poor environment for optimal brain function. You will also learn how you can use sleep and melatonin to detox the brain of many of the toxic proteins associated with degenerative neurological diseases as well as heavy metals.

To understand this better, allow me to explain by using an example of what happens in patients with Alzheimer's disease and the glymphatic system.

Our body has a glymphatic system that acts as a deep cleansing system for the brain. Like the lymphatic system throughout your body, the glymphatics removes waste from the brain. The glymphatic system is mostly only active during sleep.

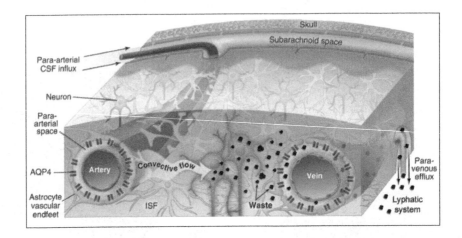

Meaning that the glymphatic system works and is active primarily during sleep and is deactivated while we are awake. The biological need of all species to get adequate sleep reflects this. It indicates that during sleep, the brain may enter the state of glymphatic activity, thus enabling the removal of potentially neurotoxic products like beta-amyloid, tau proteins, alpha-synuclein, and neurofibrillary tangles.

A good analogy to use would be to imagine your body and brain, either being a swamp or a river. Glymphatics move you more towards the river aspect keeping things clean and clear, bringing in the nutrients, and taking out the waste. Besides creating a toxic environment, the buildup of toxins makes for a better breeding ground for infections such as EBV, HHV-6, Lyme, and CMV to name just a few.

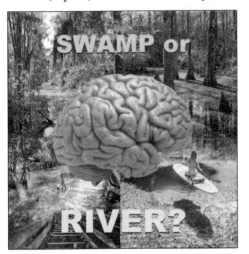

Melatonin, which is our sleep hormone, can powerfully activate your glymphatic system and allow the brain to enter the state of efficient cleansing and detoxifying activities. This is perhaps one of the more important mechanisms by which melatonin can support brain function and delay degenerative changes such as memory loss and cognitive decline.

Detoxification of your nervous system by your glymphatics would also slow down aging. And this seemingly indirect mechanism of melatonin, in reality, can be remarkably effective for preventing age-related neurological diseases such as Alzheimer's, dementia, Parkinson's, and many more.

Circling back to Alzheimer's disease, by activating and supporting the activity of glymphatics at night, melatonin can also prevent the formation of amyloid plaques and neurofibrillary tangles that cause the degeneration of neurons. Melatonin actually clears these plaques, thus making way for healthy neurons to function more efficiently.

These amyloid plaques and neurofibrillary tangles can cause degeneration of the neurons and trigger the development of Alzheimer's disease.

AMYLOID BETA PLAQUE

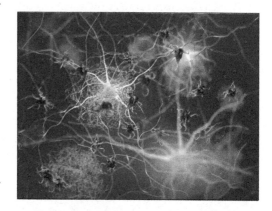

Additionally, proteins released by the immune system in response to inflammation and infection can also cause immense damage to the brain. The immune protein and pro-inflammatory agents can encapsulate the toxins in the nervous system. As a result, these toxins accumulate in the brain and cause long-term damage.

All these changes occur faster and in an uninhibited manner when your glymphatic system is not functioning optimally due to poor sleep. The detoxification of beta-amyloid plaques can occur only when you're sleeping. If you don't get enough sleep, these toxins would stay accumulated in your nervous system and keep causing damage to more and more brain cells making you more likely to develop neurodegenerative diseases like Alzheimer's and Parkinson's at a much earlier age. Nevertheless, all of this could be avoided by taking melatonin.

Melatonin can restore brain functions including memory, attention span, focus, learning, and logical thinking abilities. That's not all. As discussed earlier, it would further help you sleep better so that your glymphatic system can eliminate toxins, free radicals, and pro-inflammatory molecules from the brain.

To get a clear idea of the concept of glymphatic, beta-amyloid plaques,

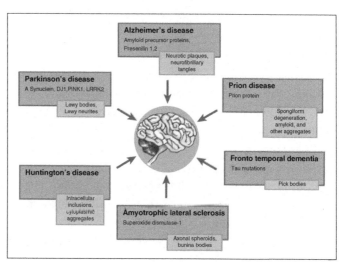

and melatonin, think of the trash at your home that is collected every day by a garbage collector.

These garbage collectors are doing the work of what glymphatics do for your body. Garbage collectors remove the trash from your home to be disposed of in a proper manner, leaving your house clean and neat so that you can stay safe from diseases and infections caused by the lack of hygiene.

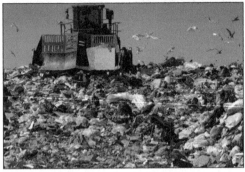

The trash we are talking about in this chapter is, of course, all the toxins released into the body during various metabolic activities. The trash also includes free radicals that cause oxidative stress and even the pro-inflammatory substances released by your immune cells. Your glymphatics can remove these toxins leaving your body clean.

Now, imagine that the garbage collectors go on strike! With no one to collect the garbage, all this trash remains accumulated in your home, in a similar way to how the toxins stay in the brain when the glymphatics aren't working properly. If the strike continues, you're going to have heaps of trash stashed in your home which is going to make your life miserable by making your environment prone to infections and many other diseases.

At the same time, the trash will also provide a perfect setting for rats to thrive. So, now you have a house with trash, plus rats.

This is similar to the beta-amyloid plaques that form in your brain when there is an accumulation of toxins. These plaques can increase your risk of Alzheimer's disease and affect the ability of your brain to function efficiently.

At this juncture, a good idea would be to have the garbage collected so that the rats eventually go away.

Yet, this is not what most modern medicines do. Most drugs prescribed to patients with Alzheimer's disease work by removing amyloid plaques. These medicines are only clearing away the rats, leaving behind the garbage that is the root cause of all the problems. We need to understand that just targeting amyloid plaques with a single chemical compound is not going to address multifactorial diseases like Alzheimer's.

The right way to treat this condition would be to check why amyloid plaques developed in the first place. And of course, it's because your glymphatics haven't been doing their work properly to remove all toxins from the brain. They have been on strike because you don't give them a chance to work peacefully, which, in turn, is because you're not getting enough quality sleep.

If you want to avoid this chain of events, you must make sure you get sound sleep by using melatonin.

In short, good sleep, which is a function of melatonin, can protect you against Alzheimer's and other neurodegenerative diseases, while bad sleep or lack of sleep can bring you closer to getting these diseases.

Is it good to eat while in bed?

Is it true that your body is eating while you're sleeping? Well, in all honesty, it's more of a cleaning and recycling process that the body goes through in different cycles. This process is called autophagy. I was first made aware of this process 15 years ago at a neurology conference, and the subject was regarding degenerative neurologic disease and how the application of fasting can help clear up protein tangles which. It was a very new and novel approach as a therapeutic, and 15 years

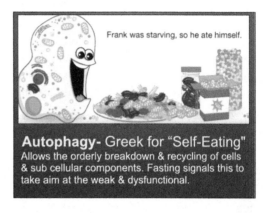

Frank was starving, so he ate himself.

Autophagy- Greek for "Self-Eating"
Allows the orderly breakdown & recycling of cells & sub cellular components. Fasting signals this to take aim at the weak & dysfunctional.

later it's starting to gain a lot of popularity. I'm in the alternative scene and this is the type of strategy I've used since I first learned about it, however, I'm starting to see neurologists locally that are beginning to embrace this methodology as well. So, let's take a bit of a dive into what this is and how you could benefit from it. Yes, you can help your body actually clean and recycle or "EAT" the unwanted harmful plaques through this process we call autophagy.

Why is autophagy so important here? Because this process can help your body clean up and recycle any old, weak, dead, or dying cellular material. This includes dysfunctional mitochondria, cancer cells, dysfunctional immune cells, all dysfunctional cells, as

well as all of the protein plaques associated with many of the diseases of aging in the brain. These protein plaques include tau, neurofibrillary tangles, beta-amyloid, and alpha's synuclein plaques!

It so happens that all tissues in our body are basically undergoing 2 processes continually which include the growth of new cells and tissues, and on the other side of this, the breakdown and recycling of old, dead, or dying, and weak tissues. This is mediated through a process called mTOR.

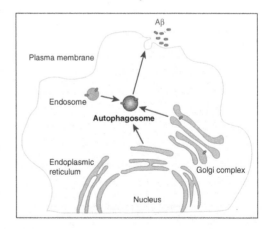

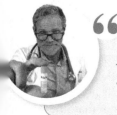

> Auto here means self, and autophagy refers to eating. So, in short, autophagy means eating the self.

This acronym stands for mammalian target of Rapimyosin. mTOR is either turned on or turned off through various stimuli. When mTOR is turned on your body is growing, and cellular growth is activated. But, when mTOR is turned off or inhibited we switch to the breakdown cleaning and recycling phase.

Growth is good, right? Or is it? It helps you build muscles; it helps you grow bigger, stronger bones; it helps us when we have an injury to repair. The growth phase can help you grow new hair, new skin cells, and all of this helps you look younger and stay healthier.

Nevertheless, let's take a look at where growth might be bad.

One of the big problems in civilized cultures is that we have way too much activation of mTOR, thus too much growth in the body. One of the key reasons for this problem is that we have quite easy access to food. When we are feeding it makes sense that our body wants to be in a growth phase. However, when we are fasting the growth switches to the cleaning and recycling phase, and mTOR is inhibited. Some of the more obvious problems associated with too much growth include cardiovascular and circulatory-related issues, where the muscular layer inside of our blood vessels thickens, choking off the flow of blood through the vessel. This is particularly a problem for the perfusion of the brain in many people as they get older. Enlargement of various organs can occur, for instance, polyps in the digestive tract as well as growths or cyst formation throughout the body. Then there's the most obvious of them all which is cancer.

The excessive multiplication of cells in the organs can initiate cancerous changes in healthy tissues. Generally, when this gets out of control the body will use a process called apoptosis, which is a formula for autophagy.

When this growth gets out of hand, the body needs to turn off mTOR and shift to the autophagy cleaning phase.

Now, there are two major influences to activate or inhibit these important cycles. Nutrient deprivation or fasting, and sleep will dial down mTOR. Ultimately, autophagy works like a recycling system in which the body eats away what is in excess but keeps what's in good condition, such as healthy cells, tissues, and even cell organelles like mitochondria. The proteins and nutrients from these cleanup cycles can then be reused to build new mitochondria, senescent cells, and dysfunctional tissues.

Senescent cells are a huge problem that are key drivers of aging inflammation and many other diseases. It's through the inhibition of mTOR and autophagy that we clear out these incredibly problematic and dangerous cells. Moreover, senescent cells have also been referred to as "zombie cells", this is because in actuality they are old dysfunctional cells that produce toxins that can be extremely inflammatory. Moreover, they also hog a lot of energy in exchange for nothing, because the cells are working. Ultimately meaning that they

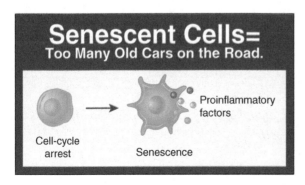

Senescent Cells=
Too Many Old Cars on the Road.

Cell-cycle arrest

Senescence

Proinflammatory factors

get fed yet you get no work out of them, only their waste product. Furthermore, it is thought that the accumulation of senescent cells is the leading cause of aging and could be a major factor in many diseases as well.

Melatonin can play an important role in limiting the number of senescent cells, decreasing the negative impact they have on your body, as well as improving the cleanup and recycling of the cells through stimulating deep sleep.

Though fasting is effective, today's generation seems to be more into overeating than into starving. Americans eat an average of 14.75 hours a day, we have mid-meal junk food, pre-meal snacks, and then, even late-night desserts.

Like I stated earlier, this is what is driving a lot of diseases in our modern society. It's an over-expression of mTOR. With the habits as explained above, we have little time where we are in a fasting state where our body goes into recycling and cleaning mode, thus enabling mTOR to be inhibited.

Besides us accumulating dysfunctional mitochondria, cells, and tissues we also don't readily have the building blocks needed to produce more healthy ones.

Valter Longo is a scientist who has brought much light to how this plays into cancer and many other diseases. He demonstrated that through decreasing our feeding window every 24 hours there can be a dramatic improvement in the body's function as well as enhanced longevity. Doing extended fasting turns on this process even more robustly when an individual would do a 3-to-5-day water fast. Longo has done experiments with consumption of fewer than 1500 calories per day for 3-to-5-day protocol where he's demonstrated that there is much benefit to gain.[1]

How does melatonin and sleep play into this process?

This is a book about melatonin, so the miracle molecule demonstrates yet another benefit with regard to sleep. Deep sleep can be a strong proponent to inhibit mTOR.

Here is research showing what a powerful regulator melatonin is for autophagy 'Therapeutic potential of melatonin related to its role as an autophagy regulator: A review'[2]

Besides the body going into a cleaning and recycling phase during sleep we also have the glymphatic system mopping up and shuffling off all of the toxins and waste products from the central nervous system. Preventing this from happening can be catastrophic to the central nervous system.

Melatonin is the primary driver for this to work properly. When melatonin levels decline as we age this problem can become much worse. We ultimately produce a buildup of dysfunctional mitochondria which then creates an energy deficiency. This then allows for a buildup of toxins that subsequently creates an environment that favors microbial overgrowth such as viruses and bacteria. Remember that the terrain is what drives microbial growth.

When you have a lack of cleanup you produce the situation that we discussed earlier, where the trash builds up and then comes the rats. What if we only focused on killing all the rats and not cleaning up all trash or if we only focused on bailing the boat and not plugging the leak? You're going to waste a lot of energy and you're not actually address-ing the core of what's driving the problem.

Anybody looking to live longer and have a more robust and vital life needs to pay close attention to these mTOR cycles!

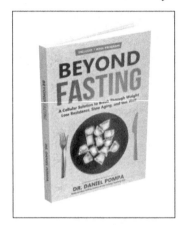

This is what I would suggest: Try starting with a 6 to 10 hour feeding window. I personally only have one or two meals per day, and generally, skip breakfast. This did not come easy for me at first and I had trouble with my blood sugar and energy when originally embarking on this process. What you're really asking the body to do is to switch into a different form of energy production using ketones as its primary fuel source. When you're sleeping and fasting you are in ketosis and your body is using these ketones as energy. Ketones are a much more efficient form of energy for the brain and body. This developed for humans over many thousands of years as when we were hunting, we were hungry, and we needed to have an edge where we functioned at a higher peak state. The problem is that because we're constantly feeding ourselves with lots of carbohydrates our body is efficient using sugars as energy and you haven't given the body an opportunity to become efficient with breaking down fats and proteins for energy, which is where you get ketones from. So, the trick is to start increasing your fat and protein intake and decreasing your carbohydrate consumption. There is, of course, a lot more to this topic and I would recommend the book from my friend Dr. Dan Pompa called Beyond Fasting.

In the next section, I want to tell you one more aspect of melatonin that's linked to the blood-brain barrier.

Understanding the role of the blood-brain barrier in melatonin production

Melatonin can stabilize and strengthen the coupling of circadian rhythms with the sleep-wake rhythms and the body's core temperature. The circadian organization such as antioxidant and immune defenses, glucose regulation, and hemostasis also depends on the biochemical signals carried by melatonin. These functions of melatonin need to be understood from the point of view of the blood-brain barrier. This is important because how the blood-brain barrier affects melatonin secretion in contrast to other hormones makes it unique and more powerful.

Interestingly, the pineal gland, in spite of being a part of the brain during its embryolog-ical stage (while it is still being formed in the fetus), is situated outside the blood-brain barrier. As a result, it loses its direct connection with the brain.

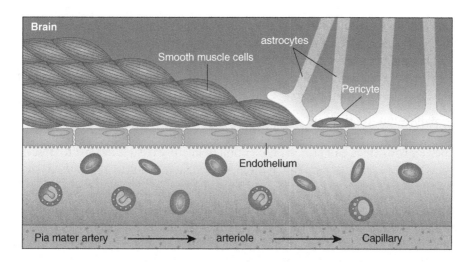

Blood Brain Barrier made of Astrocytes.

While discussing the various processes involved in the role of melatonin secretion and deep sleep, it is essential to know that the production of this hormone is somewhat independent of the blood-brain barrier, thanks to its unique location.

Why is the special ability of melatonin to escape the blood-brain barrier so important?

- It allows for a larger uptake of tryptophan, which, in turn, supports an increased melatonin production in response to darkness.

- The freedom to escape the blood-brain barrier offers relative protection to melatonin against premature enzymatic degradation leading to a 10 to 20-fold rise in melatonin levels.

- It explains why the pineal gland has to rely on stimulation by sympathetic nerves and serotonin for regulating melatonin production.[3]

These properties of melatonin make it a unique and powerful molecule that can be utilized in our fight against diseases linked to poor sleep.

Another antioxidant called glutathione should also be something to be considered. This is another nutrient that declines in many diseases as well as in age. It has been shown that low glutathione levels can contribute to a breakdown in the BBB. Moreover, it has also been shown that by supplementing with a 600 mg glutathione suppository such as GlutaMax or through intravenous administration, you can support the repair and protection of your BBB. In our clinic, we utilize supplements that enhance circulation. Which ultimately produces or allows further nutrients to support the BBB in combination with a melatonin and glutathione suppository called Sandman.

Conclusion

As I have compared before, melatonin is like the electromagnetic field of the earth. It protects our body the same way the electromagnetic field protects the earth from solar radiation. The flow of liquid metals in the outer core of our planets generates an electric current. The rotation of Earth causes these electric currents to create a magnetic field extending around the planet. This magnetic field helps to sustain life on Earth. Without it, the living species would be exposed to a high amount of radiation from the sun and cause our atmosphere to leak into space.

Besides supporting the BBB, melatonin creates an inner protective rhythm of the sleep-wake cycle that is synchronized with the activities of the glymphatics and the body's repair mechanisms. This can provide protection to healthy tissues against toxins, free radicals, beta-amyloid plaques, and much more. Consequently, allowing us to live a healthy life.

Fasting can clear up senescent cells and trigger the cleaning and recycling of cells and cellular components like mitochondria. Using the MitoFast as a technique to aid in autophagy and increase the influence of the fasting protocol might be interesting to look at if you're wanting to boost brain power and prolong brain health.

Reference

1. Wei, M., Brandhorst, S., Shelehchi, M., Mirzaei, H., Cheng, C. W., Budniak, J., Groshen, S., Mack, W. J., Guen, E., Di Biase, S., Cohen, P., Morgan, T. E., Dorff, T., Hong, K., Michalsen, A., Laviano, A., & Longo, V. D. (2017). Fasting-mimicking diet and markers/risk factors for aging, diabetes, cancer, and cardiovascular disease. *Science translational medicine, 9*(377), eaai8700. https://doi.org/10.1126/scitranslmed.aai8700

2. Boga JA, Caballero B, Potes Y, Perez-Martinez Z, Reiter RJ, Vega-Naredo I, Coto-Montes A. Therapeutic potential of melatonin related to its role as an autophagy regulator: A review. J Pineal Res. 2019 Jan;66(1):e12534. doi: 10.1111/jpi.12534. Epub 2018 Nov 26. PMID: 30329173.

3. WURTMAN RJ, AXELROD J, POTTER LT. THE UPTAKE OF H3-MELATONIN IN ENDOCRINE AND NERVOUS TISSUES AND THE EFFECTS OF CONSTANT LIGHT EXPOSURE. J Pharmacol Exp Ther. 1964 Mar;143:314-8. PMID: 14161142.

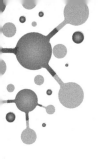

MELATONIN & IMMUNE SYSTEM

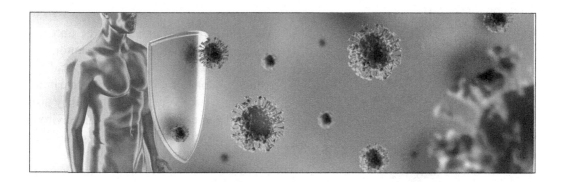

Immune Health & Autoimmune Disease

A strong immune system to fight infections has never been more important than it is today. As I write this book, we are in a global lockdown due to the COVID-19 virus and this global pandemic has created the most interest in protecting ourselves from infections I have seen in my 26 years of practice.

If only I could afford to run ads on TV for melatonin, I would educate the world on how it can be of great benefit without any risky side effects. My friend Dr. Russel Reiter has been quietly putting out the science on melatonin for COVID-19. Yet, funnily enough, I was asked to take down ALL virus-related information from my website by the FTC and FDA. It was a special operation by our government to limit the information that went against the agenda they are promoting, which is vaccines. Therapeutic options have been ignored for the most part during the COVID-19 warp speed rush for a cure. Therapeutics like mela-

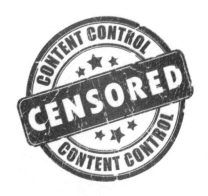

tonin without any big pharma entity pushing it into the faces of the government will surely not see its potential as useful support for COVID-19 or anything in the foreseeable future.

There are a few things more important than a properly functioning immune system. Your immune system is built on your white blood cells which circulate throughout your blood and your tissues to defend your body from foreign invaders, such as infections. But there is much more to the immune system, and we will dive into that later in this chapter.

It is important that your immune system is strong enough to be able to deal with the challenges presented to it. It's also important that your immune system, not over-respond or continue to respond, even after the challenge has been met and resolved.

Your immune system uses very toxic substances to destroy these foreign invaders. In addition to these toxic substances, the immune system also uses something called cytokines which are defined as "a number of substances, such as interferon, interleukin, and growth factors, which are secreted by certain cells of the immune system and have an effect on other cells."

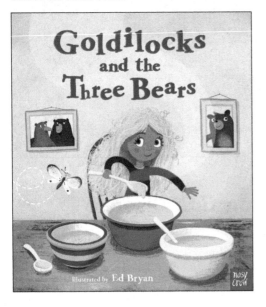

You could almost think about the immune system as a combination of a janitor, the trash collector, the recycling crew, and the maid all in one. Similarly, to how cleaning solutions can be very toxic for us, they also help to keep a sanitary and clean environment in our home and work. And just like it's important to use just enough and not too many of these services, your cleaning would be similar to the situation inside of your body with your immune system.

It's a very delicate balance between not too much not too little!

Generally, a poorly functioning immune system is due to low energy reserves as a result of bad mitochondria, which we will speak of at length in another chapter. Also, an under-functioning immune system can also be the result of not recognizing what it needs to clean up. Moreover, when the immune system is weak, it allows infections to run rampant. For instance, in cancer, the immune system recognizes the cancerous cells and cleans them up through apoptosis. Furthermore, an over-exuberant immune system lends itself to autoimmune diseases and causes out-of-control inflammation in the body with an example being severe allergies, and of course, the cytokine storm that COVID-19 has now made so infamous.

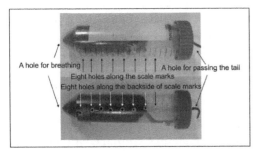

A good example that comes to mind is Goldilocks and the three bears in which the bear's porridge was either too cold or too hot, and mama's porridge was just right. Our immune system needs to be like mama's porridge.

At first glance, one would think melatonin would have no involvement in the immune system. And as mentioned in previous chapters, melatonin did not seem to have an impact when there was no stress present in the body. Remember the example we gave you where researchers were first looking at melatonin use in mice and found that the mice had no benefit with melatonin supplementation. But later, they started to subject the mice to stress which was achieved by putting them in a tube with little holes drilled in it for a few hours each day. Again, this is a common way by which they would induce stress on these laboratory animals. This is where melatonin really seemed to shine where the animals that were subjected to stress had little health consequences versus the ones that were not.

It's been more than a decade since the unique ability of melatonin to regulate and strengthen the immune system functions was discovered. Moreover, there are multiple studies that now share similar results, for example, this new study published in Behavioral Pharmacology, *'The effects of melatonin on the behavioral disturbances induced by chronic mild stress in C3H/He mice'* showed that regular treatment of stressed mice using melatonin could prevent CMS-induced disturbances. This study supported the idea that melatonin might be implicated in a homeostatic system that protects us from disruptions induced by stress.[1]

Another study, *"Effects of melatonin on stress-induced and diurnal variations of nociception in Wistar and spontaneously hypertensive rats"*, conducted by researchers at the Bulgarian Academy of Sciences reiterated that there is substantial evidence proving the antinociceptive effects of melatonin. This study proved the impact of melatonin in the modulation of nociception when the subjects were examined under acute immobilization stress as well as on

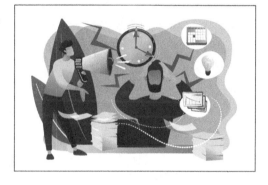

diurnal variations of spontaneously hypertensive rats and normotensive.[2]

Yet a blockbuster finding with regards to melatonin was when scientists found that the white blood cells, which, as I mentioned, are considered the main players in the defense functions performed by our immunity, have melatonin receptors. What this means, is that melatonin has a lot of involvement within the immune system and is an especially important substance for it to function optimally, particularly in states of stress where your immune system needs to react in an appropriate manner.

Melatonin appears to help the immune system function in a strong yet controlled manner.

Interesting facts about melatonin and the immune system

It's intriguing to understand how melatonin produces an ultra-specific action on the immune cells. On one hand, it stimulates the secretion of cytokines to help your body attack the invading viruses, bacteria, or other pathogens. This action helps to indicate that melatonin can STIMULATE immunity and thus, contribute to the release of proinflammatory cytokines.

But there's a twist to it. Though melatonin can activate the immune system, it does just the opposite when there's a need to reverse or prevent the damage that has occurred due to excessive inflammation. It can also STOP the immune system from producing more pro-inflammatory cytokines when they are not needed, or when they are likely to cause damage to the tissues.

It is this dual action of melatonin on the immune system that has been particularly of great interest to scientists.

Now after this quick overview of melatonin, let's move deeper and get a closer look at the action of this miracle molecule on the function of your immune system.

Role of melatonin in supporting immune system functions

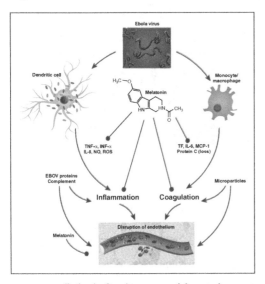

If the immune system had a gas and brake pedal, then melatonin would have a foot on each. The immune system needs to be able to accelerate and slowdown in order to protect your body, thus not becoming more of a problem than an answer to your health.

When this system isn't working, it will wind up causing diseases such as chronic infections, cancer, and autoimmune diseases.

If your immune system is functioning normally, and by normal, I mean like mama's porridge at the perfect temperature, neither too weak nor too overstimulated…Then, you can fight infections, avoid autoimmune diseases, overcome inflammatory damage, and even protect your vital organs against inflammation.

If it's a situation where you contract an infection such as COVID-19 or Ebola, where the inflammatory storm is so severe that it might kill you, then melatonin may actually protect you from the fatalities involved with these infections.

Again, is it important to look at the studies that have been conducted with melatonin as it relates to its protective action from infections and the cytokine storm.

There's a study published in the Journal of Pineal Research, "Melatonin and viral infections" in which they gave each 2 groups of mice a lethal injection of EMCV (Encephalomyocarditis V.). With the melatonin on board, the survival rate went from only 6% to 82%.[3]

Now, if you are looking for a good driver for your immune system sitting behind the steering wheel that responsibly applies the brakes and gas pedal, supplementing with melatonin might be something important to consider.

Another study published in the Current Topics in Medicinal Chemistry has demonstrated that melatonin can regulate the production of cytokines and thus, inhibit inflammation.

"There is overwhelming information demonstrating the immune-enhancing properties of melatonin."

Moreover, a 2002 study published in the Current Topics in Medicinal Chemistry, "Melatonin-Immune System Relationships", highlighted the existence of the relationship between melatonin and the immune system and revealed the rhythmic production of melatonin that works in a synchronized manner with the activities of the immune system. It also showed the effects of pinealectomy and the administration of melatonin on the variety of immune parameters, such as specific as well as non-specific immunity. The data suggested the existence of membrane and nuclear receptors for melatonin in the immune system. This study, in particular, provided overwhelming findings demonstrating the immune-enhancing effects of melatonin.[4]

But that's not all! A 2005 study published in the journal "Endocrine" talked about the effects of melatonin on cellular and humoral immune responses as well as immune mediator production and cellular proliferation. It, again, showed how this hormone can produce a direct immunomodulatory effect on cytokine production. This effect is almost always going to be a positive calming down of an activated immune system. Nevertheless, it's important to be able to apply brakes after a fast immune acceleration.

This review further highlighted melatonin's actions in immune pathologies including autoimmunity, infections, and inflammation, and emphasized its role as an immunity regulator. *"One of the main features that distinguishes melatonin from the classical hormones is its synthesis by a number of nonendocrine extrapineal organs, including the immune system."*[5]

We've mentioned this before, but it's worth repeating here that melatonin is not just released by your pineal gland, but it is also released by your immune cells. In fact, it's utilized by your mitochondria throughout all of your cells.

How does melatonin help to inhibit autoimmune disorders?

Besides controlling the brake and gas pedal, melatonin is a reliable and powerful immunopotentiating agent. In my view, it does not act directly but produces a synchronizing effect on your entire neuroendocrine system, which is how it controls and regulates the immune system.

What exactly does an autoimmune disorder mean?

An autoimmune disorder is when your body sees itself as an enemy, and consequently attacks your own cells and tissues. It so happens that sometimes, your immune cells just fail to recognize the body's healthy cells and tissues as their own.

It considers them as foreign bodies that must be killed and removed. So, the immune system activates a chain of reactions that leads to the destruction of healthy tissues:

- In your central nervous system such as in MS & ALS.
- In the thyroid gland such as in the case of Hashimoto's thyroiditis.
- In joints as in rheumatoid arthritis and ankylosing spondylitis.
- In skin such as psoriasis, lupus, and eczema.
- In the gut such as in Crohn's disease.
- In blood cells such as in autoimmune hemolytic anemia, and so on.

As a result of an immune system with a poor driver behind the wheel, you may develop rheumatoid arthritis, thyroiditis, psoriasis, eczema, lupus, and many other diseases that are categorized under the umbrella term, "autoimmune diseases". Whether you were looking to prevent or reverse these diseases, your only hope is by regulating your immune system.

Several research studies have confirmed that melatonin might be helpful in this regard. Among these, there was one research study published in the International Journal of Molecular Sciences that demonstrated the ability of melatonin to inhibit abnormal immune responses by controlling the production of cytokines and T helper cells.

It highlighted the modulatory effect of melatonin in the development of inflammatory autoimmune diseases including diabetes mellitus, systemic lupus erythematosus, multiple sclerosis, rheumatoid arthritis, and inflammatory bowel diseases. *"The effect of melatonin on the suppression of proinflammatory cytokine production has been proven in many studies."*

*Moreover, a*ccording to another research study, "Modulation by Melatonin of the Pathogenesis of Inflammatory Autoimmune Diseases" published in the International Journal Of Molecular Science, in 2013, this modulatory effect of melatonin could be effective in several inflammatory autoimmune diseases.[6]

Melatonin suppresses the production of tumor necrosis factor (TNF)-α & IL-1β. Nitric oxide has been found to be an important mediator in an inflammatory response. Melatonin also plays a role in the regulation of nitric oxide synthesis. Interestingly enough, previous studies have shown that melatonin inhibits the over-expression of inducible nitric oxide synthase (iNOS) in the liver and lungs of lipopolysaccharide (LPS)-treated rats.

There are several forms of nitric oxide and as a substance can be taken to promote a better immune system and cardiovascular function. For example, induced nitric oxide is the type you really don't want much of. It's the nasty NOS that destroys tissue and cells and you want it when you need it, but when it continues or occurs in too large amounts it is linked to many destructive diseases. Melatonin can act to modulate this so that iNOS doesn't cause damage to your body. The mechanism of melatonin in the reduction of pro-inflammatory cytokine as well as iNOS production has been suggested via the inhibition of either expression or activation of nuclear factor-κB (NF-κB).

Let's discuss how Nuclear Factor kappa for Activated B cells or NF-κB is. NF-κB plays a key role in regulating the immune response to infections. Incorrect regulation of NF-κB has been linked to cancer, inflammatory and autoimmune diseases, septic shock, viral infection, and improper immune development. NF-κB has also been implicated in processes of synaptic plasticity and memory. NF-κB is important for regulating cellular responses because it belongs to the category of "rapid-acting" immune proteins present in cells in an inactive state. This allows NF-κB to be a first responder to harmful cellular stimuli such as in a bacterial infection. It is not the bacteria itself that activates this. But it's the chemicals that are released during an infection such as pro-inflammatory cytokines, iNOS, adhesion molecules, COX-2, and matrix metalloproteinases (MMPs).

Moreover, NF-κB is widely used by eukaryotic cells as a regulator of genes that control cell proliferation and cell survival. NF-κB is a critical promoter of tumorigenesis, which creates a compelling argument for the use of antitumor therapy that is based upon suppression of NF-κB. There have been many studies showing melatonin's ability to calm down this inappropriate expression of NF-κB. For example, Gilad *et al.* showed that melatonin can suppress the expression of iNOS in white blood cells via suppression of NF-κB. Furthermore, the expression of damaging adhesion molecules by NF-κB is also suppressed by melatonin, resulting in a reduced recruitment of neutrophils to inflamed sites.

Many of the dangerous drugs being studied indiscriminately shut NF-κB down. There are important functions of NF-κB as you can see in this chapter. Modulating NF-κB is one of many reasons Big Pharma would love to patent Melatonin as it would be the biggest blockbuster drug ever. The research has shown time and time again that NF-κB activity enhances tumor cell sensitivity to apoptosis and senescence.

Remember in an earlier chapter, we talked about senescent cells that are zombie cells, which accumulate when we don't have the ability to recognize, kill, and recycle these cells. Senescent cells are cells that utilize lots of energy, produce a lot of metabolic waste, and are extremely pro-inflammatory. Also, recall that many researchers see the accumulation of senescent cells as a primary cause of aging and disease formation.

It's super important to be able to recognize tumors and produce apoptosis that essentially eats these cancer cells up like a Pac-Man. I guess the point is, you really need NF-κB as well as all of your pro-inflammatory cytokines, but you also require them at the proper amounts, and you need them to turn on and turn off on a dime! Basically, what you really want is a responsible person behind the immune wheel, controlling both the brakes and the gas pedal. That's where melatonin comes in once again.

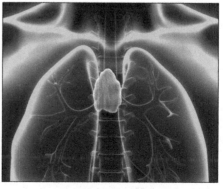

Melatonin may also help by profoundly affecting the glands and organs involved in the immune system, such as the thymus. It can also control cell-mediated immunity thereby reducing your risk of autoimmune disorders.

One study, "Melatonin rejuvenates degenerated thymus and redresses peripheral immune functions in aged mice" published in 2003 in the Immunology Letters, assessed whether melatonin rejuvenates degenerated thymus and restores immune functions in aged mice.

It showed the positive effect of melatonin on age-associated thymic degeneration and immune system dysfunctions. Exogenous melatonin administered through the drinking water to mice for 60 consecutive days reversed the age-associated thymic degeneration by the significant increase of thymus weight, the percentage of thymocyte cells at G2+S phases, and the total number of thymocytes. Spleen weight, number of splenocytes, and peripheral immune capacity including NK cell activity and mitogen responsiveness also recovered significantly by melatonin application in aged mice. These findings demonstrated that melatonin supplementation, even in late life may reverse thymic degeneration and improve peripheral immune functions. This is HUGE![7]

This benefit of melatonin may be specifically useful for those who have a family history of autoimmune diseases. Because ultimately melatonin might protect them against their genetic tendency to develop these conditions.

One study "Cytokine & Growth Factor Reviews" assessed the potential role of melatonin in autoimmune diseases linked to genetics. It showed that melatonin can regulate the cellular and humoral immune responses, and control immune mediators and cell proliferation by correcting the underlying genetic abnormalities.

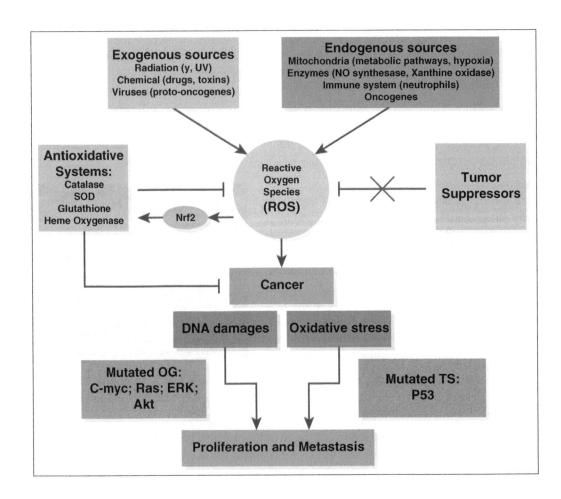

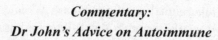

Commentary:
Dr John's Advice on Autoimmune

Besides melatonin, broccoli sprout extract supplementation should be considered to further enhance the Nrf2 gene activation.

In an article in Trends Food Sci Technol. 2017 Nov titled "KEAP1 and done? Targeting the NRF2 pathway with sulforaphane" they were able to demonstrate that supplementing with sulforaphane was a powerful activator of the Nrf2 genes.

"Broccoli, especially as young sprouts, is a rich source of sulforaphane and broccoli-based preparations are now used in clinical studies probing efficacy in health preservation and disease mitigation. Many putative cellular targets are affected by sulforaphane although only one, KEAP1-NRF2 signaling, can be considered a validated target at this time. The transcription factor NRF2 is a master regulator of cell survival responses to endogenous and exogenous stressors."

There could be an argument for using high doses of melatonin sulforaphane and broccoli-based preparations in autoimmune conditions. At our clinic we like to dig as deep as we can to discover reasons the immune might be under stress. Things like mold exposure, chronic viral infections like with EBV, CMV, HHV-6, Lyme Disease are all common core issues with autoimmune disease. The gut is a very important system to look at and will be involved in almost ALL autoimmune cases. Poor sinus and oral hygiene can also chronically activate the immune system.

Things like oil pulling for and a solid 30 day sinus protocol like with the GlutaStat line of products could be beneficial. Leaky gut due to chronic gut stress which is typically a poor microbiome, sympathetic nervous system taking blood and nutrients away from your gut, microbial infection of the gut such as candida, H.Pylori, SIBO, Clostridium P., and multiple parasitic infections.

Fasting is an important consideration to allow autophagy to clean up all the dysfunctional immune cells. Moreover, the re-feeding phase (after the fast) will trigger new health functioning immune cells to be made in your thymus gland and bone marrow.

See MitoFast here for my fasting protocol. My best advice would be to check all these factors as many cases do best when multiple aspects of these suggestions are followed at the same time to clear the system. For more on these natural approaches to health see www.UltimateCellularReset.com.

Treatment with melatonin may also promote the differentiation of type 1 regulatory T cells through the extracellular signal-regulated kinase 1/2 and ROR-α (retinoic acid-related orphan receptor-α). It would suppress the differentiation of Th17 cells through the inhibition of ROR-α and ROR-γt expressions through NFIL3. Moreover, melatonin can also inhibit NF-κB signaling pathways and reduce IL-1β and TNF-α expression while promoting Nrf2 genes. Nrf2 gene activation is a big deal! Nrf2 can protect cells and tissues from a variety of toxicants and carcinogens by increasing the expression of a number of cytoprotective genes.

NRF2 regulates the expression of antioxidant proteins that protect against oxidative damage triggered by injury and inflammation. NRF2 also plays a vital role in the regulation of metabolism, inflammation, autophagy, proteostasis, mitochondrial physiology, and immune responses. Furthermore, Nrf2 also increases intracellular glutathione, one of the more powerful antioxidants to calm down autoimmunity.

If you consider the diagram here you can see Nrf2 works closely with your antioxidant systems: Catalase, SOD, Glutathione and Heme Oxygenase. Basically, Nrf2 controls the inflammatory and oxidative states in the body responsible for worsening the symptoms of cancers and also autoimmune disorders. This suggests that melatonin could serve as a potential therapeutic target, and create opportunities for more efficient management of autoimmune diseases by regulating the novel signaling pathways involved in certain genetic expressions, such as with Nrf2 and NF-κB.[8]

Melatonin in organ transplantation

The effects of melatonin have been shown to support proper immune system functions post transplantation procedures.

We all know that organ transplantation and skin grafting have an inherent risk of rejection resulting in the failure of the procedure. This obviously occurs because the immune system considers the organ or graft as a foreign body and tries to destroy it by producing inflammatory cytokines. This is why; patients are administered immunosuppressive drugs before, during, and after the treatment to minimize the risk of rejection.

> *"We may never see the light of day within these diseases in our modern health care model though! Ahh if only melatonin was able to gain a patent. Yet another pipeline for a Pharma company like Glaxo-Smith Kline. They would spend the money for larger studies proving its effectiveness and dosages for specific diseases, and market the heck out of it on TV! That is what they do even if the drug doesn't work well or has terrible side effects. Melatonin has neither of these problems!"*

Yet in cases like these, melatonin can be of some use, thanks to its natural immunosuppressive action. Isn't it amazing how melatonin can once again be a brake pedal for the immune system when function goes the wrong way?

There was clinical research published in June 2020 in Scielo that affirmed the above, showing that melatonin administration may decrease rejection and improve transplant success.[9]

Furthermore, a research study published in the Journal of Endocrinology provided experimental evidence that melatonin can be useful in reducing graft failure, particularly in cardiac, otolaryngology, bone, ovarian, lung, pancreas, testicular, liver, and kidney transplantation. This study affirmed that melatonin can be effective in patients undergoing transplantation for end-stage organ failure. It can reduce the chances of organ rejection, and also improve bodily functions during the post-transplantation period.[10]

These immunomodulatory effects of melatonin are truly dramatic and could provide newer and more innovative ways to support the recovery of patients with end-stage organ failure.

How does melatonin affect the immunity to help you fight infections?

Let's take a look at Influenza which is the most common viral infection we face.

Influenza is one of the most common viral infections that affects nearly everyone once or several times in life. If you have weak immunity, you're likely to get influenza during every flu season.

- The protective effect of melatonin against the influenza virus has been revealed during a research study published in the Journal of Functional Foods in 2019. Melatonin was found to be effective for the pre-treatment and treatment procedures in PR8(H1N1)/Influenza A virus in infected mice.

- The severity of pneumonia was also found to be lower in mice pre-treated and treated with melatonin. This study affirmed the role of melatonin as a protective molecule against the flu.[11]

Melatonin & Sepsis

The positive effect of melatonin on the immune system has been observed in the management of viral infections in both the very young and old. Melatonin showed to help with adults as well as in newborn babies with sepsis (when an infection goes systemic).

Melatonin showed to help in preterm infants suffering from respiratory distress syndrome (ARDS), which is the common route of death from an infection that goes septic during a study "Melatonin: its possible role in the management of viral infections-a brief review" published in the Italian Journal of Pediatrics.[12]

Another study "Efficacy of Melatonin in the Prophylaxis of Coronavirus Disease 2019 (COVID-19) Among Healthcare Workers" supported by the Instituto de Investigación Hospital Universitario has shown that melatonin can be used as a prophylactic treatment. It

> *This is the definition of Sepsis: "A potentially life-threatening condition caused by the body's response to an infection. The body normally releases chemicals into the bloodstream to fight an infection. Sepsis occurs when the body's response to these chemicals is out of balance, triggering changes that can damage multiple organ systems."*

can be specifically beneficial for patients with weak immunity and healthcare workers who are regularly exposed to infectious pathogens. Again, it works best when there is stress.[13]

Melatonin can minimize the damage to healthy tissues thus providing relief from the symptoms. It also reduces the levels of lipid peroxidation products in your blood, promoting your chances of survival in the event of sepsis or septicemia. Again, sepsis or septicemia is where an infection goes systemic throughout your body and can often lead to death.

As mentioned before, sepsis is where an infection goes systemic and can be life-threatening.

In a large number of scientific experiments related to septic shock and septic disease, melatonin has reportedly exerted beneficial effects to arrest multiorgan failure and cellular damage.

Melatonin works by preventing nitric oxide synthesis and the consequent reduction in peroxynitrite formation. These are some of the most potent reactive oxygen species or ROS. In fact, peroxynitrites are linked as the most dangerous oxidants to cardiovascular disease. It's extremely corrosive to your heart and blood vessels as well as all tissues in your body, so we need something to neutralize this enemy to health.

Here is another study "Melatonin for the treatment of sepsis: the scientific rationale" published in the Journal of Thoracic Disease, demonstrating how melatonin, being one of the most premier antioxidants in your body, provides strong antioxidant defense mechanisms in order to protect your mitochondria, as well as promote mitochondrial functions.[14]

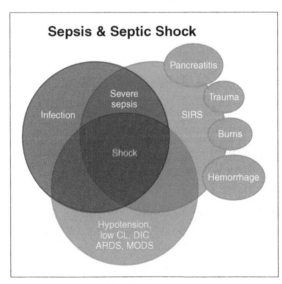

Melatonin may reverse septic shock symptoms by:

- *Preventing oxidative damage induced by lipopolysaccharide, endotoxemia, and metabolic alterations.*
- *Suppressing gene expression linked to the inducible nitric oxide synthase.*
- *Preventing apoptosis or cell death.*
- *Reducing the synthesis of proinflammatory cytokines.*

The antiseptic effects of Melatonin could protect the body against polymicrobial sepsis caused by more than one microorganism. Melatonin offers natural protection by producing an antibacterial effect on white blood cells, especially neutrophils. The research study "Protective Effect of Melatonin Against Polymicrobial Sepsis Is Mediated by the Anti-bacterial Effect of Neutrophils" published in 2019 in the Frontiers in Immunology, has further revealed that macrophages and neutrophils express melatonin receptors. The depletion of neutrophils during sepsis can be countered by melatonin. Ultimately meaning that melatonin treatment could also reduce the mortality resulting from sepsis due to multiple pathogens, where the immune system is depleted. I would suggest that this would be a large percentage of those with more than one infection.

This study suggested that melatonin could promote neutrophil formation during the middle of a major battle within your body called polymicrobial sepsis. It has an anti-bacterial effect combined with an anti-inflammatory one. Furthermore, I can tell you years ago when I was extremely sick with Lyme disease, I was finally diagnosed with this myself. Both mold toxins, as well as infections such as Lyme, can deplete your immune system creating a situation where a variety of what they call coinfections begin to take hold.

This is actually more common than many physicians appreciate, and anybody struggling with a chronic condition should be tested for this. Moreover, a large percentage will probably find this is the root cause of their disease.[15]

Melatonin & Parasitic infections

Let's look at parasites and how melatonin can support your body while one of these nasty invaders takes hold inside.

In patients with parasitic infections such as toxoplasmosis, Chagas' disease, and African trypanosomiasis, melatonin can enhance the host's immune response against the parasite by regulating the release of inflammatory mediators. These findings were proven during a study "The potential use of melatonin to treat protozoan parasitic infections: A review" published in the Biomedicine & Pharmacotherapy in 2018.[16]

Moreover, according to the study "The role of melatonin in modulating parasite infections", published in the Clinical Microbiology and Infectious Diseases, Melatonin may also reduce the amoebic lesions and induce leuco- phagocytosis, thus increasing the number of dead amoebae in patients with amoebiasis.[17]

Melatonin & Hepatitis

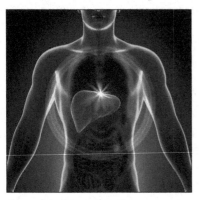

Hepatitis is a condition where the liver is inflamed, and oftentimes this can be due to a viral infection. In patients with viral-induced hepatitis, melatonin can restore the normal cellular processes in the damaged hepatic tissues. According to a research study published in The Nutrients in 2018, "Dietary Melatonin Supplementation Could Be a Promising Preventing/Therapeutic Approach for a Variety of Liver Diseases", melatonin supplementation should be considered important for preventing disease settings, particularly in the liver.[18]

When melatonin improves the ability of the immune cells to fight viruses and bacteria and control the damage during acute and chronic infective stages, it has the potential to safeguard organs like the liver in cases of hepatitis. When melatonin is supplemented in viral hepatitis researchers see reduced fatigue, body aches, and weakness, as well as normalizing blood levels of liver enzymes. In the study, "Effects of Melatonin on Liver Injuries and Diseases" published in 2017 in the International Journal of Molecular Sciences, patients suffering from hepatitis can benefit from melatonin use. The scientist postulated that the support melatonin provided was through the energy production in the mitochondria of cells.[19]

This allows the liver to do its filtering and neutralizing of the toxins in the blood. The filtration takes a lot of energy and when the mitochondria become overloaded through fighting an infection, they need the antioxidant support melatonin provides, as well as a brake system to not overheat in the battle. It's a similar story in many of these cases where melatonin does this extremely important job.[20]

We've already taken a deep dive into how melatonin regulates the over-production of oxidation through its powerful antioxidant effects. And also, how melatonin calms down the cytokine activation in order to protect the mitochondria. This prevents the mitochondria from having to shuffle out pyruvate into the cytoplasm (outside of the mitochondria, yet still within the cell) resulting in the utilization of aerobic glycolysis for energy. But remember that this energy production only gets a little over 10% of the energy (4 ATP) that you would otherwise gain through the Krebs cycle (36 ATP). This is also what happens with cancer cells. Recall the Warburg effect where the Nobel prize winner, Dr. Otto Warburg, discovered the difference between cancer cells and healthy cells and how they make energy. This is why there have been many studies showings how melatonin suppresses the growth of cancers, which we will dive into in another chapter. Let's not get sidetracked and continue to understand how melatonin protects us during infections.

EMCV and Ebola virus infections

Studies showed how amazing our miracle molecule was at protecting our body during these extremely dangerous microbial invasions. There was confirmation of the protective role of melatonin in both EMCV (Encephalomyocarditis V.) and the Ebola virus infection as was revealed in "Melatonin, the Hormone of Darkness: From Sleep Promotion to Ebola Treatment".[21]

Ebola causes severe symptoms by activating the coagulation system and thus, brings about considerable disruption in the vascular endothelium. This is becoming evident with COVID-19 as well. Yet scientific research has shown that melatonin can protect your vascular endothelium by calming down the extreme inflammation triggered by the Ebola virus.

In another study "Beneficial actions of melatonin in the management of viral infections: a new use for this molecular handyman?" published in 2012 in the

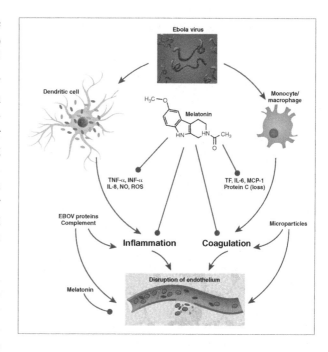

Reviews in Medical Virology, showed that melatonin produces a protective effect against EMCV (Encephalomyocarditis V.) and Semliki Forest virus (SFV).

Melatonin also appears to prevent the increase in the permeability of capillaries induced by the re-perfusion or ischemia, ultimately keeping the blood vessels intact and the capillary perfusion preserved. Likewise, with COVID-19 the lung tissue is where a lot of this endothelial damage occurs, which results in ARDS or acute respiratory distress syndrome. This is the leading cause of death, due to most infections when they go septic.

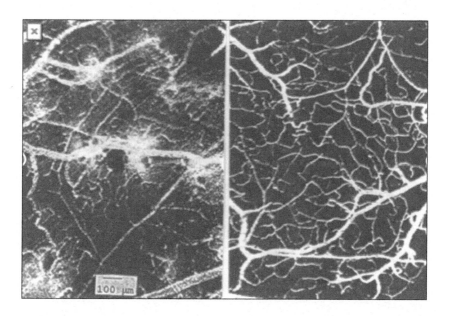

Can you imagine if Pfizer was able to get a patent on melatonin? If it could do even 10% of what melatonin can do with sepsis, with the current COVID-19 pandemic, melatonin would be the biggest blockbuster drug we've ever seen.

When the pandemic first started, I began promoting melatonin very aggressively online and was quickly shut down by the FDA. Their reasoning was that melatonin has not gone through phase 1 to 3 placebo double-blind studies and shown advocacy for COVID-19. Of course, at the time, I wasn't promoting it as a cure. However, I was pointing to all of the studies I have within this chapter, from which one can only conclude that melatonin could not be harmful but could help.

Thankfully, it seems that melatonin is starting to become more recognized and is being adopted in high doses in some of the more progressive hospitals.

Nevertheless, let's head back to the research, which brings me to one more study titled "Melatonin prevents ischemia-reperfusion injury in hamster cheek pouch microcirculation" published in 1996 revealed the beneficial effect of melatonin related to its antioxidant properties. This study highlighted that melatonin may protect the endothelial barrier integrity while further preserving the microvascular blood perfusion by dysfunctions following ischemia-reperfusion.[22]

And lastly, in the study "Ebola virus disease: potential use of melatonin as a treatment" published in the Journal of Pineal Research, it was demonstrated that the application of melatonin might prolong the patients' survival by providing adequate time for the immune system to recover and eradicate the viruses, including Ebola. Why didn't we hear about melatonin during the Ebola outbreak? Economics, pure and simple![23]

Use of melatonin in the light of COVID-19 pandemic

It is well known that melatonin levels are quite high in our younger years and then subsequently drop significantly after 30/40 years of age. Why does SARS-CoV-2 seem to

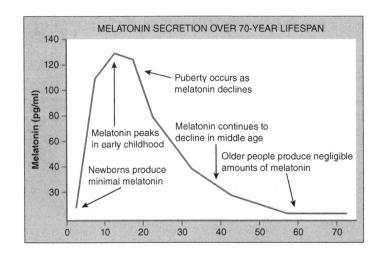

> ## Dr John's Commentary:
>
> *Melatonin and COVID-19 are an important subject right now and when you read this you may be looking back at the catastrophic results of an expedited vaccine when therapeutics were basically ignored and not funded by our government, all the while billions were thrown at vaccine development.*
>
> *Although this is not a book on vaccines, it is my opinion based on a review of the literature that there has actually been little gained by the use of vaccines over the years and much tragedy to human health has occurred. If melatonin was able to have a patent, we would be watching commercials on how great it is for COVID-19. Yet this is not the world we live in due to the economics, government cover-ups, and corruption with our CDC & FDA.*

spare younger children? The reason behind this could be that the peak melatonin levels are higher in children compared to that in adults.

We've touched on COVID in other chapters, however, let's take a deep and hard look at melatonin and how it may be an applicable treatment for COVID-19.

In this article published 6/15/2020, titled "Melatonin and COVID-19" stated the following:

In other words, all 10 patients survived and 70% of this patient base was very sick and statistically vulnerable to developing lethal ARDS.[24]

Moreover, the investigators of the previous study have also hypothesized that the peak melatonin levels achieved by using supplements may also help adults prevent COVID-19.

Another recent study published in 2020 in Melatonin Research, *"Potential utility of melatonin in deadly infectious diseases related to the overreaction of innate immune response and destructive inflammation: focus on COVID-19"* focused on assessing the effect of melatonin has revealed interesting results. It has shown:

"The high mortality of deadly virus infectious diseases including SARS, MERS, COVID-19, and avian flu is often caused by the uncontrolled innate immune response and destructive inflammation. The majority of viral diseases are self-limiting under the help of the activated adaptive immune system. This activity is cell proliferation dependent and thus, it requires several weeks to develop. Patients are vulnerable and mortality usually occurs during this window period. To control the innate immune response and reduce the inflammation during this period will increase the tolerance of patients and lower the mortality in the deadly virus infection. Melatonin is a molecule that displays respective properties, since it downregulates the overreaction of the innate immune response and

> *"In this special issue, we have reviewed as many aspects of melatonin and COVID-19 as possible. Included in this series are reports of how the CNS, heart, lungs, gut, and erythrocytes are affected by COVID-19 and what is the potential of melatonin on them. For the molecular mechanisms and signal transduction pathways, these involve effects of melatonin on CD147 binding with SARS-CoV-2 spike protein, the switch of aerobic glycolysis to mitochondrial oxidative phosphorylation in immune cells, ER stress-UPR-autophagy alterations and kynurenine and the alpha 7 nicotinic receptor activation. In addition, the melatonin doses that can be used in COVID-19 treatment have also been estimated based on the published reports. Most importantly, in this special issue, we have collected the first clinical report using melatonin to treat COVID-19 patients. Castillo et al. have successfully treated 10 patients with high doses of melatonin. Eight of these 10 patients were over 60 years old and 7 of them had the comorbidities of hypertension, diabetes and/or COPD. Advanced age and predisposed medical conditions are huge risk factors for mortality in COVID-19 patients. Fortunately, under melatonin treatment, all of the patients survived."*

overshooting inflammation, but also promotes the adaptive immune activity. Many studies have reported the beneficial effects of melatonin on deadly virus infections in different animal models and its therapeutic efficacy in septic shock patients. Furthermore, melatonin has a great safety margin without serious adverse effects. We suggest the use of melatonin as an adjunctive or even regular therapy for deadly viral diseases, especially if no efficient direct antiviral treatment is available."[25]

Ultimately, this study evaluated the possible benefits of using melatonin supplements for regulating the uncontrolled response of the innate system that causes destructive inflammation in patients with COVID-19. It further showed that melatonin may down-regulate the exaggerated response of the immune cells, control inflammation, and promote the activities of the adaptive immune system.

Can Melatonin help with allergies?

Allergies are another common problem linked with the immune system. Just like autoimmune disorders, allergies occur due to the abnormal response of the immune cells. An allergic reaction can transpire on the skin (atopic dermatitis or contact dermatitis), lungs (asthma), or upper respiratory tract (allergic rhinitis).

Does Melatonin have a use-case when it comes to allergies?

Detailed analysis and assessment of melatonin use in a study "Melatonin modulates allergic lung inflammation" which was published in the Journal of Pineal Research in 2001showed the following:

These findings were reiterated by another research study "Melatonin reduces airway inflammation in ovalbumin-induced asthma" published in Immunobiology in 2014. This study ultimately confirmed the immunomodulatory effects of melatonin that could be beneficial in the management of asthma. It proved:

Several research studies have further indicated that melatonin may minimize damage to the skin, lungs, and upper respiratory passages in patients who have had repeated attacks of allergies by regulating the response of the immune cells. It may also control the frequency and intensity of allergic reactions such as asthma, rhinitis, or dermatitis by inhibiting the exaggerated response of the immune cells to allergens.

How can Melatonin inhibit age-associated immunosenescence?

Cellular senescence is something we work on with our MitoFast Protocol. Moreover, fasting in general works to clear up senescent cells which are "zombie-like" cells that divert

> "*Asthma is an inflammatory lung disease characterized by cell migration, bronchoconstriction and hyperresponsiveness, and can be induced, as an experimental model, by ovalbumin sensitization followed by a challenge. In addition to the well-known immunostimulatory effects of melatonin, research has identified some of its anti-inflammatory properties. In this study, we evaluated the influence of pinealectomy and melatonin administration on cell migration in an experimental model of allergic airway inflammation. We evaluated, in pinealectomized rats treated or not with melatonin, cell migration into the bronchoalveolar fluid, the number of cells and their proliferative activity in the bone marrow, and plasma corticosterone levels. Pinealectomy reduces, 24 hr. after the challenge, the total cell number count in the lung and bone marrow cell proliferation, without changing the number of cells in the bone marrow or in the peripheral blood. This fact suggests that melatonin is important in the control of cell recruitment from the bone marrow and the migration of those cells to the lung. Melatonin administration to pinealectomized rats seems to restore the ability of cells to migrate from the bone marrow to the bronchoalveolar fluid. So, the development of specific inhibitors of melatonin would benefit patients with asthma.*"[26][27]

energy, thus sending out lots of pollution into your system, causing major inflammation and aging. Activating autophagy through inhibition of mTOR through fasting and use of senolytics such as with Lucitol can be helpful, however, melatonin can also aid in this fight.

When immune cells become senescent it's called immunosenescence. It's similar to the degenerative changes occurring in your immune system due to aging. Just like your joints become worn out, and your skin becomes loose due to aging, your immune system also wears out in a similar way.

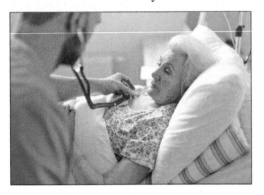

This age-associated decline in our immune functions can have a cascading effect on how all organs and tissues in your body, including the brain and heart work. Immunosenescence is characterized by a reduction in the functional activities of NK cells, macrophages, and granulocytes, all of which are immune cells that protect us against diseases and infections. Immunosenescence can also bring about a significant reduction in the production of IL-1 and a decline in the functions of monocytes. Additionally, researchers have also revealed that immunosenescence can lead to a slow rise in IL-6 production and a decrease in the activities of CD3 and CD4 cells.

But there's more! As age increases, the immune cells lose their ability to differentiate between the body's own cells from those of harmful germs, due to which any existing autoimmune diseases may become worse. Macrophages and T cells also begin to act slower than ever, allowing the symptoms of infections to become more serious before pathogens can be detected by the immune cells. Additionally, our antibodies further become less effective, putting you at an extremely high risk of severe infections.

This is why; when aged people contract infections, such as influenza and pneumonia, they develop more serious symptoms compared to younger people with the same infections.

All these changes linked to immunosenescence can do a lot of harm to your health. Research studies have shown that melatonin might play a significant role due to its immunomodulatory properties.

Melatonin would enhance the cellular and innate immunity, and stimulate the synthesis of progenitor cells of macrophages, granulocytes, and NK cells.

What are progenitor cells?

Progenitor cells are actually the descendants of stem cells that have the ability to differentiate, and form specialized cell types. There are several types of progenitor cells throughout our body, a progenitor cell is capable of differentiating into specific cells belonging to the specific organ or tissue.

"Aging is associated with a decline in immune function (immunosenescence), a situation known to correlate with increased incidence of cancer, infectious and degenerative diseases. Innate, cellular and humoral immunity all exhibit increased deterioration with age. A decrease in functional competence of individual natural killer (NK) cells is found with advancing age. Macrophages and granulocytes show functional decline in aging as evidenced by their diminished phagocytic activity and impairment of superoxide generation. There is also a marked shift in cytokine profile as age advances, e.g., CD3+ and CD4+ cells decline in number whereas CD8+ cells increase in elderly individuals. A decline in organ specific antibodies occurs causing reduced humoral responsiveness. Circulating melatonin decreases with age and in recent years much interest has been focused on its immunomodulatory effect. Melatonin stimulates the production of progenitor cells for granulocytes-macrophages. It also stimulates the production of NK cells and CD4+ cells and inhibits CD8+ cells. The production and release of various cytokines from NK cells and T-helper lymphocytes also are enhanced by melatonin. Melatonin presumably regulates immune function by acting on the immune-opioid network, by affecting G protein-cAMP signal pathway and by regulating intracellular glutathione levels. Melatonin has the potential therapeutic value to enhance immune function in aged individuals and in patients in an immunocompromised state." [28]

Melatonin, by activating and stimulating the secretion of these progenitor cells, may put the body into reverse mode, and slow down aging. Just like stem cells, progenitor cells can later be differentiated to form new healthy cells that can replace the old, dead, and damaged cells, thus restoring optimum health. Moreover, progenitor cells also help to slow down the effect on immunosenescence.

There's more to melatonin and immunosenescence:

- Melatonin can also stimulate the production of IL-2, -6, and -12 and support T-helper cell production, particularly of the CD4+ cells.

- At the same time, melatonin may reduce CD8+ cells by acting through the immuno-opioid network. All these changes melatonin can bring about in your immune system would have a positive effect on your health by slowing down immunosenescence.

These findings were revealed during a research study "Melatonin, immune function and aging" published in Immunity & Ageing in 2005. This study confirmed the following findings:

I personally know many people that fly to Mexico to get their NK cells expanded and the cost is approximately $40-50,000. Could it be that taking high doses of melatonin could do that same thing for a fraction of the cost?

Melatonin can offer special help for lung injuries

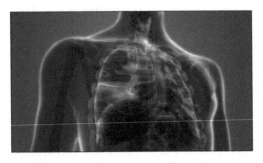

Lungs are highly vulnerable to damage caused by inflammation and infections. Breathing in environmental pollutants, smoking – both active and passive – and inhaling chemical fumes and gases, can do a lot of damage to your lung tissues putting you at the risk of emphysema, bronchitis, and bronchiectasis. In case the damage is severe, patients may develop chronic obstructive lung disease and lung cancer.

Recent clinical research has shown that melatonin could provide potential benefits for preventing lung damage. It can bind to the receptors on the lungs called the NLRP3 inflammasomes that are associated with several infections, including COVID-19. Melatonin, by getting to these receptors first, would help in blunting the injuries from infectious pathogens and other harmful toxins.

The research published in the journal, Life Sciences, in 2020 has also explored this in detail. Moreover, others have shown that melatonin may limit virus-related damage and could be beneficial for minimizing lung injuries.[29]

Conclusion

The immune system is the real backbone of your health. It can determine how efficiently all the organs of your body function, and how well you are able to fight and even avoid diseases. Melatonin offers a safe and effective way to allow your immune system to function more efficiently. It would not just strengthen the immunity but also regulate the activities of the immune cells. The immune-boosting and immunoregulatory properties of melatonin could provide a huge breakthrough in the management of autoimmune diseases, infections, allergies, and immunosenescence.

Furthermore, in addition to using melatonin, I suggest a regular fasting routine, such as with MitoFast where you do a 24hr fast weekly and a 3-5 day fast several times a year. Ozone therapy can also help strengthen the immune system, as it activates autophagy or cleaning and recycling of dysfunctional immune cells. For viral immunity, I further suggest supplementing with glutathione, zinc, quercetin, and selenium.

Moreover, it is also my opinion that poor sinus health can be a major drain on many people's immune systems, so a 30-day sinus cleanse is good to do at least once a year.

Dosing melatonin is supra-physiologic dosing, in a manner that absorbs better than the traditional oral route is a good idea. Using suppository or liposomal in the 100's of milligrams is my suggestion to many of my patients, and even the most knowledgeable scientist on melatonin, Russel Reiter, MD, PH.D., takes 100-200 per night himself.

Reference

1. Kopp C, Vogel E, Rettori MC, Delagrange P, Misslin R. The effects of melatonin on the behavioural disturbances induced by chronic mild stress in C3H/He mice. Behav Pharmacol. 1999 Feb;10(1):73-83. doi: 10.1097/00008877-199902000-00007. PMID: 10780304.

2. Pechlivanova, Daniela & Dzhambazova, Elena & Kolev, Georgi & Nenchovska, Zlatina & Tchekalarova, Jana. (2016). Effects of melatonin on stress-induced and diurnal variations of nociception in Wistar and spontaneously hypertensive rats. Comptes rendus de l'Académie bulgare des sciences: sciences mathématiques et naturelles. 69. 1223 - 1230.

3. Bonilla, E., Valero, N., Chacín-Bonilla, L., & Medina-Leendertz, S. (2004). Melatonin and viral infections. *Journal of pineal research*, *36*(2), 73–79. https://doi.org/10.1046/j.1600-079x.2003.00105.x

4. Guerrero JM, Reiter RJ. Melatonin-immune system relationships. Curr Top Med Chem. 2002 Feb;2(2):167-79. doi: 10.2174/1568026023394335. PMID: 11899099.

5. Carrillo-Vico, A., Guerrero, J.M., Lardone, P.J. *et al.* A review of the multiple actions of melatonin on the immune system. *Endocr* **27,** 189–200 (2005). https://doi.org/10.1385/ENDO:27:2:189

6. Lin, G. J., Huang, S. H., Chen, S. J., Wang, C. H., Chang, D. M., & Sytwu, H. K. (2013). Modulation by melatonin of the pathogenesis of inflammatory autoimmune diseases. *International journal of molecular sciences*, *14*(6), 11742–11766. https://doi.org/10.3390/ijms140611742

7. Tian YM, Zhang GY, Dai YR. Melatonin rejuvenates degenerated thymus and redresses peripheral immune functions in aged mice. Immunol Lett. 2003 Aug 5;88(2):101-4. doi: 10.1016/s0165-2478(03)00068-3. PMID: 12880677.

8. Zhao CN, Wang P, Mao YM, Dan YL, Wu Q, Li XM, Wang DG, Davis C, Hu W, Pan HF. Potential role of melatonin in autoimmune diseases. Cytokine Growth Factor Rev. 2019 Aug;48:1-10. doi: 10.1016/j.cytogfr.2019.07.002. Epub 2019 Jul 16. PMID: 31345729.

9. Haddad, Carolina F. et al. Melatonin and organ transplantation: what is the relationship?. Revista da Associação Médica Brasileira [online]. 2020, v. 66, n. 3 [Accessed 15 November 2021] , pp. 353-358. Available from: <https://doi.org/10.1590/1806-9282.66.3.353>. Epub 03 June 2020. ISSN 1806-9282. https://doi.org/10.1590/1806-9282.66.3.353.

10. **Esteban-Zubero, E., García-Gil, F. A., López-Pingarrón, L., Alatorre-Jiménez, M. A., Iñigo-Gil, P., Tan, D., García, J. J., & Reiter, R. J. (2016). Potential benefits of melatonin in organ transplantation: a review, *Journal of Endocrinology*, *229*(3), R129-R146. Retrieved Nov 15, 2021, from https://joe.bioscientifica.com/view/journals/joe/229/3/R129.xml**

11. Huang, Shing-Hwa & Liao, Ching-Len & Chen, Shyi-Jou & Shi, Li-Ge & Lin, Li & Chen, Yuan-Wu & Cheng, Chia-Pi & Sytwu, Huey-Kang & Shang, Shih-Ta & Lin, Gu-Jiun. (2019). Melatonin possesses an anti-influenza potential through its immune modulatory effect. Journal of Functional Foods. 58. 189-198. 10.1016/j.jff.2019.04.062.

12. Silvestri, M., Rossi, G.A. Melatonin: its possible role in the management of viral infections-a brief review. *Ital J Pediatr* **39**, 61 (2013). https://doi.org/10.1186/1824-7288-39-61

13. Efficacy of Melatonin in the Prophylaxis of Coronavirus Disease 2019 (COVID-19) Among Healthcare Workers. - Full Text View - ClinicalTrials.gov

14. Colunga Biancatelli, R., Berrill, M., Mohammed, Y. H., & Marik, P. E. (2020). Melatonin for the treatment of sepsis: the scientific rationale. *Journal of thoracic disease*, *12*(Suppl 1), S54–S65. https://doi.org/10.21037/jtd.2019.12.85

15. Xu, L., Zhang, W., Kwak, M., Zhang, L., Lee, P., & Jin, J. O. (2019). Protective Effect of Melatonin Against Polymicrobial Sepsis Is Mediated by the Anti-bacterial Effect of Neutrophils. *Frontiers in immunology*, *10*, 1371. https://doi.org/10.3389/fimmu.2019.01371

16. Ahmad Daryani, Mahbobeh Montazeri, Abdol Satar Pagheh, Mehdi Sharif, Shahabeddin Sarvi, Azam Hosseinzadeh, Russel J. Reiter, Ramtin Hadighi, Mohammad Taghi Joghataei, Habib Ghaznavi, Saeed Mehrzadi, The potential use of melatonin to treat protozoan parasitic infections: A review, Biomedicine & Pharmacotherapy,Volume 97,2018,Pages 948-957,ISSN 0753-3322,https://doi.org/10.1016/j.biopha.2017.11

17. França-Botelho AC (2020) The role of melatonin in modulating parasite infections. Clin Microbiol Infect Dis 5: DOI: 10.15761/CMID.1000170

18. Bonomini, F., Borsani, E., Favero, G., Rodella, L. F., & Rezzani, R. (2018). Dietary Melatonin Supplementation Could Be a Promising Preventing/Therapeutic Approach for a Variety of Liver Diseases. *Nutrients*, *10*(9), 1135. https://doi.org/10.3390/nu10091135

19. Zhang, J. J., Meng, X., Li, Y., Zhou, Y., Xu, D. P., Li, S., & Li, H. B. (2017). Effects of Melatonin on Liver Injuries and Diseases. *International journal of molecular sciences*, *18*(4), 673. https://doi.org/10.3390/ijms18040673

20. Zhang, J. J., Meng, X., Li, Y., Zhou, Y., Xu, D. P., Li, S., & Li, H. B. (2017). Effects of Melatonin on Liver Injuries and Diseases. *International journal of molecular sciences*, *18*(4), 673. https://doi.org/10.3390/ijms18040673

21. Masters, A., Pandi-Perumal, S. R., Seixas, A., Girardin, J. L., & McFarlane, S. I. (2014). Melatonin, the Hormone of Darkness: From Sleep Promotion to Ebola Treatment. *Brain disorders & therapy*, *4*(1), 1000151. https://doi.org/10.4172/2168-975X.1000151

22. S. Bertuglia, P.L. Marchiafava, A. Colantuoni, Melatonin prevents ischemia reperfusion injury in hamster cheek pouch microcirculation, *Cardiovascular Research*, Volume 31, Issue 6, June 1996, Pages 947–952, https://doi.org/10.1016/S0008-6363(96)00030-2

23. Tan DX, Korkmaz A, Reiter RJ, Manchester LC. Ebola virus disease: potential use of melatonin as a treatment. J Pineal Res. 2014 Nov;57(4):381-4. doi: 10.1111/jpi.12186. Epub 2014 Oct 14. PMID: 25262626.

24. Archives | Melatonin Research (melatonin-research.net)

25. Tan, D.X. and Hardeland, R. 2020. Potential utility of melatonin in deadly infectious diseases related to the overreaction of innate immune response and destructive inflammation: focus on

COVID-19. *Melatonin Research*. 3, 1 (Mar. 2020), 120-143. DOI:https://doi.org/https://doi.org/10.32794/mr11250052.

26. Marseglia, L., D'Angelo, G., Manti, S., Salpietro, C., Arrigo, T., Barberi, I., Reiter, R. J., & Gitto, E. (2014). Melatonin and atopy: role in atopic dermatitis and asthma. *International journal of molecular sciences*, *15*(8), 13482–13493. https://doi.org/10.3390/ijms150813482

27. Wang, W., & Gao, J. (2021). Effects of melatonin on protecting against lung injury (Review). *Experimental and therapeutic medicine*, *21*(3), 228. https://doi.org/10.3892/etm.2021.9659

28. Srinivasan V, Maestroni GJ, Cardinali DP, Esquifino AI, Perumal SR, Miller SC. Melatonin, immune function and aging. Immun Ageing. 2005 Nov 29;2:17. doi: 10.1186/1742-4933-2-17. PMID: 16316470; PMCID: PMC1325257.

29. Zhang, R., Wang, X., Ni, L., Di, X., Ma, B., Niu, S., Liu, C., & Reiter, R. J. (2020). COVID-19: Melatonin as a potential adjuvant treatment. *Life sciences*, *250*, 117583. https://doi.org/10.1016/j.lfs.2020.117583

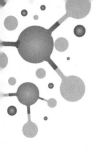

6

MELATONIN & INFECTIONS

Cytokine Storm, ARDS & COVID-19

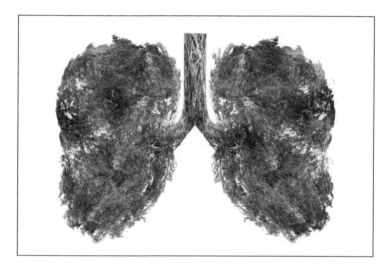

We already discussed various mechanisms through which melatonin can help to manage infections. Now, let's take a deeper look into how melatonin can help you avoid injury and death from infection by inhibiting the cytokine storm.

A cytokine storm is when there is a poor *brake system* in place, and the defense mechanisms run out of control. Without brakes, these defense mechanisms turn against our own bodies by bringing about a severe inflammatory process known as the cytokine storm.

To know why this happens and what melatonin can do in this regard, let's first take a closer look at what the cytokine storm is and means to your body.

What exactly is a cytokine storm?

Cytokine storm is actually an immune reaction that has gone wild. It seems to be linked with some of the most severe infections humans have ever faced such as EBOLA, ZIKA virus, MERS (Middle East Respiratory Syndrome), SARS (Severe Acute Respiratory Syndrome) and, of course, the recent and ongoing pandemic COVID-19.

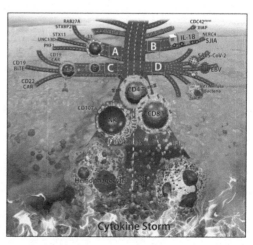

Cytokine Storm

Here's what happens.

During an inflammatory episode such as with an infection, cytokines are released in response to the infection, some of which are IL1B, IL6 seen in the image below. These cytokines affect our immune cells in a way that disables the ability of these cells to both produce energy efficiently, as well as make their own melatonin. The mitochondria within these immune cells, as in any other cell in our body, are the way in which we make the APT from glucose, we need this energy during infections more so than in normal situations.

The cytokines will have a direct impact on an enzyme called pyruvate dehydrogenase kinase (PDK) which will inactivate the pyruvate dehydrogenase complex (PDC) which is necessary to convert pyruvate into acetyl Co-A. Acetyl Co-A subsequently then allows the mitochondria to normally make energy through the TCA or the Krebs cycle (producing 36 ATP) as well as create melatonin.

As a side note, this melatonin is made through the conversion of Acetyl Co-A to N-Acetylserotonin (NAS) then to melatonin from the NAS. When the PDK is upregulated by too many cytokines, it causes energy to be made through aerobic glycolysis which is where pyruvate is shuffled outside of the mitochondria into the cytosol and used to make ATP.

Remember, aerobic glycolysis makes only 4 ATP. So, now we are really running low on gas in a time of need. It's like running out of gas while driving through an alligator alley in Florida. Not a good day to be stranded on this dangerous stretch of road. On top of this, we now cannot produce melatonin to calm this storm; so, things run *wild* and out of control.

Those who suffer from recurrent infections due to a weak immune system and individuals who are more likely to develop serious complications due to COVID-19 and other infections are people whose immune systems tend to react in a rather catastrophic way. Moreover, "weak immune system" situations are simply weak mitochondria within our immune cells, allowing for poor melatonin and inefficient ATP due to chronic inflammation resulting in too much chronic cytokines upregulation of PDK.

What happens in patients with COVID-19 once the body is exposed to the viruses, is that the immune cells flood the respiratory system. They attack the lungs, which they should actually be protecting. Even the blood vessels begin to leak and the blood itself starts forming clots within the vessels.

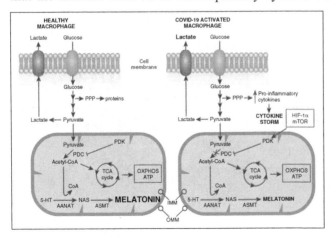

The lungs are particularly vulnerable due to the fact this is where we have a large volume of oxygen which is very reactive and oxidative.

Slowly, the blood pressure plummets, and this is when

the organs begin to fail, resulting in the life-threatening complications responsible for the risk of morbidity. Scientists and doctors increasingly believe that these changes occur due to the immune system losing the brakes, so much so that it harms instead of providing protection.

Melatonin when present allows more production from your macrophages to fight infections, interleukins IL6, IL1, IL8 & TNF alpha from the macrophage. It's signaling and telling the macrophage *"Hey, calm down and apply a little brake before you have a car accident"*. So, one aspect is that melatonin calms down the interleukins and secondly it acts as an antioxidant for the macrophages, monocytes, and neutrophils.

Why does your immune system need an antioxidant during an infection?

When your immune cells are active, they are "eating" the pathogens, further bringing these into the cells and placing them into vesicles within the cells. Let's call these "Hot Tubs".

These pathogens within the Hot Tubs are killed through the cell, basically by injecting bleach into this vesicle. This process produces a lot of reactive oxygen species or ROS. This requires a massive amount of oxidation from the miracle molecule to quench this process as your premier antioxidant.

What is the difference between Interleukin and Cytokine?

Cytokines are proteins that are made in response to pathogens and other antigens that regulate inflammatory and immune responses. Interleukin production is a self-limited process. The messenger RNA encoding in most interleukins is unstable and causes a transient synthesis.

What goes wrong while fighting infections to cause a cytokine storm?

Normally, when the body encounters a pathogen, your immune system is entrusted with the responsibility of attacking the invader, followed by which it is expected to stand down. But this doesn't happen all the time. Sometimes, the orderly army of immune cells wielding their molecular weapons goes out of control, just like the obedient soldiers morphing into an unruly mob.

While there are several tests and treatments, which may help to identify and tame this form of self-destruction by immune cells, it can also be too early to be sure of the best course of treatment for those who are already too weak and suffering from COVID-19.

CYTOKINES
VERSUS
INTERLEUKINS

CYTOKINES	INTERLEUKINS
A number of substances, such as interferon, interleukin, and growth factors, which are secreted by certain cells of the immune system and have an effect on other cells	Any of a class of proteins produced by leucocytes for regulating immune responses
A large group of signaling molecules	A subfamily of cytokines
Can have either autocrine, paracrine or endocrine action	Have either autocrine or paracrine action
Regulate the nature, intensity, and duration of the immune response	Induce the proliferation, differentiation, maturation, migration, and adhesion of cells of the immune system

Common variants of such a hyperactive immune reaction may occur in an array of other infections, as well as other conditions that are triggered by faulty genes and autoimmune disorders. In patients with these conditions, the body considers its own tissues as invaders, attacks them, and then, destroys these healthy tissues by producing a cytokine storm.

This is why; all of these diseases are categorized under one umbrella term "cytokine storm". It is named after the proinflammatory cytokines that rampage through your bloodstream. Yet cytokines are nothing but small proteinaceous compounds — there are dozens of them — which serve as the messengers for the immune system, transiting between different cells and tissues, producing a variety of effects, with some asking for more severe immune activity and some requesting less.[1]

Which conditions can trigger a cytokine storm?

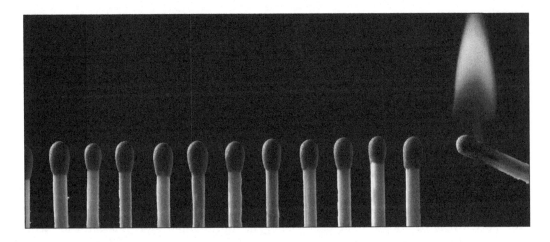

A cytokine storm can occur in a variety of conditions such as:

- Viral infections like COVID-19, influenza, Epstein-Barr virus, herpes viruses, and cytomegalovirus, can all trigger a cytokine storm. It is, sometimes, referred to as the reactive MAS or HLH.[2]

- Cytokine release syndrome may develop in people who suffer from leukemia and are receiving immunotherapy or treatment with infused immune cells or antibodies.[3]
- Hemophagocytic lymphohistiocytosis is a genetic disorder that may cause excessive stimulation of immune cells. While this condition can be deadly, especially in infants, it can be treated by taming cytokine storms with a bone marrow transplant that replaces the improperly functioning immune cells with healthy ones.[4]
- Macrophage activation syndrome may occur in patients with autoimmune disorders such as juvenile arthritis, lupus, or Still's disease.
- Blood infections such as sepsis can also trigger a cytokine storm and bring about widespread destruction of healthy tissues.[5]
- Lymphoma and leukemia are types of blood cancers that may create a cytokine storm.[6]

Graft-versus-host disease can occur when transplanted stem cells produce immune cells, which attack the healthy tissues in the recipient's body. Scientists suspect a cytokine storm to underlie this condition.[7]

How can melatonin help?

According to a research study, "Melatonin: Roles in influenza, Covid-19, and other viral infections" published in the Reviews In Medical Virology, melatonergic pathways can play a role in calming the cytokine storm. This study has postulated:

The study confirms the role of melatonin in taming the cytokine storm with its ability to regulate the functions of the immune system.

In another recent research study, "Melatonin Inhibits COVID-19-induced Cytokine Storm by Reversing Aerobic Glycolysis in Immune Cells: A Mechanistic Analysis" published in the Medicine in Drug Discovery in June 2020, it was proved that exogenously administered

66

"The regulation of the melatonergic pathways, both pineal and systemic, may be an important aspect in how viruses drive the cellular changes that underpin their control of cellular functions. The role of the melatonergic pathways in viral infections, especially influenza and COVID-19, needs to be emphasized to control the outbreaks. Viral or preexistent suppression of pineal melatonin disinhibits neutrophil attraction, thereby contributing to an initial cytokine storm. Virus - and cytokine-storm-driven control of the pineal and mitochondrial melatonergic pathway can regulate immune responses against infectious pathogens."[8]

melatonin could inhibit cytokine storm induced during viral infections. It further showed how melatonin could help to reverse aerobic glycolysis by repressing HIF-1α and mTOR, thus disinhibiting PDC activity and promoting acetyl-coenzyme. The reinstated, mitochondria-generated melatonin in combination with the parenteral melatonin may provide a formidable weapon to reduce the cytokine storm, as well as its damaging consequences, thereby relieving the signs of a COVID-19 infection.[9]

These studies suggest that melatonin can calm the cytokine storm and can help to minimize the damage caused due to infections.

Damage caused by the rising cytokine storm

The damage caused by the rising cytokine storm is not limited to how it affects you during infections. When the cytokines that stimulate immune activities become abundant, the immune system may lose its ability to stop it by itself. And this is a highly grave situation it simply means even the patient's own immune system would be rendered helpless when the cytokine storm gets out of hand. The immune cells will then continue to spread beyond the infected body part, and start attacking even the healthy tissues.

For example, the cytokines would gobble up white and red blood cells, thus damaging the liver. It will cause the blood vessel walls to open up to allow immune cells to enter the surrounding tissues. And in severe cases, the blood vessels may get so leaky that the air passages and lungs might fill with fluids, causing serious difficulty in breathing.

The loss of fluids from the bloodstream into the tissue spaces will cause blood pressure to drop, putting more strain on the heart that will find it more and more difficult to pump blood. At the same time, the blood will begin to form abnormal clots throughout the body, thus choking the blood flow further.

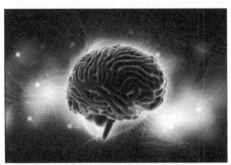

When the vital organs don't get enough blood, the person can go into a state of shock, thereby risking multiple organ failures or in worst cases, even death.

According to the expert immunologist and rheumatologist at the University of Alabama in Birmingham, "Most patients with infections only have a fever initially, and about half of them develop some sorts of nervous system symptoms like headaches, seizures, and even coma." The findings of this research study have shown that the development of symptoms from a simple fever to seizures or coma can occur rather rapidly if the patient's immunity is poor or when the body's own defense mechanisms fail to function optimally, as it occurs due to low melatonin production due to the lack of sleep.[10]

It is only recently that doctors are coming to understand why and how the cytokine storm develops. While there are no fail-safe tests to detect the cytokine storm brewing, there are some signs that might indicate it could be underway.

For example, the levels of the protein ferritin in the blood may rise in patients with severe infections who are at risk of cytokine storm and multiple organ failure. This may occur as the concentrations of the inflammation indicators, like C-reactive protein secreted by the liver increase in the blood.

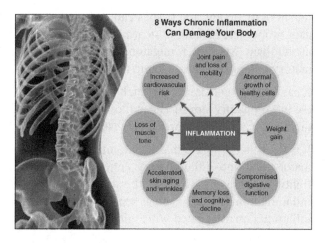

So, one of the ways to make sure your immune system is working efficiently to fight the virus without going out of control to cause a cytokine storm is to keep a check on the protein ferritin and C-reactive protein levels in the blood.

What melatonin can do to tame the cytokine storm?

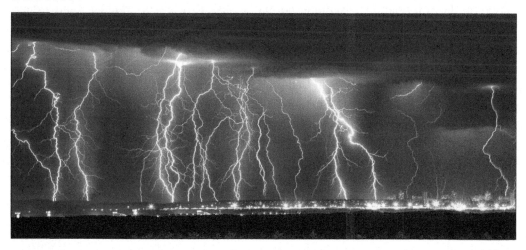

It is possible to stay safe and avoid the serious consequences linked to cytokine storms when your body has enough melatonin. Several research studies have already been conducted to assess the effects of different medications, supplements, and hormones on the cytokine storm specifically in patients with COVID-19 and influenza. Among the many supplements assessed, it is melatonin that has shown promise.

One research study "Melatonin is a potential adjuvant to improve clinical outcomes in individuals with obesity and diabetes with the coexistence of Covid-19" published in the European Journal of Pharmacology in 2020 showed how melatonin could be effective for calming the cytokine storm. The researchers confirmed that the increased accumulation of fats in body organs and tissues can cause several metabolic disorders. Due to its antioxidant properties, melatonin treatment can improve inflammatory mechanisms and energy metabolism. Moreover, melatonin efficiently decreases the production of blood inflammatory cytokines such as leptin and resistin.

It has been demonstrated that melatonin has a remarkable therapeutic action in decreasing the inflammatory storm. The authors anticipated that melatonin can be used as a low-cost therapeutic agent to improve the disorders associated with cytokine storm and obesity.

It was further reported that melatonin has immunomodulatory roles with dual proinflammatory and anti-inflammatory actions. The proinflammatory effect is exhibited while fighting pathogens, whereas the anti-inflammatory action is manifested in high-grade inflammation. In cases such as sepsis, oxidative stress, organ injury, and also in low-grade inflammation associated with aging and neurodegenerative diseases.

This double-edge blade of melatonin is attributed to several mechanisms. Besides its ability to downregulate proinflammatory cytokine production and upregulate anti-inflammatory cytokine production, melatonin exhibits high antioxidant capacity. It can downregulate inducible nitric oxide synthases (the bad one) and cyclooxygenase-2, and prevent the activation of the inflammasomes NLRP3, and NF-κB.[11]

The overall effect of these activities of melatonin would be reduced inflammation.

Based on this information, sustaining normal levels of melatonin in elderly individuals and people with weak immunity, like diabetic and obese patients, is suggested to be an important strategy to strengthen the body's defense systems."

Lastly, another research study "Melatonin Inhibits COVID-19-induced Cytokine Storm by Reversing Aerobic Glycolysis in Immune Cells: A Mechanistic Analysis" published in the Medicine in Drug Discovery in 20202 which has shown that: *"Because of melatonin's potent antioxidant and anti-inflammatory activities, it would normally reduce the highly pro-inflammatory cytokine storm and neutralize the generated free radicals thereby preserving cellular integrity and preventing lung damage."*[12]

Melatonin & Vaccines

Considering the COVID 19 vaccine?

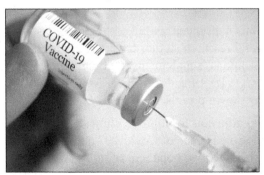

Because melatonin enhances the immune response to vaccines by increasing peripheral blood CD4+ T cells and IgG-expressing B cells, scientists feel it's smart to dose 2 weeks prior and 4 weeks post-vaccine. Based on the prior knowledge from the influenza vaccine, up to 50% in lack of effectiveness would be found among healthy adults receiving vaccines against SARS-CoV-2. Evidence that insufficient sleep may be a causal factor accounting for this variability. Thus, individuals experiencing total or partial sleep loss exhibit markedly reduced antigen-specific antibodies as compared to healthy sleepers.

This article suggests using melatonin pre and post to gain a healthier effect from the vaccine:

"Exogenous melatonin as a potential adjuvant in anti-SarsCov2 vaccines". Administration of exogenous melatonin might boost the potency of the immune response, and duration of the vaccine-induced immunity. Moreover, melatonin administration might be especially useful in elderly males, but the existing evidence point to a general capacity of melatonin to enhance both cell-mediated and humoral immune responses irrespective of sex and age. The author suggests a very low dose of 2 mg of a long-acting form of melatonin and references (Maestroni et al. 1987) regarding the administration of supra-pharmacological doses, stating it might be wisely avoided surrounding a vaccine as such doses may decrease the immune response (Maestroni et al. 1987).[13] Yet, there's no denying this is a little controversial, and more research should be done in this area. Here, another researcher who penned the paper "An urgent proposal for the immediate use of melatonin as an adjuvant to anti- SARS-CoV-2 vaccination", references the use of 10-20 mg daily as a dose to follow.

"Melatonin enhances the immune response to vaccines by increasing peripheral blood CD4+ T cells and IgG-expressing B cells. Administration of exogenous melatonin could increase the potency of the immune response and the duration of the immunity induced by the vaccine. Besides, melatonin could also prevent adverse effects of the vaccination due to its antioxidant and immunomodulatory properties."[14]

Conclusion

These studies have provided enough evidence for doctors and physicians to be sure of the powerful anti-inflammatory, and immunomodulatory activities of melatonin that could be effective for calming the cytokine storm. By now, you must be wondering why melatonin isn't more well known for its ability to save lives with infections from the worst pathogens known to mankind, based on a large body of research.

And the answer to that boils down to just one word… Patent.

There is no economic upside for a large pharma company to promote nor take it through placebo double-blind studies for an indication. The way our FDA works is that one drug (one molecule usually) is taken through 3 levels of study and it has various endpoints that the company and the FDA see as reasonable. This allows the drug to be used for a narrow and specific application.

Of course, drugs can then be used off-label after that. However, many times they will need to do another phase 3 study for new indications for insurances to pay. It generally costs many tens of millions to do this. If there is no patent to protect the company from competition selling the same drug, they have a much more difficult time recouping their money.

This is a huge problem for many natural remedies that would be far safer and effective than most drugs on the market.

This is why melatonin will, most likely, never be widely spoken about for cytokine storm usage, or any other indication it works for. And it's up to you to share this with your doctor and use this information for yourself. If you're a healthcare practitioner, it's time to recognize the shortcomings of our "Big Parma" health system and start looking at melatonin as well as other natural nutrients as safe and efficient therapies for your patients. These alternatives options and information sources are all around you these days on podcasts, YouTube, Google, PubMed, and seminars.

Anybody at a high risk of a cytokine storm needs to consider supplementing with melatonin.

Sometimes supraphysiologic doses are needed and we will be discussing this a little later.

Reference

1. Definition of cytokine - NCI Dictionary of Cancer Terms - National Cancer Institute

2. Dulek D., Thomsen I. (2019) Infectious Triggers of Cytokine Storm Syndromes: Herpes Virus Family (Non-EBV). In: Cron R., Behrens E. (eds) Cytokine Storm Syndrome. Springer, Cham. https://doi.org/10.1007/978-3-030-22094-5_14

3. Definition of cytokine release syndrome - NCI Dictionary of Cancer Terms - National Cancer Institute

4. Familial hemophagocytic lymphohistiocytosis | Genetic and Rare Diseases Information Center (GARD) – an NCATS Program (nih.gov)

5. Chousterman BG, Swirski FK, Weber GF. Cytokine storm and sepsis disease pathogenesis. Semin Immunopathol. 2017 Jul;39(5):517-528. doi: 10.1007/s00281-017-0639-8. Epub 2017 May 29. PMID: 28555385.

6. Wang, H., Xiong, L., Tang, W., Zhou, Y., & Li, F. (2017). A systematic review of malignancy-associated hemophagocytic lymphohistiocytosis that needs more attentions. *Oncotarget*, *8*(35), 59977–59985. https://doi.org/10.18632/oncotarget.19230

7. James L.M. Ferrara, Cytokine dysregulation as a mechanism of graft versus host disease, Current Opinion in Immunology,Volume 5, Issue 5, 1993,Pages 794-799,ISSN 0952-7915, https://doi.org/10.1016/0952-7915(93)90139-J.

8. Bahrampour Juybari K, Pourhanifeh MH, Hosseinzadeh A, Hemati K, Mehrzadi S. Melatonin potentials against viral infections including COVID-19: Current evidence and new findings. Virus Res. 2020 Oct 2;287:198108. doi: 10.1016/j.virusres.2020.198108. Epub 2020 Aug 5. PMID: 32768490; PMCID: PMC7405774.

9. Reiter, R. J., Sharma, R., Ma, Q., Dominquez-Rodriguez, A., Marik, P. E., & Abreu-Gonzalez, P. (2020). Melatonin Inhibits COVID-19-induced Cytokine Storm by Reversing Aerobic

Glycolysis in Immune Cells: A Mechanistic Analysis. *Medicine in drug discovery*, *6*, 100044. https://doi.org/10.1016/j.medidd.2020.100044

10. Faigen baum D, June, C, Cytokine Storm, N Engl J Med 2020; 383:2255-2273, 2020 DOI: 10.1056/NEJMra2026131

11. El-Missiry, M. A., El-Missiry, Z., & Othman, A. I. (2020). Melatonin is a potential adjuvant to improve clinical outcomes in individuals with obesity and diabetes with coexistence of Covid-19. *European journal of pharmacology*, *882*, 173329. https://doi.org/10.1016/j.ejphar.2020.173329

12. Reiter, R. J., Sharma, R., Ma, Q., Dominquez-Rodriguez, A., Marik, P. E., & Abreu-Gonzalez, P. (2020). Melatonin Inhibits COVID-19-induced Cytokine Storm by Reversing Aerobic Glycolysis in Immune Cells: A Mechanistic Analysis. *Medicine in drug discovery*, *6*, 100044. https://doi.org/10.1016/j.medidd.2020.100044

13. Regodón S, Martín-Palomino P, Fernández-Montesinos R, Herrera JL, Carrascosa-Salmoral MP, Píriz S, Vadillo S, Guerrero JM, Pozo D. The use of melatonin as a vaccine agent. Vaccine. 2005 Nov 16;23(46-47):5321-7. doi: 10.1016/j.vaccine.2005.07.003. Epub 2005 Jul 18. PMID: 16055232.

14. Ramos, E., López-Muñoz, F., Gil-Martín, E., Egea, J., Álvarez-Merz, I., Painuli, S., Semwal, P., Martins, N., Hernández-Guijo, J. M., & Romero, A. (2021). The Coronavirus Disease 2019 (COVID-19): Key Emphasis on Melatonin Safety and Therapeutic Efficacy. *Antioxidants (Basel, Switzerland)*, *10*(7), 1152. https://doi.org/10.3390/antiox10071152

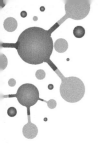

7

MELATONIN & AUTOIMMUNE DISEASES

Autoimmune diseases are conditions in which the body's immune system mistakenly attacks healthy cells, tissues, or organs. This results in different disease conditions such as type 1 diabetes mellitus, ALS (Amyotrophic lateral sclerosis), SLE (systemic lupus erythematosus), multiple sclerosis, inflammatory bowel disease, and rheumatoid arthritis.

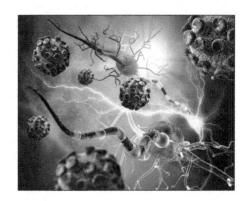

Biological effects of melatonin

Melatonin is considered a pleiotropic molecule with both pro-inflammatory and anti-inflammatory properties. It is immunomodulatory, meaning that it reduces excessive immune functions in inflammatory conditions while improving immune response in immunocompromised individuals. So, you could say melatonin is truly adaptogenic, meaning that it is ready to meet whatever needs it is called for.

Melatonin receptors are seen in a wide variety of immune cells. That means melatonin has an influence on almost your entire immune system including the cells like CD4+ T cells, CD8+ T cells, and B cells.[1] These cells are used to kill invading pathogens and help you to produce antibodies to protect you from future infections. I am going to get a little bit deep here with studies; so, if this isn't your interest, skip to the next section.

Here is a study showing that treatment with melatonin enhances the production of natural killer cells and monocytes in the bone marrow of mice. Other studies also show that mice treated with melatonin have decreased expression of interleukin (IL)-2 and interferon (IFN) gamma. At the same time, there is an increase in the production of T helper cell cytokines like IL-4 and IL-10.

Melatonin is also essential in the development of T helper cells. The balance of T helper cells is crucial in regulating cellular immune responses.

T helper 1 (Th1) is important for inflammatory responses by producing pro-inflammatory cytokines such as IFN-y and IL-2.

However, T helper 2 (Th2) is anti-inflammatory and produces cytokines such as IL-4, IL-5, IL-10, and IL-13.

Studies show that low doses of melatonin increase Th1 cytokines, thereby increasing inflammation[2], while high doses of melatonin reduce pro-inflammation, thereby reducing inflammation.

Melatonin & Autoimmune Diseases

Autoimmune diseases could be classified as either organ-specific, as is found in type 1 diabetes mellitus, or systemic as in systemic lupus erythematosus. In the United States, autoimmune diseases are said to affect about 5% of the population. This results from the activation of immune cells, T and B cells, discussed earlier, by antigens on the body tissues, which the body mistakenly sees as a threat.

The activation of these immune cells by this antigen results in damage to target tissues by the activated cells. This is where I need to interject my personal opinions:

Autoimmune conditions don't just happen for no reason. Some of the factors at the root of this include chronic toxicity, chronic infections, and imbalances in the digestive tract leading to either dysbiosis or leaky gut syndrome. All of these cause inflammations which regulates cytokines which then break down your cells ability to make energy and this results in the ability to have a properly regulated immune system.

Besides having an improperly regulated immune system, there are also specific triggers to the immune system whereby the immune system gets confused, and the information is encoded in order to attack a specific tissue in the body.

Although we are diving into melatonin in this article, these considerations need to be addressed along with melatonin supplementation, in my opinion. Without addressing the root cause, it will be like bailing a leaking boat or painting over rust. You can reference ultimate-cellularreset.com for more up-to-date information about melatonin as well as other strategies for autoimmune conditions. So, as it indicates that melatonin is an immunomodulatory hormone. Melatonin has been shown to have a regulatory impact on the pathophysiology of these disease conditions. Understanding this mechanism can help in the use of melatonin supplements in alleviating symptoms and slowing the progress of the disease.

We're going to take a look at a variety of different autoimmune conditions and consider the latest research using melatonin and how it might affect the specific conditions. Conditions such as Type 1 Diabetes mellitus, Multiple sclerosis, Systemic lupus erythematosus, inflammatory bowel diseases, and Rheumatoid arthritis.

Pathophysiology of Type 1 Diabetes Mellitus

Type 1 diabetes mellitus (T1D) is also known as insulin-dependent diabetes mellitus. This autoimmune disease results from the destruction of beta cells in the pancreatic islets, which are responsible for producing insulin. It is also called childhood or juvenile-onset diabetes because it usually starts during childhood with symptoms of polydipsia (increased thirst), polyphagia (increased eating), and polyuria (increased urination) with associated weight loss.

This autoimmune disease is T cell-mediated. There is hyperglycemia, ketosis, insulitis, and the presence of anti-islet antibodies, including anti-glutamic acid decarboxylase (GAD) antibodies, anti-insulin antibodies (AIA), and IA-2 autoantibodies.

Melatonin Modulation of Type 1 Diabetes Mellitus

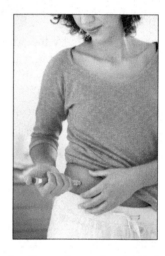

On your pancreas, you have MT1 & MT2 receptors for melatonin. They are called "G-coded melatonin receptors".[3] That means this is a direct link to diabetes and melatonin. When you go to sleep these receptors are activated by melatonin and insulin is lowered and glucose is increased via these MT1&2 receptors. These receptors have a direct link through cAMP and cGMP which is a massive signal to your metabolism. This is so you can have more glucose to make repairs needed within the body. Although eating late might increase serotonin which helps to increase building blocks for melatonin it might not be best for your health long term. Especially if you're leaning towards Type 2 diabetes. In this section, we will discuss how melatonin assists in the autoimmune form of diabetes which is type 1. In type 1 Diabetes mellitus, the destruction of insulin-producing beta cells results from the activation of pro-inflammatory cytokines such as TNF-alpha and IFN-gamma, which are mediated by Th1 cells.

Studies carried out on non-obese diabetic mice, an animal model of T1D, show that prolonged administration of melatonin resulted in increased survival and delayed onset of diabetes.[4] Melatonin helps shift the immune response from Th1 cells to Th2 cells, thereby reducing TNF alpha and IFN gamma production, which protects against beta-cell destruction.

Studies also show that pancreatic islet grafts done for diabetic mice increased survival rate from 7 days to 17 days when melatonin was administered. This pancreatic islet graft is a potential surgical therapy for T1D by administering melatonin to prevent the graft from attack by the immune cells or rejection.

In chapter 16 we'll be learning more about how melatonin can be useful in cases of diabetes, both type 1 and 2.

Pathophysiology of Multiple Sclerosis

Multiple sclerosis is a chronic inflammatory demyelinating disease of the central nervous system. It results from the loss of the neuronal myelin sheath due to an attack by autoantigen-specific immune cells. This leads to pain, fatigue, body weakness, and even vision loss at times. The onset of the disease is usually between the age of 20 and 40 years.

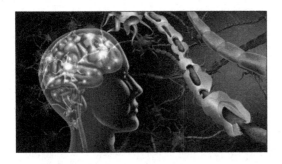

The pathogenesis of multiple sclerosis involves both the adaptive and innate immune cells. Experimental autoimmune encephalomyelitis (EAE) is the commonly used animal model for multiple sclerosis due to its close similarities.

Findings show that animals with EAE have T cells and macrophages infiltrating the CNS lesions. This autoimmune process is initiated by the adaptive immune CD4 T cells, which results in the production of inflammatory cytokines by the innate immune cells like macrophages. These pro-inflammatory cytokines result in severe inflammation and damage to the myelin sheath and neurons seen in EAE.[5] The production of reactive oxygen species in the affected areas as markers of oxidative stress is increased in the neurons of Multiple sclerosis patients.

Melatonin Modulation of Multiple Sclerosis

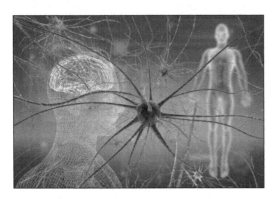

Findings show that there is dysregulation of melatonin production in patients with multiple sclerosis. There is an excretion of a high amount of melatonin metabolites in such individuals' urine at night.[6] This means that such patients have a reduced level of melatonin. This is correlated to the fluctuation of multiple sclerosis symptoms.In multiple sclerosis, there is the activation of Th17 cells, which worsens the inflammation. Melatonin suppresses the Th17 cells, which helps slow down or stop the progression of the disease.

Pathophysiology of Systemic Lupus Erythematosus

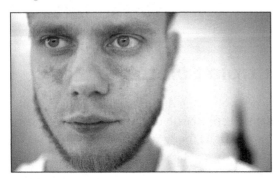

Systemic lupus erythematosus (SLE) is an autoimmune disease characterized by malar (butterfly) rash, photosensitivity, nephritis, and arthritis. It results from damage to tissues by immune cells. SLE affects more women than men and can manifest at any age.

In SLE, there is an activation of autoreactive T cells, resulting in B cell hyperactivity. This leads to the production of Th1 cytokines such as IL-2 and IFN-gamma as well as TH2 cytokines IL-4. SLE also shows increased levels of inflammatory cytokines TNF-alpha and IL-6.

Melatonin Modulation of Systemic Lupus Erythematosus

Research shows that melatonin administration can be helpful in the treatment of SLE.[7] The mice model of SLE shows improvement in the symptoms after the administration of melatonin. However, the effects of melatonin administration are time-dependent as well as gender-sensitive.

When melatonin is administered to female mice in the morning, there is an increase in survival rate, and symptoms improve. However, when administered in the evening, there is no noticeable improvement.

For male mice, however, the effect of melatonin is different. Melatonin treatment of SLE in male mice worsens the symptoms by increasing inflammatory cytokines and auto-antibodies.[8] This effect in males may be due to testosterone in males, which increases proinflammatory cytokines when combined with melatonin. Therefore, for patients with SLE, melatonin supplements will benefit female patients and should be used in the morning.

ALS and Melatonin

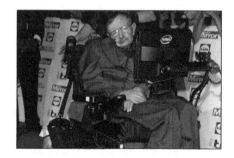

In ALS oxidative stress is a common molecular denominator of the disease progression. Melatonin shows a unique spectrum of antioxidative effects not conveyed by classical antioxidants. Due to this unique antioxidant property, it shows effectiveness against ALS in super-physiological doses.

"In a clinical safety study, chronic high-dose (300 mg/day) rectal melatonin was well tolerated during an observation period of up to 2 yr. Importantly, circulating serum protein carbonyls, which provide a surrogate marker for oxidative stress, were elevated in ALS patients, but were normalized to control values by melatonin treatment. This combination of preclinical effectiveness and proven safety in humans suggests that high-dose melatonin is suitable for clinical trials aimed at neuroprotection through antioxidation in ALS." [18]

A study performed in 2006 called "Reduced oxidative damage in ALS by high-dose enteral melatonin treatment" used 300 mg melatonin suppositories dust once a day for ALS.[9] This is a section reported in the study.

Safety of melatonin in the management of autoimmune disorders

Another concern related to the use of melatonin for autoimmune disorders is the higher doses used in several experiments. However, melatonin has exhibited a high level of safety even in clinical trials when used in higher doses.

According to a clinical trial 'Modulation by Melatonin of the Pathogenesis of Inflammatory Autoimmune Diseases' published in the International Journal of Molecular Sciences in 2013, participants with amyotrophic lateral sclerosis, who were administered a daily dose of 30 to 60 mg of melatonin orally tolerated it without any side effects.[10]

It has also shown that patients who received daily melatonin treatment in the form of rectal suppositories at a higher dose of 300 mg per day also showed no complications while exhibiting significant improvement in the symptoms.

Other than the oral doses and the suppositories, the safety and efficacy of intravenous melatonin have also been proven.

The report has also demonstrated that the treatment of patients undergoing aortic surgery can be combined with intravenous melatonin administration in a dose of 60 mg to improve the outcomes.

Therefore, the application of higher pharmacological doses of melatonin in the management of autoimmune disorders can be considered acceptable.[11]

In another research study, 'Reduced oxidative damage in ALS by high-dose enteral melatonin treatment' published in the Journal of Pineal Research has suggested combining the conventional treatment in patients with amyotrophic lateral sclerosis (ALS) with melatonin to support faster recovery.

This study was focused on assessing the effectiveness of melatonin in the management of ALS, which is a collective term used for the fatal motor neuron diseases of different etiologies, having oxidative stress or free radical damage as a common molecular precursor to disease progression.

This study showed that the antioxidant effect of melatonin remains active even when it is administered in the form of rectal suppositories.

The potential role of melatonin as a neuroprotective compound was also established in this study. It showed that melatonin could attenuate glutamate-induced cell death in the cultured motoneurons. Additionally, the higher doses of oral melatonin also worked significantly by delaying disease progression and extending the survival of the participants.

The clinical safety of melatonin was also demonstrated in this study. It shows that the long-term use of high doses (300 mg) of rectal melatonin in the form of suppositories could be well tolerated. It also helped produce the desired results. The research study was conducted over a period of 2 years during which no adverse effects were noticed in participants.

Importantly, the melatonin uses also helped to reduce the circulating levels of serum protein carbonyls, which is a marker for oxidative stress in ALS patients. The serum protein carbonyls levels returned to control values following melatonin treatment. The combination of proven safety and preclinical effectiveness of melatonin suppositories reiterate the usefulness of high doses of melatonin for neuroprotection and antioxidation in patients with autoimmune disorders such as ALS.[12]

I suspect there would be considerably better results in many of the studies where the dosing was performed poorly, if the original study had been performed similarly to this one using a suppository. Studies show that oral absorption of melatonin is only 2.5% whereas a suppository bypassing the gut and digestive enzymes, as well as, passing through the liver would have a much higher absorption.

Conclusion

In conclusion, anyone with an autoimmune condition should seriously consider supplementing with quality melatonin. The question is how much melatonin should one use? Will it shut down my normal production of melatonin and if I take high doses of melatonin is that dangerous? Anyone that is looking to deal with sleep issues, as long as they're not trying to reset their circadian rhythm in a separate time zone, will be fine with doses of melatonin from 3 to 20 mg.

There's something called super-physiological dosing of melatonin where doses up above 40 mg all the way up to 200-300 mg are taken. These doses are both safe as studies show that even up to 150,000 mg, melatonin would not cause any toxicity. In addition to that, unlike most hormones, melatonin does not create negative feedback on your brain's production of melatonin. Anyone suffering from an autoimmune condition may consider taking higher doses of melatonin. Due to melatonin only being 2 1/2% absorbed orally, some may consider the use of suppositories or even a liposomal delivery such as with Sandman.

In addition to melatonin supplementation, it is advised to seek the care of a functional and or naturopathic practitioner that can run the right laboratory tests to determine what's at the root cause of the autoimmune condition. Once they have this knowledge, they can work on correcting the underlying problem, wherein you start and continue your melatonin protocol. This commentary in the conclusion of chapter 5 is worth repeating here:

The immune system is the real backbone of your health. It can determine how efficiently all the organs of your body function, and how well you are able to fight and even avoid diseases. Melatonin offers a safe and effective way to allow your immune system to function more efficiently. It would not just strengthen the immunity but also regulate the activities of the immune cells. The immune-boosting and immunoregulatory properties of melatonin could provide a huge breakthrough in the management of autoimmune diseases, infections, allergies, and immunosenescence.

Furthermore, in addition to using melatonin, I suggest a regular fasting routine, such as with MitoFast where you do a 24hr fast weekly and a 3-5 day fast several times a year. Ozone therapy can also help strengthen the immune system, as it activates autophagy or cleaning and recycling of dysfunctional immune cells. For viral immunity, I further suggest supplementing with glutathione, zinc, quercetin, and selenium.

Moreover, it is also my opinion that poor sinus health can be a major drain on many people's immune systems, so a 30-day sinus cleanse is good to do at least once a year.

Dosing melatonin is supra-physiologic dosing, in a manner that absorbs better than the traditional oral route is a good idea. Using suppository or liposomal in the 100's of milligrams is my suggestion to many of my patients, and even the most knowledgeable scientist on melatonin, Russel Reiter, MD, PH.D., takes 100-200 per night himself.

Reference

1. Yoo, Y. M., Jang, S. K., Kim, G. H., Park, J. Y., & Joo, S. S. (2016). Pharmacological advantages of melatonin in immunosenescence by improving activity of T lymphocytes. *Journal of biomedical research*, *30*(4), 314–321. https://doi.org/10.7555/JBR.30.2016K0010

2. Kühlwein E, Irwin M. Melatonin modulation of lymphocyte proliferation and Th1/Th2 cytokine expression. J Neuroimmunol. 2001 Jul 2;117(1-2):51-7. doi: 10.1016/s0165-5728(01)00325-3. PMID: 11431004.

3. Mulder H, Nagorny CL, Lyssenko V, Groop L. Melatonin receptors in pancreatic islets: good morning to a novel type 2 diabetes gene. Diabetologia. 2009 Jul;52(7):1240-9. doi: 10.1007/s00125-009-1359-y. Epub 2009 Apr 18. PMID: 19377888.

4. Mok JX, Ooi JH, Ng KY, Koh RY, Chye SM. A new prospective on the role of melatonin in diabetes and its complications. Horm Mol Biol Clin Investig. 2019 Nov 6;40(1):/j/hmbci.2019.40.issue-1/hmbci-2019-0036/hmbci-2019-0036.xml. doi: 10.1515/hmbci-2019-0036. PMID: 31693492.

5. Yeganeh Salehpour M, Mollica A, Momtaz S, Sanadgol N, Farzaei MH. Melatonin and Multiple Sclerosis: From Plausible Neuropharmacological Mechanisms of Action to Experimental and Clinical Evidence. Clin Drug Investig. 2019 Jul;39(7):607-624. doi: 10.1007/s40261-019-00793-6. PMID: 31054087.

6. Gholipour T, Ghazizadeh T, Babapour S, Mansouri B, Ghafarpour M, Siroos B, Harirchian MH. Decreased urinary level of melatonin as a marker of disease severity in patients with multiple sclerosis. Iran J Allergy Asthma Immunol. 2015 Feb;14(1):91-7. PMID: 25530144.

7. Medrano-Campillo P, Sarmiento-Soto H, Álvarez-Sánchez N, Álvarez-Ríos AI, Guerrero JM, Rodríguez-Prieto I, Castillo-Palma MJ, Lardone PJ, Carrillo-Vico A. Evaluation of the immunomodulatory effect of melatonin on the T-cell response in peripheral blood from systemic lupus erythematosus patients. J Pineal Res. 2015 Mar;58(2):219-26. doi: 10.1111/jpi.12208. Epub 2015 Feb 4. PMID: 25612066.

8. Zhou LL, Wei W, Si JF, Yuan DP. Regulatory effect of melatonin on cytokine distur-
    bances in the pristane-induced lupus mice. Mediators Inflamm. 2010;2010:951210. doi:
    10.1155/2010/951210. Epub 2010 Jul 20. PMID: 20706659; PMCID: PMC2913856.

9. Weishaupt JH, Bartels C, Pölking E, Dietrich J, Rohde G, Poeggeler B, Mertens N, Sperling
    S, Bohn M, Hüther G, Schneider A, Bach A, Sirén AL, Hardeland R, Bähr M, Nave KA,
    Ehrenreich H. Reduced oxidative damage in ALS by high-dose enteral melatonin treatment.
    J Pineal Res. 2006 Nov;41(4):313-23. doi: 10.1111/j.1600-079X.2006.00377.x. PMID:
    17014688.

10. Lin, G. J., Huang, S. H., Chen, S. J., Wang, C. H., Chang, D. M., & Sytwu, H. K. (2013).
    Modulation by melatonin of the pathogenesis of inflammatory autoimmune diseases.
    International journal of molecular sciences, *14*(6), 11742–11766. https://doi.org/10.3390/
    ijms140611742

11. Lin, G. J., Huang, S. H., Chen, S. J., Wang, C. H., Chang, D. M., & Sytwu, H. K. (2013).
    Modulation by melatonin of the pathogenesis of inflammatory autoimmune diseases.
    International journal of molecular sciences, *14*(6), 11742–11766. https://doi.org/10.3390/
    ijms140611742

12. Weishaupt JH, Bartels C, Pölking E, Dietrich J, Rohde G, Poeggeler B, Mertens N, Sperling
    S, Bohn M, Hüther G, Schneider A, Bach A, Sirén AL, Hardeland R, Bähr M, Nave KA,
    Ehrenreich H. Reduced oxidative damage in ALS by high-dose enteral melatonin treatment.
    J Pineal Res. 2006 Nov;41(4):313-23. doi: 10.1111/j.1600-079X.2006.00377.x. PMID:
    17014688.

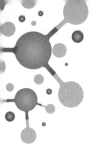

8

MELATONIN & CARDIOVASCULAR

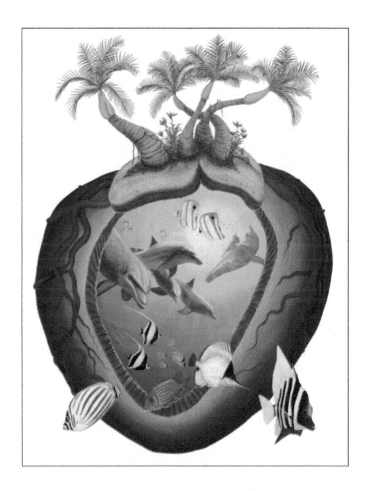

"An Open Heart" by John Lieurance

Heart Health, Cholesterol & Blood Pressure.

Much of your health depends on how efficiently your heart functions. A poorly functioning heart is the beginning of most diseases, as it would simply mean a lack of efficient supply of blood, oxygen, red cells, white cells, and vital nutrients to all organs of the body.

We need to take special care of our hearts as we only get one for our entire lifetime. Besides, the brain and the heart are among the top two most metabolically sensitive organs in the body, meaning that, any disruption in energy production from the cell will manifest in both these organs first. Of course, the mitochondria are at the core of this energy production, and we've already discussed in subsequent chapters how melatonin is very important during stressful situations to protect the mitochondria and our vital energy production.

There are a variety of different actions where melatonin improves the functions of the heart and the entire cardiovascular system. In fact, melatonin produces many favorable effects for your heart, blood vessels, and even helps to lower blood pressure and cholesterol.

In this chapter, we will learn how melatonin helps to improve heart functions and protects you from the disorders linked to high blood pressure, poor cardiac output, and irregular heart rhythm.

Melatonin and cardiovascular diseases

Atherosclerosis is one of the most common chronic vascular diseases in which oxidative stress and inflammation are implicated to be the major causative factors. The early stages of the development and deposition of cholesterol plaques involve endothelial activation, which is induced by the oxidized low-density lipoproteins, inflammatory cytokines, and the modifications in endothelial shear stress.

The research study "Melatonin and Cardiovascular Disease: Myth or Reality?" published in the Cardiologia in March 2012 has shown that melatonin can help to reduce the risk of atherosclerosis by decreasing the levels of LDL or bad cholesterol and increasing the levels of HDL, the good cholesterol.[1]

The study suggested that the antioxidant effects of melatonin on low-density lipoprotein oxidation may depress the plasma level of total cholesterol and VLDL (very low-density lipoprotein) cholesterol. This action of melatonin is linked to improved heart health. It indicates that this hormone would protect the heart against atherosclerosis that basically occurs due to the deposition of cholesterol plaques along the walls of the arteries.

Basically, these plaques are formed when your diet comprises foods rich in unhealthy, pro-inflammatory fats, like trans fats and saturated fats, but lacks healthy fats like mono-unsaturated fats (MUFA) and polyunsaturated fats (PUFA). Heated up vegetable oils are the main culprit that needs to be avoided. These are the primary oils used in restaurants to cook food, therefore it's almost impossible to eat out regularly and avoid them. Plaque buildup can also be indirectly related to when your liver is not efficient enough to metabolize fats.

These unhealthy fats oxidize very easily then tend to remain circulating in the bloodstream without being utilized to supply energy to the body. The high level of oxidation and inflammation will erode the protective layer within the blood vessels making it easier for this plaque to accumulate. These circulating fats, over a period of time, form thick plaques that get deposited at various places along the inner walls of the blood vessels, thus clogging them. In younger individuals, these plaques are generally softer and can dislodge, creating a higher risk of stroke. As we get older, they harden and become more calcified, with less risk of a stroke but lead to poor circulation. These plaques can lodge themselves in the arteries that supply blood to the heart or your brain. The result would be a heart attack or stroke, respectively.

These dangerous consequences of high cholesterol levels could be avoided if your body has sufficient melatonin. Melatonin may reverse the hypercholesterolemic states by increasing an endogenous cholesterol clearance effect.[2]

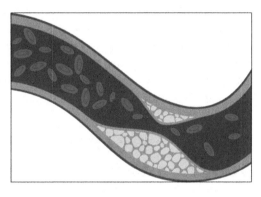

This means melatonin would stimulate the rate at which cholesterol in the bloodstream and tissues is cleared from the body through various mechanisms, like being burnt up for energy or broken down to be eliminated. Due to its lipophilic nature, melatonin can also enter the lipid phase of low-density lipoprotein particles readily and prevent lipid peroxidation. To confirm this hypothesis further, this study even showed the association between nocturnal raised levels of oxidized LDL (low-density lipoprotein) and the reduced melatonin levels in patients with atherosclerosis-induced myocardial infarction.

These findings support the theory that melatonin has the potential to lower total cholesterol levels and stimulate the levels of good or high-density lipoprotein cholesterol levels. And these changes would be protective against the development of cardiovascular diseases.

The study showed that the administration of melatonin in pharmacological doses would also reduce blood pressure as a consequence of different mechanisms, including the direct hypothalamic effect it can produce.[3]

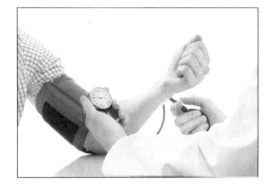

For example, melatonin would act on the hypothalamus and regulate its activities to ensure your blood pressure stays within normal limits. Similarly, it may also help to lower catecholamine levels, cause relaxation of the smooth muscles in the walls of blood vessels, and most importantly, produce antioxidant effects. So, here's the dichotomy, as we get older, we have lower melatonin levels, and our blood pressure goes up. Doctors then give us blood pressure-lowering medications that have a negative effect on our melatonin levels. If more doctors were aware of how melatonin works with blood pressure, there would be fewer prescriptions for blood pressure medications and many more for melatonin supplementation.

Catecholamines are hormones secreted by your adrenal glands, located at the top of your kidneys. Some examples of catecholamines include norepinephrine, dopamine, and epinephrine (which was earlier called adrenalin). Your adrenal glands secrete and release catecholamines into the blood when you are emotionally or physically stressed. Some of the typical effects of catecholamines include increased heart rate, blood pressure, and blood glucose levels.

Melatonin, with its ability to downregulate catecholamines, could bring your blood pressure within normal limits and prevent the serious consequences related to hypertension, such as stroke and heart attacks. If you are currently taking blood pressure medication it might be a good subject to bring up to your doctor, regarding starting melatonin and having him monitor your blood pressure in order to taper off if you have less of a need for the medication. Please keep in mind, none of the suggestions in this book are meant as medical advice and you should always get the approval of your healthcare provider before you make any changes to your medicines or supplement regime.

How do Mitochondrial dysfunctions affect your heart?

We've discussed the mitochondria in detail and how it's the powerhouse of the cell. Without healthy mitochondria, the cells in your body would no longer be able to produce the energy they need to survive or function.

So, what happens to your heart when stress from inflammation cripples these mitochondria?

You may want to go back and review the section on how inflammation regulates cytokines which then has a negative effect on how the cell produces energy. How almost all stressful conditions have a commonality where this inflammation and cytokines are upregulated and thus have a negative impact on the mitochondria. How we start to produce only 4 ATPs versus 36, which is less than 10% of the energy efficiency we would otherwise have. The heart and brain are the 2 most metabolically active organs of your body. So, they also need a continuous source of energy. The functions of these 2 vital organs are highly vulnerable to low energy supply.

And this is why; when your body is struggling with inflammation, the damage it brings to the mitochondria at the cellular level would have a very bad impact on how efficiently your heart works? Let me explain why.

Mitochondria play a crucial role in the normal functioning of your heart and in the pathogenesis of various types of heart diseases. Specific mitochondrial dysfunctions may trigger the development of cardiomyopathies simply by affecting the energy supply to heart muscles.[4]

According to a research study published in the Texas Heart Institute Journal in 2013, the heart depends highly on the generation of oxidative energy in mitochondria to receive the large number of ATPs it requires for its continuous, contractile pumping activities. Additionally, cardiac mitochondria also perform other cellular functions like generating reactive oxygen species (ROS) and regulating cellular apoptosis.[5]

The mitochondria also play a role in the regulation and growth of cardiac bioenergetic arrangement.

> *Doctor John's Advice: Many people live in this stressful chemistry their entire life or for many many years. This stressful chemistry could be a consequence of your diet, the exercise you're not getting, too much exercise, stressful mental-emotional states, toxic exposure from pesticides and herbicide, work-related toxic exposure, mold and biotoxin exposure or accumulation, microwave stress from 4G and 5G, acute or chronic unresolved infections in the body to include cavitation's in the jaw and poor oral and sinus hygiene, and heavy-metal exposure in accumulation. Many of these things can be dealt with once we understand what they are and how detrimental they are to our health and well-being. This is where a solid functional doctor uses natural and practical methods to isolate these things and to begin to make positive changes in your life. Of course, measuring the results along the way is important.*

Disruptions in energy production due to the impairment of mitochondrial functions have been implicated in a wide range of metabolic, degenerative, neoplastic, and age-related diseases affecting the heart and other organs.

Mitochondrial cardiomyopathies are characterized by impaired heart-muscle functions, structure, or both. It may present in various forms such as hypertension, coronary artery disease, and valvular diseases. The presentation of mitochondrial cardiomyopathies may also include dilated hypertrophic left ventricular non-compaction, ventricular tachyarrhythmia, and heart failure.

This just goes to show the severity or the extent to which mitochondrial dysfunctions can affect the heart.

Is it possible to restore healthy functions of the heart by eliminating the root cause of inflammation-causing mitochondrial dysfunctions? If you can ensure your heart muscles are not deprived of energy during stressful chemistry in the body, much of these complications could be avoided.

The potential use of melatonin as an antioxidant during myocardial infarction

There is evidence suggesting the cardioprotective benefits of melatonin in patients with myocardial infarction. The extent of the ischemic reperfusion injury to the heart could be decreased to some extent when exogenous melatonin is included in the treatment protocol.

Melatonin would reduce the infarct size and the risk area, plus minimize the incidences of reperfusion arrhythmias.

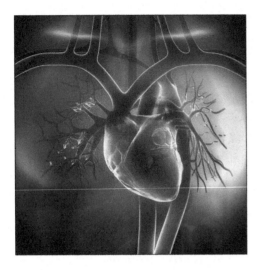

Also, ischemia is associated with the formation of reactive oxygen species from residual molecular oxygen molecules. So, it is suggested that the cardioprotective effect of melatonin is probably associated with its ability to scavenge and destroy free radicals and stimulate the expression of antioxidant enzymes.

The scavenging action of melatonin occurs in both physiological and larger pharmacological doses. Not just melatonin but several of its metabolites have the ability to detoxify free radicals and restore healthy heart functions. Yet melatonin is believed to work by stimulating essential enzymatic intracellular antioxidant enzymes such as superoxide dismutases (SOD) within both mitochondrial and the cytosol of the cell. It may also induce the activities of another powerful intracellular antioxidant called glutathione. Moreover, it might also protect mitochondria against oxidative stress and thus, ensure the heart muscles receive a good supply of energy needed to perform pumping action and other functions. This indicates the role of melatonin as a bioenergetic agent and its ability to improve mitochondrial functions. Research data suggests that patients with a history of myocardial infarction and angiographic no-reflow tend to have a low level of intra-platelet melatonin and higher systemic oxidative stress than people without this phenomenon.

This data suggest that melatonin may act as a potent antioxidant agent, thus reducing myocardial damage induced by ischemia or reduced oxygen supply to the heart muscles.

Intravenous melatonin in myocardial infarction patients

Interestingly, there have also been attempts to demonstrate the inhibition of ischemic damage to the heart muscles after the administration of melatonin intravenously, especially in patients who have undergone treatments like a percutaneous coronary intervention.

These studies have shown that intravenous, as well as intracoronary injections of melatonin, might limit myocardial damage and help patients recover faster after having suffered a heart attack.

Let's make a quick note here about what makes melatonin particularly beneficial in acute cases of cardiac emergencies.

The molecules of melatonin can be distributed quickly throughout the body; whether it is administered orally, through a suppository, or oral liposomal as with Sandman. It can cross all physiological barriers and enter the cardiac cells with ease and produce the desired effect to repair the damaged muscles.[6]

Taking care of your heart and cardiovascular system through disease prevention and treatment is where melatonin can really help. The heart has to work harder, and the pressure puts more stress on the blood vessels potentially leading to thickening of these blood vessels, therefore, causing more restriction of blood flow.

As stated, before melatonin keeps blood pressure low and melatonin declines as we get older. So, could it be that it's the lack of melatonin that is in part causing blood pressure to be elevated? It's also been documented that blood pressure medication has a negative effect on our production of melatonin, as well as the quality and duration of our sleep. Most patients with cardiac diseases have to fight the various side effects of blood pressure medications. Balancing the blood pressure first with melatonin and then second with anti-hypertensive medications makes the most sense to me.

Combined therapy using antihypertensive drugs with melatonin may help to relieve these side effects to a great extent as well. Maybe in a large number of cases simply just adding in melatonin may do the trick. It's certainly worth trying but it's important that you do this with the guidance of your healthcare provider and not try to do it by yourself.

How does melatonin help to relieve the side effects of blood pressure medications?

Patients with high blood pressure often suffer from poor sleep quality as a result of the negative effects of medications called beta-blockers.

According to a research study, patients treated for hypertension, who also use melatonin, have an improved quality of sleep compared to those who use only anti-hypertensive drugs. The improvement in sleep quality is in the forms of a shorter sleep onset period, reduced awakening during sleep, and more restful sleep.

This is an important finding considering beta-blockers are widely prescribed to patients with hypertension. These drugs are also used for the treatment of several other cardiovascular diseases, as well as anxiety disorders, migraine, and post-traumatic stress disorder.

It's known that the lack of sleep can worsen hypertension, by contributing to mental stress and impairing the natural healing mechanisms of the body. Sleep deprivation has also been linked to a higher risk of mortality in patients with heart diseases. And with insomnia being the most common side effect of these drugs, it becomes vital to include melatonin in the treatment protocol when one fully considers all of the research presented in this chapter.

According to another study "Night-time exogenous melatonin administration may be a beneficial treatment for sleeping disorders in beta-blocker patients" published in the Journal of Cardiovascular Disease Research in 2011, a clear improvement in sleep quality can be achieved along with better control over blood pressure by combining the use of beta-blockers and exogenous melatonin.

Also, unlike sedatives that are commonly prescribed to patients with sleep problems, melatonin didn't produce a "rebound" effect. This means, even after patients stop using melatonin, the improvement in their sleep pattern persists. It does not deteriorate even after going off the supplement, as it happens with several sedatives or sleep drugs.[7]

Remember as stated in previous chapters, there's no negative feedback loop where or when you take melatonin, no matter how much you take, it does not shut down your own production of melatonin. In fact, it may actually do the opposite and provide a carry-over benefit. So, even after you stop taking melatonin, you may continue to enjoy the benefits of improved sleep. Additionally, the use of melatonin did not show any sign of rising tolerance that would otherwise necessitate the use of higher doses. This shows that melatonin could provide multifactorial benefits by reducing the sleep problems caused due to the side effects of beta-blockers.

Melatonin as a heavy metal chelating agent for heart

According to a research study "*Protection of Metal Toxicity by Melatonin -Recent Advances* "published in the *Research Gate*, melatonin has a widespread subcellular distribution that enables it to interact with several toxic metals and molecules, thereby reducing the damage to the organs at the cellular level.

This property of melatonin makes it a powerful chelating agent, moreover, these qualities have been related to the reduced toxicity in the heart and other vital organs by heavy metals. It contributes to the prevention of toxicity induced by heavy metals such as mercury and lead. Melatonin may also alleviate cadmium-induced endoplasmic reticulum and cellular stress, regulate unfolded protein response, influence germ cell apoptosis, and prevent neurotoxic effects.

The protective effects of melatonin against mercurial toxicity may help in the prevention of myocardial toxicity, neurotoxicity, renal toxicity, thyrotoxicity as well as reproductive toxicity. It may also act as a chelating agent against arsenic toxicity as is manifested through its natural anti-oxidative mechanisms. Furthermore, it might also induce mitochondrial biogenesis and autophagy to eliminate these toxins from the heart muscles and valves, thereby restoring the healthy functions and higher efficiency of this organ to pump blood.

This is a huge reason to take melatonin in and of itself. Mitochondrial biogenesis to create new fresh healthy energy-producing cellular components and clearing out all of the weak, damaged, and dysfunctional mitochondria which are just spewing inflammatory and oxidative substances.

Melatonin has also been found to protect the heart against copper, chromium, and aluminum by exhibiting anti-inflammatory, pleiotropic, anti-lipidic, antioxidative, and other therapeutic effects. Moreover, melatonin may also mediate both intrinsic and extrinsic pathways for apoptotic cell death and exhibit anti-metastatic effects through the regulation of NFkB. These pleiotropic functions of melatonin make it a powerful cardioprotective molecule especially for men and women at risk of metal toxicity.[8]

Emerging further studies indicate the possibility that the cholesterol plaques blamed to be the major precursor to most cardiovascular diseases may actually contain microbes. The cholesterol plaques having microbes can create a biofilm on the endocardium (the inner walls of the heart), as well as the heart valves that regulate the flow of blood through different chambers like the atrium and ventricles.

And this new emerging idea makes melatonin more important considering its ability to boost your immune system's response against infections. The antioxidant property of melatonin would also destroy reactive oxygen species and down-regulate inflammation that would cause damage to cardiac muscles. This in combination with the chelating effect of heavy metals, improved restorative sleep, lowering of the blood pressure, and an improved cholesterol profile, would protect and can even restore heart health to a great extent.

How do you know if you are at a higher risk due to metal toxicity?

You can do testing to determine what type of heavy metal load you have in your body, and it's important to take into consideration risk factors such as mercury amalgam fillings. Especially if you have mercury amalgam fillings and you drink a lot of hot coffee or tea which will leach the mercury out of the amalgam more rapidly. Other heavy metal risk factors include eating a lot of fish, especially larger predatory fish, vaccinations, and environmental exposure.

For this reason, I think it's a good idea to take binders when one first starts to embark on melatonin supplementation. You can reference ultimatecellularreset.com for more information about what type of binders, when to take them etc.

Conclusion

Cardiovascular health is incredibly important and the simple fact that melatonin can improve gut function and microbiome health, as well as blood sugar and metabolic disorders makes it unsurprising to see how beneficial melatonin can be in this arena. However, melatonin goes a step further and improves your energy through the mitochondria.

Remember the brain and the heart are the two most metabolically sensitive organs and any challenges with energy are going to show up in both of these places early. Improving sleep will improve stress management, as well as down regulate the sympathetic nervous system which drives blood pressure.

Time and time again, I have seen in the clinic how melatonin improves blood pressure and lipid profiles with my patients. Anyone interested in improving cardiovascular function should seriously consider melatonin supplementation.

Reference

1.   Dominguez-Rodriguez A, Abreu-Gonzalez P, Reiter RJ. Melatonin and cardiovascular disease: myth or reality? Rev Esp Cardiol (Engl Ed). 2012 Mar;65(3):215-8. English, Spanish. doi: 10.1016/j.recesp.2011.10.009. Epub 2012 Jan 13. PMID: 22245066.

2. Karolczak, K., & Watala, C. (2019). The Mystery behind the Pineal Gland: Melatonin Affects the Metabolism of Cholesterol. *Oxidative medicine and cellular longevity*, *2019*, 4531865. https://doi.org/10.1155/2019/4531865

3. Pechanova, O., Paulis, L., & Simko, F. (2014). Peripheral and central effects of melatonin on blood pressure regulation. *International journal of molecular sciences*, *15*(10), 17920–17937. https://doi.org/10.3390/ijms151017920

4. Mitochondria and Heart Disease | IntechOpen

5. Meyers, D. E., Basha, H. I., & Koenig, M. K. (2013). Mitochondrial cardiomyopathy: pathophysiology, diagnosis, and management. *Texas Heart Institute journal*, *40*(4), 385–394.

6. Dominguez-Rodriguez A, Abreu-Gonzalez P, Reiter RJ. Melatonin and cardiovascular disease: myth or reality? Rev Esp Cardiol (Engl Ed). 2012 Mar;65(3):215-8. English, Spanish. doi: 10.1016/j.recesp.2011.10.009. Epub 2012 Jan 13. PMID: 22245066.

7. Fares A. (2011). Night-time exogenous melatonin administration may be a beneficial treatment for sleeping disorders in beta blocker patients. *Journal of cardiovascular disease research*, *2*(3), 153–155. https://doi.org/10.4103/0975-3583.85261

8. Rana, Suresh. (2018). Protection of Metal Toxicity by Melatonin -Recent Advances. 6.

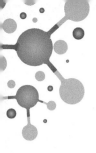

MELATONIN & SEX HORMONES

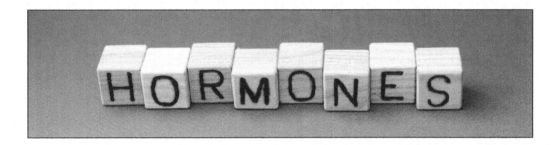

Who doesn't want to improve their sex life? I'm sure the answer is pretty obvious! Your overall vitality is ultimately a reflection of your sexual vitality. When you're stressed, you're not typically aroused. I'm sure anyone reading this has experienced being pushed too far in some way, whether physically, mentally, or emotionally, where they have found themselves lacking sex drive. Since melatonin works on stress it

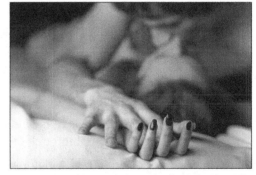

should be no surprise that there is also a body of research on melatonin in this specific area of health as well. Think about how sexy YOU feel after a great night's sleep, well guess what? That's melatonin doing its work on your sex hormones.

Your body relies on cycles and rhythms. The sleep-wake cycle is the most obvious, and this cycle is wired into steroid hormones released by both the testes and ovaries.

Through puberty, these steroid hormones help you grow and develop. After puberty and in our later years the female hormones, estrogen and progesterone, and the male hormone, testosterone influence metabolism, healing, proper weight and muscle mass, reproduction, sexual functions, appetite control, urine secretion, motivation, proper cardiovascular function, and overall physical conditioning.

The imbalances in the levels of these hormones can trigger the development of diseases. Melatonin has been found to be effective in the management of disorders linked to imbalances in sex hormones.

The discovery of hormone-balancing effects of melatonin

The possible role of melatonin in maintaining the balance of sex hormones was postulated when several studies showed abnormal melatonin secretion in patients with sexual dysfunctions and infertility. The research study "Melatonin and sex hormone interrelationships-a review" published in the Journal of Pediatric Endocrinology and Metabolism in 1999 revealed that there is evidence supporting the relationship between melatonin and reproductive hormones.

The evidence relies on the findings of abnormal levels of melatonin in patients with reproductive disorders and the pathologies of the pineal gland that were also associated with clinical manifestations of abnormal levels of reproductive hormones.

What these studies have suggested is the change in the levels of melatonin and the dysfunctions related to the pineal gland are more common in patients with hormonal disturbances linked to sexual and reproductive disorders. This raises the possibility that correcting melatonin levels could be an effective strategy for restoring normal levels of sex hormones in men and women.

Also, this study pointed out that the normal rhythmic secretion of melatonin is closely related to the rhythmic secretion of reproductive hormones in infants. The same has been found to be reciprocally related to hormonal levels during puberty. This indicates that the secretion of melatonin and sex hormones are closely interlinked. They can influence each other, both positively and negatively.

So, maintaining optimum levels of melatonin could prove to be effective for maintaining normal levels of sex hormones through these interlinked mechanisms.

Moreover, the demonstration of melatonin receptors in reproductive organs as well as in the brain, coupled with the localization of the receptors for sex hormones in the pineal gland have further strengthened these relationships. It indicated that the presence of receptors for sex hormones and melatonin in common organs and tissues could be one of the factors for why and how they influence each other.

The findings of these studies have formed a basis on which the link between melatonin and sex hormones can be further established.[1]

So how does the secretion of melatonin affect the levels of male and female sex hormones and how can the use of exogenous melatonin provide relief from the symptoms of sexual and reproductive dysfunctions?

Melatonin can help in the management of ED

When the moment arises, yet other "male parts" don't, this is called ED or erectile dysfunction and is actually pretty common. Sexual problems like erectile dysfunctions (ED) can be highly frustrating for men. According to the National Institutes of Health (NIH), ED has been found to affect nearly 30 million men in the United States.

It has also been estimated that about 4% of men in their 50s and 17% of men in their 60s develop a complete lack of ability to get an erection.[2]

While there are several different causes that can lead to sexual dysfunctions, melatonin is considered by some as one of the most effective ways to manage it.

How does melatonin affect ED?

Before diving into this section, you should understand that both men and women rely on testosterone levels for sex drive. There is also an erection that takes place in the clitoris which is linked to testosterone. Porn or nerve function is one of the common causes of ED. Research studies have shown that correcting nerve functions and improving nerve health could help to restore sexual functions in men.

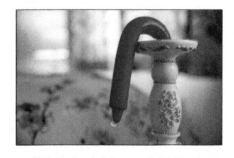

According to a research study, "Melatonin and tadalafil treatment improves erectile dysfunction after spinal cord injury in rats" published in the Clinical and Experimental Pharmacology and Physiology, using large doses of melatonin might help to heal the damaged nerves and relieve the sexual dysfunctions linked to nerve injuries.

This study involved the use of melatonin in a dose of 10 mg per kg body weight. This would be 700mg to an average-sized male human. The results of this study indicated that the antioxidant capabilities of melatonin might help to restore and prevent tissue damage.[3]

This study goes on the report the use of melatonin is also linked to an improved balance of hormones in the body. Since the production of all hormones in the body is interlinked and based on a cycle, "Circadian Rhythm". Maintaining healthy levels of melatonin and the natural rhythm of hormone production is considered one of the ways to improve levels of testosterone.

They concluded that melatonin supplementation might help to slow the age-related decline in the production of testosterone in men and thus, help them avoid ED linked to hormonal imbalances.

In a separate study 'melatonin improves erectile dysfunction with lower body ischemia' it is discovered that melatonin has a positive impact on circulation and can improve erectile dysfunction when it's linked to vascularity.[4]

The fight or flight side of your nervous system or sympathetic is anti-erectile. However, the resting and digesting side or the parasympathetic pathways are pro-erectile.[5]

As we discussed in other chapters melatonin has a positive effect on the parasympathetic nervous system. Put plainly, melatonin supports the parasympathetic nervous system that is an opposing force to the stress-induced sympathetic nervous system. Without this opposition, there would be a tremendous amount of stress as the body would be in a constant state of fight, flight, or hide. This chronic state is a common cause of many diseases as we've discussed in this book. Because melatonin works to balance this, it improves the ability to have an erection.

When we say that erectile dysfunction could be neurological, we mean that it could be both neurological: through the autonomic nervous system and the parasympathetic nervous system, as well as neurologic meaning that the nerves in and around the penis are weak and not functioning properly.

It appears that melatonin addresses erectile dysfunction from both of the most common causes, neurogenic and vascular. I feel it's more probable that most cases of ED have both neurogenic and vascular causes involved, as the circulation will affect fuel delivery to the nerves and subsequently, poor nerve function will affect the autonomics in the blood vessels which can disrupt blood flow.

Melatonin has a supportive effect on the female reproductive system

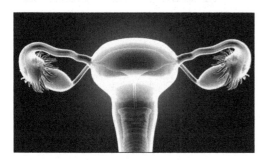

Sex hormones are stimulated through a primary hormone from the brain which then creates a cascade leading to the sex glands producing the sex hormones. Melatonin affects the functions of the female reproductive system by acting on the ovaries both directly and indirectly. By indirect support, melatonin acts on the primary signaling hormone GnRH. Thereby stimulating the release of gonadotropins.

It should be noted that GnRH is responsible for the release of LH (Luteinizing hormone) and FSH (Follicle Stimulating Hormone) from the anterior pituitary gland in women. It is common for treatment plans using hormone replacement therapy to cycle using luteinizing hormones in order to maintain and preserve the sex glands. Moreover, when you're given exogenous hormones, meaning from outside, it tends to shut down your endogenous production.

Remember, melatonin doesn't have a negative feedback loop like many other hormones do. Nevertheless, your sex hormones have an extraordinarily strong negative feedback loop and this needs to be considered when giving hormone replacement therapy.

By pulsing luteinizing hormones you'll stimulate your own hormones to produce, therefore keeping them working when they would otherwise be inhibited by continuing to take the exogenous hormones. Since melatonin works to invigorate all of your sexual organs through this pathway, it seems to be a logical adjunct to any hormone replacement therapy protocol.

Melatonin can also act on the ovaries directly through its anti-apoptotic and antioxidant properties, as well as through its regulation of LH and signaling molecules in the ovaries.

Since FSH and LH both play a vital role in the reproduction and menstrual cycles in women, melatonin is believed to influence these functions as well, thanks to its ability to regulate FSH and LH through GnRH. Furthermore, MT-1 and MT-2 receptors for melatonin have been detected on both the ovaries and testes. Increasing evidence shows that melatonin acts at the level of the ovary to modify ovarian functions via a receptor-mediated process on the ovarian melatonin receptors.[6] [7]

Ultimately, there is a complex interplay between melatonin, GnRH, LH, and FSH on the other sex hormones in women, their reproductive functions, and menstrual cycles.[8]

Melatonin in the management of infertility

Melatonin supplementation may be a great therapy in the management of infertility in women with endometrial dysfunctions.

This study demonstrates just that. "Melatonin Promotes Uterine and Placental Health: Potential Molecular Mechanisms" published in the International Journal of Molecular Sciences in 2019.

Researchers wanted to determine the effect of melatonin on endometrial morphology and embryo implantation. They found that melatonin can produce a positive effect on the endometrium. It can allow for better implantation of the embryos on the endometrial lining of the uterus possibly by raising progesterone levels.

The results of this study suggested that the use of melatonin could improve the chances of conception in women struggling with fertility issues. It may also be used during ART (Assisted Reproductive Techniques) like IVF (In-vitro fertilization) to improve the chances of successful outcomes of infertility treatment.

During IVF, an embryo fertilized in a laboratory is implanted into the uterus through artificial means. The successful implantation of the embryo on the endometrial wall of the uterus is crucial for conception. Melatonin might support the implantation of the embryo to the endometrial lining, thereby improving the chances of pregnancy in this case.[9]

To improve implantation, melatonin also modifies the epithelial and endometrial thickness by lowering estradiol levels while improving its glandular density. This, in turn, would result in the attenuation of reactive oxygen species with increased production of TAS (total antioxidant substances).

This means the antioxidant capacity of melatonin would be further enhanced allowing it to protect the endometrial tissues, making it more efficient to perform the function of implantation essential for successful conception.

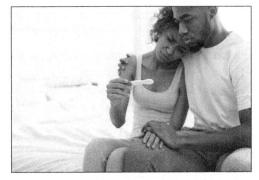

Another research study 'Melatonin and female reproduction' published in the Journal of Obstetrics and Gynecology

Research in 2014 showed that Melatonin can be successfully used to improve ovulation and promote embryo implantation. Moreover, it might be helpful in overcoming the deficiencies in fertilization, implantation, and conception during in vitro fertilization.[10]

These studies have affirmed the role of melatonin in the management of infertility, even in women who need to undergo advanced ART treatments.

Melatonin effects on breast cancer

Melatonin appears to have a protective effect on the development of breast cancer. Some research studies have shown that women with a lower level of melatonin hormone such as those who sleep fewer hours or work in shifts have a higher risk of breast cancer.

The use of melatonin in such cases appears to slow down the growth of cancer. It might improve the chances of survival of women with breast cancer by minimizing the multiplication and spread of cancer cells. This effect could be attributed to its ability to regulate the production of female reproductive hormones like estrogen.

It may also modify the functions and activities of estrogens receptors on the breast cells, thereby influencing the development of breast cancer. Therefore, the use of melatonin is believed to be potentially useful in the management of estrogen-dependent breast cancer.

The anticarcinogenic effect produced by melatonin could also be linked to its antioxidant properties. It can protect the tissues against free radical damage and thus, prevent cancerous changes. Moreover, this antioxidant activity of melatonin could be considered effective not just for the management of breast cancer but even ovarian, prostate, uterine, and endometrial cancers that are triggered due to oxidative stress and the imbalances in the levels of sex hormones.[11]

Researchers believe melatonin can also be used to improve the quality of life in women who have been diagnosed with cancer. It may be used alone or in combination with other conventional treatments.

Stress is the killer of sex

It's well documented that there is a process called "pregnenolone steal" where we lose many of our sex hormones due to excessive stress. When our bodies shift to this fight or flight mode, or sympathetic dominant state, to deal with stress our endocrine system prioritizes dealing with this emergency over the support to your endocrine system.

Pregnenolone steal is when DHEA after having converted into pregnenolone and when it would normally then convert into sex hormones, is shifted into making cortisol to deal with stress. Due to melatonin's ability to shift from sympathetic to parasympathetic, it can have a positive impact on preventing this pregnenolone steal.

> **Dr John's Comment:**
>
> Some of the other methodologies in natural medicine to address ED is the use of shockwave technology, which is a device that creates sound and light energy into areas in and around the penis. The device can stimulate nerves and blood vessel growth. Also, platelet-rich plasma and stem cell injections into the penis can be very helpful. Besides melatonin, these are some additional therapeutics that can be done with great effectiveness that we have utilized at Advanced Rejuvenation for many years.

Melatonin's ability to buffer stress seems to be the common theme throughout this book if you're not already noticing. Stress is nothing to hide from, it is a positive in the sense that our body can become stronger if it's able to deal with and be resilient to stress. Melatonin allows for this to happen which is why it has such a wide reach as far as health benefits.

Conclusion

There is a major difference between sex hormones and melatonin, in the sense that melatonin does not have a negative feedback loop where sex hormones have a very strong negative feedback loop. This negative feedback loop needs to be considered when giving hormone replacement therapy.

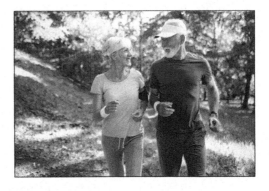

In this chapter, we looked at studies showing the positive impact melatonin has on gonadotropin-releasing hormone and luteinizing hormone. It is common for treatment plans using hormone replacement therapy to cycle using a luteinizing hormone to maintain and preserve the sex glands. Moreover, when you're given exogenous hormones meaning from outside, meaning from outside it tends to shut down your endogenous production. Yet, by pulsing luteinizing hormones you'll stimulate your own hormones to produce, therefore, keeping them working when they would otherwise be inhibited by continuing to take the exogenous hormones. Since melatonin works to invigorate all of your sexual organs through this pathway, it seems to be a logical adjunct to any hormone replacement therapy protocol.

In summary, melatonin seems to be a safe and effective treatment for the management of sexual problems linked to hormonal imbalances which translates into so many health benefits related to low hormone statuses such as poor injury healing, low energy, poor quality of skin and hair, low motivation and sex drive, poor muscle volume and strength, and poor cardiovascular function, are just a few common problems associated with low testosterone.

When I think of vitality I think of strong male and female hormone status. In our clinic, we test for these and strive to balance them through various strategies including hormone replacement therapy but also by improving sleep usually with super physiological melatonin dosing. Isn't the wide net melatonin casts in order to improve our health span and lifespan impressive?

Reference

1. Luboshitzky R, Lavie P. Melatonin and sex hormone interrelationships--a review. J Pediatr Endocrinol Metab. 1999 May-Jun;12(3):355-62. doi: 10.1515/jpem.1999.12.3.355. PMID: 10821215.

2. Erectile dysfunction - Symptoms and causes - Mayo Clinic

3. Tavukçu HH, Sener TE, Tinay I, Akbal C, Erşahin M, Cevik O, Cadirci S, Reiter RJ, Sener G. Melatonin and tadalafil treatment improves erectile dysfunction after spinal cord injury in rats. Clin Exp Pharmacol Physiol. 2014 Apr;41(4):309-16. doi: 10.1111/1440-1681.12216. PMID: 24552354.

4. Sawada N, Nomiya M, Zarifpour M, Mitsui T, Takeda M, Andersson KE. Melatonin Improves Erectile Function in Rats With Chronic Lower Body Ischemia. J Sex Med. 2016 Feb;13(2):179-86. doi: 10.1016/j.jsxm.2015.12.018. Epub 2016 Jan 20. PMID: 26803454.

5. Giuliano F, Rampin O. Neural control of erection. Physiol Behav. 2004 Nov 15;83(2):189-201. doi: 10.1016/j.physbeh.2004.08.014. PMID: 15488539.

6. Tamura H, Jozaki M, Tanabe M, Shirafuta Y, Mihara Y, Shinagawa M, Tamura I, Maekawa R, Sato S, Taketani T, Takasaki A, Reiter RJ, Sugino N. Importance of Melatonin in Assisted Reproductive Technology and Ovarian Aging. Int J Mol Sci. 2020 Feb 8;21(3):1135. doi: 10.3390/ijms21031135. PMID: 32046301; PMCID: PMC7036809.

7. Allan F. Wiechmann, David M. Sherry,Neurotransmitters and Receptors: Melatonin Receptors, Reference Module in Neuroscience and Biobehavioral Psychology,Elsevier,2017, ISBN 9780128093245,https://doi.org/10.1016/B978-0-12-809324-5.01447-4.

8. Starr, J. (2011). The Effect of Melatonin on the Ovaries. The Science Journal of the Lander College of Arts and Sciences, 5(1). Retrieved from ttps://touroscholar.touro.edu/sjlcas/vol5/iss1/6

9. de Almeida Chuffa LG, Lupi LA, Cucielo MS, Silveira HS, Reiter RJ, Seiva FRF. Melatonin Promotes Uterine and Placental Health: Potential Molecular Mechanisms. *International Journal of Molecular Sciences*. 2020; 21(1):300. https://doi.org/10.3390/ijms21010300

10. Tamura H, Takasaki A, Taketani T, Tanabe M, Lee L, Tamura I, Maekawa R, Aasada H, Yamagata Y, Sugino N. Melatonin and female reproduction. J Obstet Gynaecol Res. 2014 Jan;40(1):1-11. doi: 10.1111/jog.12177. Epub 2013 Oct 7. PMID: 24118696.

11. Melatonin (breastcancer.org)

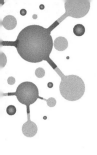

MELATONIN & DEGENERATIVE NEUROLOGIC DISEASE

Stroke, Mental Illness & Mood

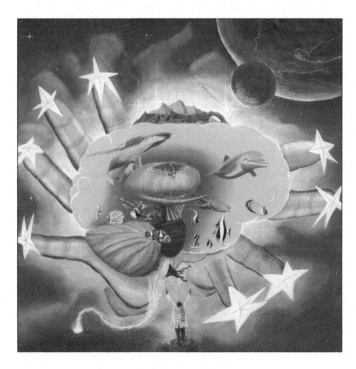

"Neurological Paradise"

Art by John Lieurance

Poor brain function can show up as minor forgetfulness or brain fog all the way to severe end-stage degenerative neurological disorders where our memories are lost or movement disorders where there's an inability to control one's movements.

These diseases are some of the most devastating as well as challenging to treat. I started specializing in these types of treatments through functional chiropractic neurology early on in my career, then one day I was on the other side of the equation as a patient with neurological complaints myself.

It started in 2007 with depression and debilitating arthritis in my left shoulder, then with the economic turndown in 2008 I had to close my practice and try to heal myself. It was a perfect storm that had great consequences on my health, spiraling me into a worse situation over the following 10 years that resulted in several symptoms that would come and go such as vertigo, POTS, cognitive issues like word finding and memory challenges, emotional instability, blurry vision, sensitivity to light and sound (photophobia, hyperacusis), hearing loss and my inflammatory arthritis began to get much worse.

I was eventually diagnosed with ankylosing spondylitis or AS by a rheumatologist and prescribed lots of drugs to cope with my condition. I really had no diagnosis I believed to be accurate as I felt like I had an infection, however, I was relying on the standard medical establishment and even though I was very much into alternative medicine myself, I could not figure out my own illness. You can only imagine how difficult this was as I was the doctor who folks came to see, even flying in from far away to seek my expertise but fixing myself or even figuring out what was wrong with me remained elusive for many years.

I lost my practice and the prestigious building I once owned was foreclosed on and I went from being a robustly healthy multi-millionaire to being in debt and looking like I was homeless due to the toll the illness was taking my physical body. See more about my story here.

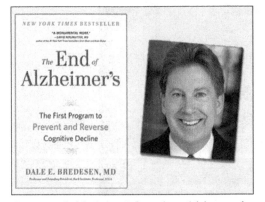

As painful as this was, it was my "Pain to Purpose" story ultimately and led me to find out what was wrong, and even writing this book may never have happened. I finally tested myself for Lyme disease and viral infections and the markers were literally off the chart. Some of my EBV titers were among the highest a viral expert had ever even seen! Why did numerous other doctors both medical and alternative miss this? I was loaded with infection!

On top of this later I found mold in my home and then found I tested positive for many mold illness markers. What happened to me is that my immune system was depleted with the entourage of these infections and all of the toxins they were releasing. It's not just about the infections, but also these same infections release these fat-soluble toxins that can have a devastating effect on health.

I bring the story up in this chapter because many neurological diseases can have biotoxin illness and CIRS as part of the clinical picture. Melatonin works on multiple aspects of both of these complications. I didn't know of the benefits of melatonin early on, however, I found glutathione suppositories helped me more than any other supplement and this was the beginning of my interest in suppositories.

With my case and many others, we see in our clinic we have found that there are very few mono strategies that can have a significant improvement in brain function. There must be a combination of several therapeutics in order to get a measurable response.

Dr. Dale Bredesen in his book *The End to Alzheimer's* brought chronic infections and toxicity as a primary culprit. This has caught the attention of the vast majority of the medical community. He broke down the causes of Alzheimer's disease into three main categories; infection and toxicity are 2 of them. After discovering the stressor that was the cause leading to the inflammation in the brain that resulted in Alzheimer's he then had various strategies and combinations to address one or more of them.

I personally feel like these are the most prevalent, non-vascular or traumatic, causes of most neurologic conditions. All causes of any degenerative neurological disorder have inflammation as part of its consequence. Dr. Bredesen also talks about the importance of deep sleep and how that keeps the brain healthy and clear of toxins that can build up. Because melatonin works on the glymphatics to detoxify the brain, neutralizes toxins, protects the brain during infections, and works to repair the brain. Melatonin hits all sides to act as a powerful medicine for brain support and it has the brightest application in this area of medicine.

Melatonin is one of those therapeutics that if I had only one, I would use this on all of my neurologic cases. Because melatonin affects so many different aspects of metabolism, mitochondrial health, inflammation, regeneration, sleep, and immune functions, it is no surprise that there's been loads of research demonstrating that melatonin can help in a wide range of neurologic conditions.

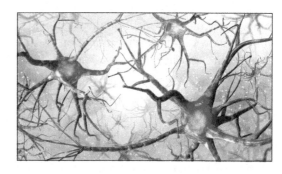

I was at a conference in Fort Lauderdale called "Brain Regeneration" where I sat next to some of the lead alternative doctors in the country such as Dr. Joe Mercola. At the conference, we were presented data regarding super physiological melatonin dosing. During the presentation, the doctor sitting next to me leaned over and said, "We started doing this a couple of months ago and this is one of the most significant treatments I've discovered". Well, that got my attention! And that was the beginning of my journey to understand melatonin.

In regard to having a healthy brain and slowing or reversing some of the devastating damage from many degenerative neurological disorders, melatonin is one important molecule that needs to be taken seriously. Leading researchers have discovered that melatonin can guard against brain degeneration brought about by aging, toxic exposure, and environmental factors. New studies have also uncovered the ability of melatonin to protect against the common age-related neurological diseases affecting the brain, including Parkinson's and Alzheimer's.

Melatonin is so beneficial at protecting the brain that scientists have found an age-related decline in the production of melatonin could be one of the factors for the concomitant increase in the development of neurodegenerative diseases. In fact, obvious signs of melatonin deficiency can be seen in patients with Alzheimer's, like disruptions in the day/night pattern, delirium, and mood changes.

Supplementing with high doses of melatonin starting from middle age and continuing through older age has been shown to protect people against Alzheimer's, as well as Parkinson's disease.

One research study 'Practical Evaluation and Management of Insomnia in Parkinson's Disease: A Review Published in the Movement Disorders' has revealed that the dysfunctions of the circadian system in patients with Parkinson's could be a consequence of neurodegeneration. In advanced cases of Parkinson's disease, behavioral factors like limited sunlight exposure can weaken circadian rhythm and promote faster degeneration of the brain tissues. The use of melatonin might be beneficial in such cases to reset the circadian rhythm and thus, slow down the degeneration.[1]

This finding was proven during a research study 'Usefulness of Early Treatment With Melatonin to Reduce Infarct Size in Patients With ST-Segment Elevation Myocardial Infarction Receiving Percutaneous Coronary Intervention' that was published in the American Journal of Cardiology in 2017. It showed that melatonin might limit the extent of the ischemia-reperfusion injury and increase the efficacy of the mechanical reperfusion in patients with myocardial infarction or stroke. The study also found that the infarct size reduced in size when melatonin was administered early following the onset of symptoms.[2]

Discoveries have validated melatonin's potential to protect the brain from oxidative stress. Remember that oxidative stress is like the smoke coming out of the coal-burning train. Well, the brain being one of the most metabolically active organs in the body is going to produce a lot of smoke a.k.a. oxidation. With this fact, it is no surprise that melatonin allows the brain to function at a much more efficient level. Besides, the powerful antioxidant melatonin is also responsible for deeper stages of sleep which stimulate the detoxification of the brain. With these findings, it seems melatonin deserves a new title: "The brain hormone."

Melatonin has been proven to protect you against Alzheimer's, Parkinson's, Stroke, Traumatic Brain Injuries, and much more.

The role of melatonin in neurodegenerative diseases

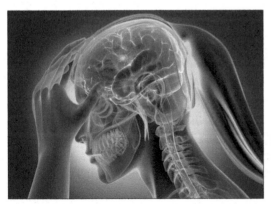

The following study titled 'Melatonin Antioxidative Defense: Therapeutical Implications for Aging and Neurodegenerative Processes' published in Neurotoxicity Research in 2013 revealed that the decline in melatonin production in aged men and women is a major factor contributing to the development of age-associated neurodegenerative diseases.[3]

The application of melatonin in preventing oxidative stress in neuronal cells or the brain of animals treated with neurotoxic agents has revealed its use as a neuroprotective agent. The results of this study suggested that melatonin could play a valuable therapeutic role in the prevention and treatment of Parkinson's disease, Alzheimer's disease, amyotrophic lateral sclerosis, stroke, Huntington's disease, and brain trauma.

Melatonin's efficacy in reducing free radical damage in the brain shows that it could also reduce swelling in the brain or cerebral edema that occurs following brain injuries and stroke.[4]

Another study 'Retardation of brain aging by chronic treatment with melatonin' published in the Annals of The New York Academy of Sciences has reiterated similar findings. This study has shown that slowing of the functional decline in the aging brain is highly relevant for non-pathological senescence as well as a broad range of neurodegenerative diseases. Aging of the brain associated with cumulative oxidative stress in macromolecules and the abnormal levels of inflammatory activities in brain cells could be ameliorated by using melatonin.

Maybe you remember us discussing cellular senescence where the old dysfunctional cells which are normally cleaned up and recycled continue to operate and create a lot of inflammation and oxidation. Well, supplementation with melatonin would elucidate the key intracellular targets associated with age-related inflammatory events and thus, protect the brain against degenerative changes linked to Alzheimer's and Parkinson's disease.[5]

Another study 'Early melatonin supplementation alleviates oxidative stress in a transgenic mouse model of Alzheimer's disease' published in the Free Radical Biology and Medicine in 2006 demonstrated the increased brain oxidative stress can be reduced through the use of melatonin.

The potent antioxidant and free radical scavenging effect of melatonin were applied in a mouse model for Alzheimer's disease to mimic the neuronal loss, accumulation of senile plaques, and memory impairment. The mice were treated with melatonin in a dose of 10 mg per kg body weight (comparable to 700 mg for an average male human adult) for 4 months and the long-term influence of melatonin was assessed before amyloid plaques were deposited.

The results of this study have shown that patients with Alzheimer's disease have an increase in the level of TBARS (thiobarbituric acid-reactive substances) in the brain and a decrease in GSH (glutathione) content.

Let me explain what TBARS means to the health and functions of the brain.

Thiobarbituric acid reactive substances (TBARS) are formed in the body as a by-product of lipid peroxidation or degradation products of fats. TBARS are generated as a result of damage to the brain tissues in patients with Alzheimer's or due to heart attacks or stroke.

Glutathione also plays a paramount role in improving the antioxidant defenses in the brain and maintaining redox homeostasis. The reduction in glutathione levels in the brain has also been observed as a result of aging and neurological disorders such as Alzheimer's and Parkinson's disease. In fact, reduced levels of Glutathione can worsen the neurodegenerative changes in the brain and contribute to the faster development of Alzheimer's disease and Parkinson's.

When melatonin was administered to Alzheimer's and Parkinson's patients, it was found that it helped reduce TBARS levels and improved glutathione levels in the brain. This indicates the efficacy of melatonin for reversing the abnormal changes in the nervous system and slowing down the pathogenesis of Alzheimer's.

In addition, mice administered melatonin also showed a significant decline in some factors that indicated inhibition of neuronal apoptosis, which is basically neuronal self-destruction. These results have supported the hypothesis that oxidative damage is an early event in the pathogenesis of neurodegenerative brain disorders and that antioxidant therapy using melatonin might be beneficial.

This study has recommended the use of melatonin as a potential therapeutic candidate in the treatment of Alzheimer's disease. It may also be used as a preventive measure to inhibit the development of this condition.[6]

What happens to the brain when there is melatonin deficiency?

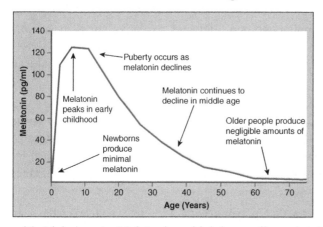

What's interesting, is if you look at the decline of melatonin as we age in this graph it makes sense that as we get older, we are more vulnerable to problems occurring with our brain and nervous system. It would therefore make sense how melatonin deficiency is playing a role in the aging of the brain.

Profound reduction in melatonin levels has been found in patients with Alzheimer's. Melatonin, which is usually maintained at a high level in the brain and spinal fluid during young and middle age starts to decline sharply as age increases in a fashion that parallels closely to the risk of Alzheimer's incidence.

Research study 'Role of melatonin in Alzheimer-like neurodegeneration' published in the Acta Pharmacologica Sinica in 2006 has revealed that Melatonin secretion decreases with aging. Patients with Alzheimer's disease or other neurodegenerative disorders like dementia and Parkinson's may have a more profound reduction in the secretion of this hormone.

Data from clinical trials have indicated that melatonin supplementation in such cases could ameliorate sundowning and slow down the progress of cognitive impairment. Melatonin has been found to efficiently protect the neuronal cells from Abeta-mediated toxicity with its antioxidant, anti-inflammatory, and anti-amyloid properties. Moreover, melatonin would not just inhibit Abeta generation, but also arrest the formation and deposition of amyloid fibrils by the structure-dependent interactions with Abeta.

> ## Dr John's Clinical Note:
>
> We have been using glutathione in our clinic for neurologic conditions for over 20 years with great responses. Glutathione acts on improving the immune system, decreasing oxidation as an antioxidant, it improves sleep and lastly, it also detoxifies chemicals and heavy metals out of the body and brain. Like melatonin, glutathione is one of those substances that is poorly absorbed when taken orally therefore we have traditionally been giving glutathione as an IV or as a suppository. I have found better results with suppository because I can provide this to our patients to do at home and to do them regularly, whereas the intravenous approach is more expensive and is usually more sporadic. I think ultimately both glutathione and melatonin and a suppository would provide better support than either of them individually

Recent studies have further suggested that abnormal hyperphosphorylation of tau protein in the brain plays a vital role in the molecular pathogenesis of AD and in neurodegeneration.[7]

Tau is a necessary protein that helps nerve cells communicate through microtubules. Tau is modified pathologically through abnormal phosphorylation, glycosylation, ubiquitination, glycation, polyamination, nitration, truncation, and aggregation. We need tau, but when it misbehaves it creates major problems! Researchers have found that the major component where tau misbehaves is hyperphosphorylation.

Recent studies have demonstrated that melatonin can attenuate hyperphosphorylation of tau! A direct regulatory effect of melatonin on the activities of the key chemistry in the brain that protects us from this hyperphosphorylation of tau through antioxidant pathways using protein phosphatases and protein kinases.[8]

Cholinergic nerves are the key nerves responsible for memory and work with the neurotransmitter acetylcholine. Most of the AZ drugs work on acetylcholine receptors. Things like phosphatidylcholine can be beneficial supplements to boost brain function and is helpful for brain fog all the way to later stage degenerative neurological disorders.

> Basically, tau does rancid just like many vegetable oils do when heated which also create lots of problems for our body and nervous system. As a side note this is why I never eat vegetable oils especially when used for cooking. Vegetable oils are cheap so most all restaurants use them to cook with so ask next time you dine out and see if you can find a restaurant that doesn't use vegetable oil for cooking!

I have found Alpha-GPC to work very well for both AZ and just boosting cognition with many of my clients as well. The benefit of using high and regular dosing of phosphatidylcholine is the cell membrane flushing effect. Since many toxins find themselves settling there a constant flush of PTC or phosphatidylcholine can be of great benefit for many people with neurological challenges, as well as chronic infections with Lyme, EBV, and CIRS in general, which is related to biotin illness. In our clinic, besides melatonin, we use a "Membrane Resolution" protocol which involves using good fats, PTC, butyrate, and dietary changes.

If melatonin can do this for Alzheimer's, then what do you think melatonin would do for someone with brain fog? Do things need to get that bad before we start considering melatonin?[9]

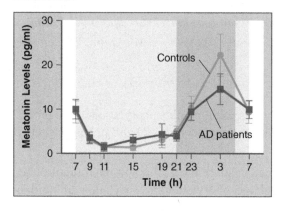

Moreover, another study was focused on evaluating sleep disruptions, sundowning, nightly restlessness, and other disturbances in the circadian rhythm seen frequently in patients with Alzheimer's disease. The changes in the pineal gland and suprachiasmatic nucleus were thought to be the biological precursors for these behavioral disturbances. Melatonin is the primary endocrine messenger for circadian rhythmicity therefore the major factor influencing the pathogenesis of Alzheimer's.

This study compared the melatonin levels in healthy people, both younger and older. It also compared melatonin levels in old people: with and without Alzheimer's disease.

The results were as follows:

The first comparison showed that the melatonin levels in the spinal fluid of HEALTHY older people above 80 years of age were just half of that in younger people. This showed that as age increases, the melatonin levels can reduce EVEN IN HEALTHY PEOPLE.

The second comparison showed that the age-related decline in melatonin can become much worse once neurodegenerative changes start to occur due to Alzheimer's disease. It was found that the melatonin levels in the CSF of older patients WITH Alzheimer's disease were just one-fifth of that in the people of the same age WITHOUT Alzheimer's disease.

This means the age-related decline in the CSF levels of melatonin can become more severe in patients with Alzheimer's. This study suggests that melatonin supplementation might be an effective strategy to restore healthy melatonin levels in the brain and CSF. They state that melatonin supplementation should reduce and slow down the degenerative changes in the brain and even reduce the risk of developing Alzheimer's disease.[10]

How does melatonin work in the management of Parkinson's diseases?

It is common for patients with Parkinson's disease to develop sleep-related symptoms. Several studies have already confirmed the efficacy of melatonin in improving sleep quality, decreasing night-time activity, and shortening the sleep latency period.

Researchers believe that melatonin could be beneficial for patients who suffer from reduced sleep due to Parkinson's.

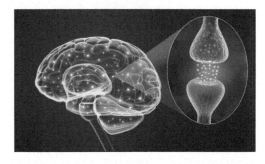

A study 'Melatonin for sleep disturbances in Parkinson's disease' published in Sleep Medicine in 2005 revealed the therapeutic role of melatonin in the management of Parkinson's disease. It showed that supplementing with melatonin in a dose of 50 mg per day produced a significant improvement in the total night-time sleep. There was also a significant decline in the sleep disturbances experienced after they started using melatonin. They also reported having better sleep which further helped to improve their daytime alertness. Being able to sleep well at night allowed the participants to feel fresh during the daytime and reduced sleepiness and drowsiness during morning hours. This means melatonin supplements given to Parkinson's sufferers could improve the duration of sleep.[11]

The role of melatonin in the management of Parkinson's is not limited to improving sleep quality.

Considering melatonin's effects on the brain's detox mechanisms, the glymphatics, might be playing an important role in the outcome of these Parkinson's disease cases. Also, the disease is characterized by the degeneration of neurons in a part of the brain called substantia nigra. Melatonin is believed to inhibit these abnormal changes in the brain by acting as a powerful antioxidant and neuroprotective agent.

Animal studies have demonstrated that melatonin supplementation may prevent or even reverse the change in behaviors and motor functions induced by Parkinson's disease. This finding was proven during a study 'Melatonin attenuates tyrosine hydroxylase loss and hypo-locomotion in MPTP-lesioned rats' published in the European Journal of Pharmacology in 2008.

The study was aimed at assessing the effects of melatonin on the loss of tyrosine hydroxylase and hypo-locomotion. Before we learn how melatonin helps in this case, let me first explain what the loss of tyrosine hydroxylase and hypo-locomotion mean in terms of the development of Parkinson's disease.

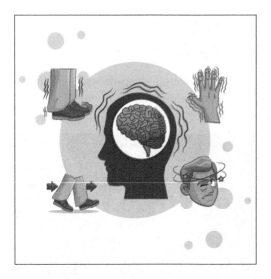

Hypo-locomotion or Bradykinesia, as seen in Parkinson's disease, refers to the reduced ability of patients to perform physical movements due to the degeneration or damage to the nerves that produce dopamine. It often slows them down, making their walk slow and erratic, causing them to lose balance, slow speech, or lose normal facial expressions. This explains what hypo-locomotion means.

The loss of tyrosine hydroxylase is a consistent neurochemical abnormality related to Parkinson's disease. Tyrosine hydroxylase plays a role in converting tyrosine to dopamine, which, in turn, is needed for communication between nerves and muscles. Patients with Parkinson's have a low level of dopamine due to the loss of tyrosine hydroxylase. As a result, the nerve functions involved in muscle movements are affected. This is one of the reasons why patients with Parkinson's experience tremors, inability to maintain balance, and unsteady gait.

The loss of tyrosine hydroxylase can also accelerate the degeneration of some neurons called the dopaminergic neurons in the part of the brain located within the substantia nigra. This explains why it is important to improve or protect levels of tyrosine hydroxylase in order to prevent the development of these movement disorders.

Coming back to the study we were discussing, it showed that the administration of melatonin in a dose of 50 mg per kg bodyweight could inhibit hypo-locomotion and neuronal damage. It further showed that melatonin could also reduce the risk of cognitive deficit linked to Parkinson's disease.

Ultimately, the results of this study revealed that the use of melatonin could be highly effective in the management of Parkinson's. *It would not just slow down but also reverse and inhibit the brain damage caused due to this disease.*[12]

The similarities between Parkinson's and Alzheimer's where melatonin can strike

Parkinson's has multiple similarities to Alzheimer's. Both of these diseases can lead to dementia, and both are linked to out-of-control oxidative damage.

In the case of Parkinson's, oxidative stress is focused more on those regions of the brain that control movements and balance (substantia nigra). And in both these diseases, brain dysfunctions and cell death are brought about by the accumulation of abnormal, inflammatory, and oxidizing proteins. In Alzheimer's, it's beta-amyloid whereas in Parkinson's it's called the alpha-synuclein.

Researchers have demonstrated how melatonin can attack the development of Parkinson's disease at each of its vital junctures. Let me explain some of these mechanisms that involve the action of melatonin in inhibiting the activities of alpha-synuclein.

A study, "Effect of melatonin on α-synuclein self-assembly and cytotoxicity", published in the Neurobiology of Aging in 2012, implicated the accumulation of alpha-Synuclein (αS) in the brain tissues as a critical step in the development of Parkinson's disease. This study revealed that melatonin can reduce the build-up of alpha-Synuclein by producing antioxidant and neuroprotection activities.

This anti-assembly effect on α-synuclein by melatonin is evident in the form of reduced cytotoxicity in the brain cells as was assessed following the use of melatonin supplements. It showed that melatonin would act as a neuroprotective agent and further enhance the brain functions thereby protecting a person against the age-related memory decline. It is believed to work by preventing the production of alpha-synuclein in brain cells, while at the same time attacking the existing molecules of this toxic protein making them available for faster cellular cleanup.[13]

In another study published in the Journal of Pineal Research in 2011, melatonin was shown to reduce the expression of alpha-synuclein in the dopamine-containing neuronal regions of amphetamine-treated postnatal rats. This study showed that melatonin can restore the normal activities of key enzymes involved in the production of dopamine specifically by reducing cytotoxicity induced by Amphetamine (AMPH).

AMPH is a psychostimulant drug that has been abused very commonly in recent years. It is known to induce severe neurotoxicity in the central dopaminergic pathways associated with increased oxidative stress in the brain. Recently, AMPH has also been shown to increase the level of alpha-synuclein in dopaminergic neuroblastoma cell cultures significantly.

This study has revealed that the neuroprotective and antioxidant properties of melatonin could help to attenuate the adverse effects of AMPH on the accumulation of alpha-synuclein in the dopaminergic pathways. Melatonin supplementation before the use of AMPH decreased the accumulation of alpha-synuclein to 70 to 90% of the base values.

Moreover, they saw an increased immunological hyper-reactivity in the brain linked to the accumulation of alpha-synuclein following the use of AMPH. This was restored to normal following melatonin supplementation. Just like another study demonstrated that melatonin could protect our brain against heavy metals. It seems it's like melatonin is like the ozone layer protecting life on the earth.

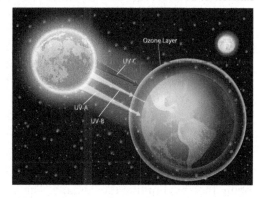

This showed that melatonin has direct or indirect effects in controlling the expressions of alpha-synuclein and prevents neurotoxicity linked to the abuse of Amphetamine.

Melatonin is also believed to slow down, prevent, or reverse the changes in behaviors and motor functions by enhancing the survival of the dopamine-producing cells which were destroyed or damaged in Parkinson's disease.[14]

Does melatonin reduce stroke risk?

As you age, lower and lower melatonin levels make your brain more vulnerable to damage!

Your brain without adequate melatonin levels to protect your precious neurons places you at higher risk for short as well as long-term neurological stresses. Decreased melatonin levels have even been associated with a higher risk of stroke, with the odds appearing to increase more than 2 percent for each 1 pg./mL reduction in the melatonin production as was revealed by this study: 'Impaired Nocturnal Melatonin in the Acute Phase of Ischemic Stroke: A cross-sectional matched case-control analysis' Published in the Journal of Neuroendocrinology in 2009.[15]

One study, 'Pineal calcification is associated with symptomatic cerebral infarction' published in the Journal of Stroke and Cerebrovascular Diseases in 2014 showed that people whose pineal gland had become non-functional and calcified had their risk of stroke increased by nearly 35%![16]

Plenty of evidence is available to support and explain this increased risk. The damage is done due to both types of stroke – ischemic (insufficient blood supply) and hemorrhagic (bleeding inside the brain tissues) – which is basically considered to be the result of excessive free radical production. From the endothelial lining of your blood vessels to the oxidizing of the lipids floating in your blood it doesn't take much imagination to realize that buffering this oxidation can lower these risks.

In animal models of ischemic stroke, melatonin has been shown to improve repair of the brain resulting in the return of cognition. Again, scientists consider the antioxidant effect of our miracle molecule, neutralizing and scavenging free radical oxidation. They proved this during the research 'Direct Measurement of Free Radical Levels in the Brain After Cortical Ischemia Induced by Photothrombosis' Published in the Physiological Research in 2016.[17]

Moreover, according to the study 'Melatonin and the cardiovascular system' published in the Neuroendocrinology Letters in 2002, melatonin may also inhibit the indirect risk factors for stroke, including elevated cholesterol, and high blood pressure. It has been shown to reduce cholesterol plaque formation by 38%, reduce LDL cholesterol by 42%, and decrease blood pressure to the normal range. Again, most experts on cholesterol will agree that cholesterol is not the bad guy. Fat is not the enemy; it is oxidized fat that is bad. Rancid fat due to too much oxidation and not enough antioxidant buffering capacity is generally the recipe for disaster - Setting you up for cardiovascular damage such as stroke and heart disease.[18]

Furthermore, these studies have shown that once a stroke begins to develop, melatonin might minimize the damage by inhibiting the death of neurons in the affected part of the brain, thereby, limiting the damage. The neuroprotective effects of melatonin along with the vascular protection make melatonin the best defense against a stroke along with a healthy diet and exercise.

I started looking at MMP-9 years ago with my patients and it is a great marker for inflammation and can be elevated due to biotin illness such as from CIRS due to mold or chronic infections like EBV or Lyme. Stroke has also been shown to elevate MMP-9. In fact, a study looking at MMP-9 'Melatonin decreases matrix metalloproteinase-9 activation and expression and attenuates reper- 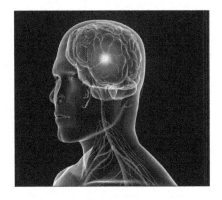 fusion-induced hemorrhage following transient focal cerebral ischemia in rats' was published in the Journal of Pineal Research in 2008. It showed that the melatonin-mediated reduction in the ischemic brain damage and reperfusion-induced hemorrhage could be partly attributed to the ability of this hormone to reduce post-ischemic activation of MMP-9.

MMP-9 (Matrix metallopeptidase 9) is a type of matrixin that belongs to a class of enzymes involved in the degradation of the extracellular matrix. The activation of MMP-9 following an ischemic stroke can promote injury of the blood-brain barrier, worsen edema in the brain tissues, and increase infarct size. The reduced MMP-9 levels by melatonin would minimize degradation of the extracellular matrix, thereby protecting the brain against further damage.

It's my opinion that stroke may often be an effect of things like a chronic infection or toxic exposure such as biotin illness. Melatonin has been shown to support detoxification of the brain, support the immune system during infections, support glymphatic detox, and even neuroprotection. It's no wonder we see things like MMP-9 decreasing with our miracle molecule as it works on so many routes!

One of the important determinants of recovery from a stroke is the extent of "plasticity" in the healthy and surviving neurons. Plasticity indicates how well the surviving neurons would be able to shift their functions and take on some of the activities of destroyed and damaged brain cells. Plasticity is key to learning as well as the brain's ability 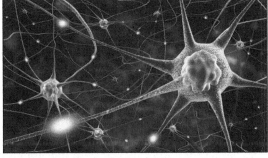 to re-route pathways that have been damaged.

This is the main reason why Chiropractic Neurologists are able to correct so many neurological conditions. We use targeted therapies to activate the brain and promote new connections to be made in order to allow the brain to rewire itself. One of my favorite therapies for post-stroke is mirror exercises, where the good side is used and viewed by the patient. This tricks the brain into activating the nerves to rewire in order to gain function for the nerves going to the damaged side of the body.

This study 'Melatonin improves presynaptic protein, SNAP-25, expression, and dendritic spine density and enhances functional recovery following transient focal cerebral ischemia in rats' published in the Journal of Pineal Research in 2009 has shown that Melatonin might increase the plasticity of the neurons on both the sides of the brain, including the affected side and the unaffected opposite side. And this effect is likely to speed the recovery. The dendrites are the outgrowing arms that form when neurons make these nerve connections related to plasticity. The connection point that the dendrites make when they fuse is called the synapse. Our miracle molecule works on this which is a major part of the healing post-stroke or even after any type of neurologic damage.[19]

Another way melatonin might help to reduce the damage caused due to a stroke is by preventing the activation of harmful "protein-melting" enzymes. An ischemic stroke can trigger a rise in the levels of "protein-melting" enzymes that can further impair the integrity of the blood-brain barrier, resulting in brain swelling, increased intracranial pressure, occasionally transforming the ischemic stroke into a hemorrhagic stroke.

What do these enzymes damage?

These melting enzymes have a negative effect on the protection layer that keeps things from the outside from getting into the brain, the BBB, or blood-brain barrier.

This study 'When melatonin gets on your nerves: its beneficial actions in experimental models of stroke' published in the Experimental Biology and Medicine in 2005 showed that melatonin administration during and after ischemia would reduce the activation of these destructive enzymes and thus, tightened the blood-brain barrier, reduced tissue swelling, and prevented hemorrhagic transformation.

Moreover, a breakthrough in melatonin research has revealed the unique potential of this molecule to protect the brain against ischemia/reperfusion injury by controlling endoplasmic reticulum stress. This study, "Melatonin protects the brain against ischemia/reperfusion injury by attenuating endoplasmic reticulum stress" was published in the Internal Journal of Molecular Medicine in 2018 showing how melatonin could be effective in the management of neurodegenerative diseases of the brain by its ability to attenuate endoplasmic reticulum stress.

Endoplasmic reticulum (ER) stress is known to play a key role in mediating ischemic-reperfusion damage to the brain. This study was aimed at evaluating whether melatonin could inhibit ER stress in neurons that were exposed to glucose and oxygen deprivation and in patients exposed to transient focal cerebral ischemia.

The participants were treated with melatonin in a dose of 5 mg per kg body weight (30-40mg) at the onset of reperfusion after transient occlusion (obstruction to induce loss of blood supply) of one artery in the brain for about 90 minutes. This mechanism is similar to what happens when a patient suffers a cerebrovascular stroke due to the loss of blood supply to a part of the brain. The loss of blood supply leads to brain infarction just the way myocardial infarction or heart attack occurs when the blood supply to cardiac muscles is interrupted.

The results of this study have demonstrated that treatment with melatonin could significantly reduce the extent of infarction and reduce the size of the lesion while increasing the number of surviving neurons. This suggests that prior supplementation with melatonin could play a key role in protecting the brain against stroke, and ER stress. It may also reduce the extent of damage caused to the brain due to the loss of blood supply as a result of which the severity of symptoms of stroke would be reduced considerably. The increased number of surviving neurons following melatonin supplementation could enable patients to recover faster by ensuring the infarcted part of the brain is able to heal in a shorter period. I think we have provided enough evidence showing all the way melatonin helps prevent or support faster and more robust recovery after ischemic and hemorrhagic stroke.

If you have a family history of stroke or you have risk factors like high cholesterol, especially the LDL and you have high oxidation which can be seen with a variety of inflammatory markers such as TGF-Beta, MMP-9, CRP (cardiac high sensitivity best), diabetes with dis-regulated insulin resistivity usually with a Hemoglobin A1C over 5, Ferritin and high iron are some of the lab markers I like. There are even urine tests you can do at home to test oxidation, one of which is called the oxidata.

Besides melatonin supplementation, one should look for causes that can drive up excessive oxidation. Also, keep in mind, oxidation is not all bad, it's a cycle and it needs to be balanced. Oxidation in the right amounts can be beneficial and actually work to kill infections and stimulate your antioxidant system to become more efficient.

Another consideration is carbohydrates and sugars. Eating higher carb meals with fats is much more dangerous than keeping your meals to a slow-burning carb (like Brussel sprouts) due to the oxidation the sugar and insulin bring, which then oxidizes the fats in your bloodstream. See it's not fats that are the enemy, it's actually the type of fats and the foods eaten with them, such as fast-burning carbs that place you more at risk for stroke. I will often suggest to my patients to fast until lunch and use a ketogenic diet 4-5 days a week. Keeping fast-burning carbs to a minimum most days.

You should find a doctor who understands these concepts and won't just place you on a statin that's toxic to your mitochondria when it's a much more complicated issue and can be treated much more eloquently with some basic dietary changes and supplementing with melatonin.[20]

Is ISRIB and melatonin related?

ISRIB or (integrated stress response inhibitor) is another molecule that could work wonders just like melatonin.

The discovery of this molecule by the scientist Peter Walter has created a scientific whirlwind. It has been looked up to as a highly effective neuroprotective agent that could blunt the effect of neurodegenerative diseases including Alzheimer's or Parkinson's, and reverse injuries caused due to brain trauma. ISRIB is believed to hold the power to regenerate, heal, and rejuvenate the damaged or aging brain.

The discovery of ISRIB has been rather interesting. It is known that the cells in our body are continually streaming out proteins to perform different functions, including fighting off bacteria and making new memories. Proteins are able to perform these functions due to their highly specific shapes. If a cell begins to stream out misshapen proteins, these unfolded proteins could trigger an abnormal response that would lead to the slowing down of the production of new proteins while destroying the abnormal or sloppy ones.

If such errant proteins keep forming, the cell is unable to survive, and this is what happens when the brain begins to age leading to neuronal death and brain atrophy. In simple words, when the cell is unable to fix the problem of protein synthesis, it dies.

If this response is overactive, it may lead to the death of too many cells leading to the faster development of diseases like Alzheimer's, and Parkinson's. If the process goes awry in other ways, it may lead to the proliferation of cancer cells.

Peter Walter was interested in modifying the unfolded protein response so that the ability of the cell to survive could improve.

But this mechanism of altering unfolded protein response was too complex as it involved multiple cellular pathways. So, Walter needed a molecule that had the potential to stimulate or regulate these mechanisms. After screening a vast number of compounds, he was able to find that one molecule he was looking for, and that molecule was ISRIB.

It was Walter who named this molecule as ISRIB (integrated stress response inhibitor) for its potential to inhibit the integrated stress response. He found out that ISRIB not only modified the unfolded protein response, but also affected other critical chemical pathways when cells were exposed to major stressors like UV light, iron deficiencies, and viruses. In all these situations that are triggered by the excessive creation of sloppy proteins at the cellular level, the cells tend to respond by switching off the activities of a protein called eIF2 alpha. This protein is also linked to memory functions.

These links between ISRIB, eIF2 alpha, and memory functions were intriguing enough to set off more research on the neuroprotective effect of ISRIB.

Research has shown that partial restoration of the protein synthesis rate could be regulated by the small molecule ISRIB that prevents neurodegeneration without causing pancreatic toxicity. This is a major advancement that the medical field has witnessed in recent times. The discovery of the unique effects of ISRIB molecules could provide answers to reversing neurodegenerative disorders and protecting the aging population against the decline in cognitive functions due to Alzheimer's and Parkinson's.

This study, 'Partial restoration of protein synthesis rates by the small molecule ISRIB prevents neurodegeneration without pancreatic toxicity' was published in the Cell Death & Disease in 2015. It suggested that endoplasmic reticulum (ER) stress might result in the transient repression of protein synthesis. This form of dysregulation has been increasingly associated with a broad range of diseases, especially neurodegenerative disorders. This study further found that the treatment with the small molecule ISRIB could restore protein synthesis without creating any adverse effect on the pancreatic functions. ISRIB treatment could lead to the partial restoration of protein synthesis. It is also likely to provide a sufficient boost to protein synthesis adequate to support neuronal survival, allowing some protective functions of the unfolded protein response to persist in the secretory tissues.

Similar mechanisms might also be observed following melatonin supplementation, which has got researchers excited about the possibility of using small molecule ISRIB or melatonin against Endoplasmic reticulum (ER) stress as an answer to brain degeneration.

These studies on ISRIB have provided great insights into the pathways that could be modified for inhibiting the development of Parkinson's and Alzheimer's. Activating the functions of eIF2 alpha could also be mediated by melatonin which is why melatonin too is considered a vital molecule that could protect the older population against the development of neurodegenerative diseases just like ISRIB does.[21]

Other considerations besides melatonin for neurological health

NAD+ An Important Nutrient Related to Brain Health, Aging & Circadian Rhythm Adaptations

NAD+ is a good nutrient to replenish when you age, as its loss is linked to aging and poor brain function as well as degenerative neurological conditions.

Nicotinamide adenine dinucleotide (NAD+) is an essential pyridine nucleotide that plays a critical role in many cellular processes associated with energy production, development, mitochondria function, and cellular protection against stress, and longevity. Studies show that cellular levels of NAD+ reduce with aging at a rate of 50% every 20 years. Modulation of NAD+ usage or production can help prolong both health span and lifespan. NAD+ is found in abundance in the mitochondria, nucleus, and cytoplasm. It is important for key cellular energy-producing or metabolic pathways such as glycolysis, tricarboxylic acid cycle, and fatty acid beta-oxidation.

First, let's discuss why you might want to supplement w*ith NAD+*.

NAD+ is a sister to Niacin, which is a vital vitamin that you cannot live without. NAD+ is a critical coenzyme found in every cell in your body, and it's involved in hundreds of metabolic processes. Maintenance of an optimal NAD+/NADH ratio is essential for mitochondrial function. In fact, the maintenance of the mitochondrial NAD+ pool is of crucial importance. From plants to metazoans, an increase in intracellular levels of NAD^+ directs cells to make adjustments to ensure survival, including increasing energy production and utilization, boosting cellular repair, and coordinating circadian rhythms.

By the time we are middle-aged, levels of NAD^+ will have fallen to half of the youthful levels. In recent years, several studies have shown that the treatment of old mice with

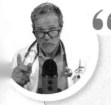

Euler-Chelpin, in his 1930 Nobel Prize speech said, "NAD+ is one of the most widespread and biologically most important activators within the plant and animal world."

NAD+ supports your cells and supports senescent cells.

precursors to NAD$^+$ can greatly improve health. Observed effects include increased insulin sensitivity, a reversal of mitochondrial dysfunction, reduced stem cell senescence, and lifespan extension.

Doctors in the know and scientists in the field all conclude that molecules that maintain NAD$^+$ levels, will allow people to celebrate many more anniversaries. Inflammation is not just linked to aging but is present and involved in almost all disease processes.

NAD+ levels naturally decline with age, and various stressors can deplete your NAD+ at a more rapid rate. Poor restorative sleep and alcohol use are the top two stressors that deplete NAD+; however, any stressor will drain away NAD+ as well. Anytime you have a higher energy demand, immune activation due to infections stress, mental stress, emotional stress, physical stress, structural stress, electromagnetic (EMF's) stress, and chemical stress are the main "Stress" categories. We cannot avoid these completely, and so, inevitably, our NAD+ levels will be taxed, creating a need to replace NAD+.

Researchers show that increased NAD+ will likely make the inflammatory signaling of senescent cells worse. Senescence typically occurs in response to damaging stimuli and stress. Senescent cells increase with age and disease states, resulting in inflammation and age-related diseases such as cancer, cardiovascular and metabolic diseases, and neurodegenerative diseases. NAD+ and senescent cells are good reasons to pulse NAD+ and not take this nutrient daily. This is why in our Mito Fast protocol we include a couple of days in Phase 1 of NAD+ loading prior to fasting in phase 2.

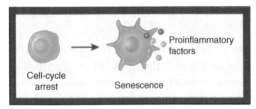

Moreover, one study suggests that chromatin structures change in a circadian manner and that NAD+ is the key metabolite for circadian chromatin remodeling. 'The Circadian NAD+ Metabolism: Impact on Chromatin Remodeling and Aging.'

Basically, this means, during time changes and seasonal changes, or even sleep-wake changes your NAD+ levels might be important to consider for you to adapt to the changes more efficiently!

Here is a more detailed article I wrote on NAD+.

How to take NAD+?

NAD+ can be taken using intravenous injections, IM injections, patches, nasal spray (like NeuroNAD+), liposomal, or suppository (like NAD+Max). Both NAD+, as well as the precursors (NR & NMN), can be taken in the aforementioned forms.

Some products like NAD+Max have all three, yet there is much controversy about absorption of NAD+ or its two precursors. Suppositories make the most sense, and an IV is the next best choice but usually a 5–8-hour drip and can cost $500-$1,500 USD. Versus placing a suppository with the same amount of NAD+ that slowly releases over 5-7 hours for $15-$20 with no inconvenience of time.

Senolytic plant extracts inhibit mTOR, activating autophagy & mitophagy

There are a few extracts worth mentioning that have been reported to inhibit mTOR signaling.

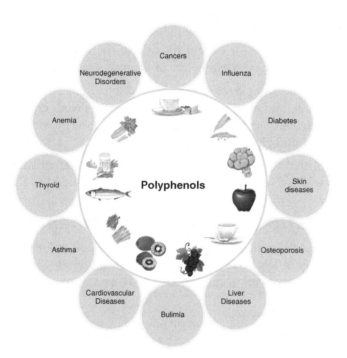

- *Apigenin*, a family member of flavonoids, is abundant in fruits (oranges, apples, cherries, grapes), vegetables (onions, parsley, broccoli, sweet green pepper, celery, barley, tomatoes), and beverages (tea, wine)[22].

- *Cryptotanshinone* is one of the major tanshinones isolated from the roots of the plant *Salvia miltiorrhiza Bunge* (Danshen.[23].

- *Curcumin* (diferuloylmethane), a natural polyphenol product of the plant *Curcuma longa*[24].

- *Fisetin* might be the more powerful of all polyphenols, a family member of flavonoids, that occurs in fruits and vegetables, such as strawberries, apples, persimmons, and onions[25].

- **Indoles** are natural compounds in cruciferous vegetables such as broccoli, cauliflower, cabbage, and brussels sprouts[26].

- **Isoflavones**, a class of flavonoid phenolic compounds, are rich in soybean[27].

- **Quercetin**, a polyphenolic compound, is mainly from tea consumption, onions, red grapes, and apples[28].

- **Pterostilbene** from blueberries.[29]

- **Resveratrol**, a natural polyphenol-rich in red grapes and red wine[30] suppresses mTOR signaling.

- **Tocotrienols**, members of vitamin E superfamily[31].

- Finally, it is worth mentioning that many other natural products, such as caffeine, epigallocatechin gallate (EGCG, in green tea), celastrol, butein, capsaicin, and β-elemene a class of terpenes such as Beta Pinene from the pine tree family can all inhibit mTOR and upregulate autophagy.

You can't possibly get all this or even a fraction of the dosage of each of these plant extracts in a standard diet or even eating lots of the plants high in them.

Research shows that for example, curcumin can't absorb well. You need to take piperine to aid in its absorption, and even then, it's little that you absorb compared to what you ingest. This is why delivery methods other than oral might be considered to get the most robust autophagy and mitophagy.

Taking these polyphenols during fasting may have an even better effect than during feeding times. This is why we suggest Lucitol during phase 2 of the Mito Fast.

Nicotine benefits for brain enhancement

Nicotine therapy might also be an interesting nutrient to look at for the aging brain. The first clue that nicotine might have positive effects on the brain was the discovery that smoking *reduces* the risk of Parkinson's disease (PD), a progressive neurological disorder that affects movement.[32]

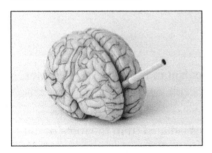

Current smokers have almost half the risk of developing PD than non-smokers.[33]

This disease is caused by the loss of brain cells that produce the neurotransmitter dopamine, which is responsible for movement. According to world-renowned nicotine expert Neil L. Benowitz, MD, *isolated* nicotine exhibits few documented health risks.[34]

In his book *Nicotine Safety and Toxicity* (Oxford University Press), he points out that nicotine, in fact, is undergoing evaluation as a possible treatment for numerous medical and neurological disorders including Alzheimer's, Parkinson's, attention deficit disorder, ulcerative colitis, and sleep apnea.

Investigative journalist Dan Hurley extensively studied the effects of nicotine on the brain while researching his book *Smarter: The New Science of Building Brain Power.*

Using nicotine in a nasal spray like with Zen avoids all the damaging effects of smoking. See Zen here for more on Zen Meditation Mist

CIRS, melatonin & neurological health

CIRS was first described by Dr. Richie Shoemaker, who has pioneered many aspects of diagnosing and treating CIRS due to mold illness. Lyme disease, Breast Implant Illness, and Mold Illness share similar phenomena, where toxins are not adequately cleared from the cell. This is due to the exposure and or build-up of these primary fat-soluble toxins, such as biotoxins from viruses, bacteria, and mold.

Biotoxins are substances that are both toxic and have a biological origin. They come in many forms and can be produced by nearly every type of living organism. There are mycotoxins (made by fungi), zootoxins (made by animals), and phytotoxins (made by plants). What I have found clinically, is that there are genes some individuals do not have, such as the immune response genes (HLA-DR genes) that are required to eventually form an antibody to a given foreign antigen. In these cases, the biotoxins are not 'tagged' and remain in the body indefinitely, free to circulate and wreak havoc. This applies to a subset of the population (about 22%), which prevents them from clearing these biotoxins from the cells.

The accumulation of these biotoxins occurs particularly within the cell membranes, which is a fat-soluble area of the cell and has a slow turnover of about 18 months to allow these toxins to remain for long periods of time. The accumulation of these toxins within the cell is the primary cause of CIRS. This is the primary way the cells communicate with the environment, where it strives to balance itself based on what it's exposed to.

When the messages through the cell membrane become altered, or they are not able to properly make these communications, the cell will begin to relate to its environment with inflammation, and nerve cells won't be able to transmit impulses properly.

Clearing the cell membrane within your brain from biotoxin is not an easy task and cannot occur quickly due to the turnover rate. Therefore, it is important for any CIRS sufferer to focus on a long-term care program to deal with this specific issue. (4-6 months at least). I have outlined a protocol for what I call ***"Membrane Resolution",*** where specific oils and Phosphatidylcholine (PTC) are given IV and or orally to help flush the cell membranes.

Another important compartment is the hepato-biliary-enteric system where these fat-soluble toxins circulate through the liver-gallbladder-gut over and over again triggering inflammation. Using specific binders, to pull these toxins out of circulation in the gut and liver is as important as addressing the cell membranes. I prefer natural toxin binders as well as cholestyramine —to lessen the toxic load.

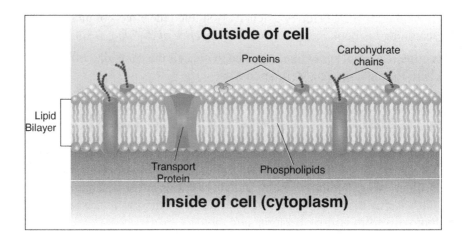

These binders are taken both first thing in the morning with fresh organic lemon juice, stimulating the liver and gallbladder to release the toxic build-up into the gut, as well as before bed as the gallbladder secretes bile the first 2 hours of sleep.

Your sinuses are a filter, and that filter needs to be checked and serviced.

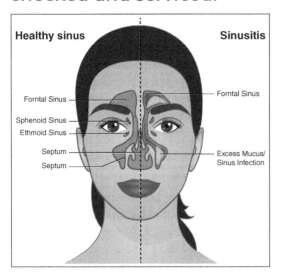

Sinuses are another place infection can outgas biotoxins and in fact, MARCoNS infection is quite common with neurological cases as part of the clinical picture. This connection is not surprising considering how close this toxic reservoir is to your brain.

MARCoNS nasal infection is a Multiple Antibiotic Resistant Coagulase Negative Staphylococcus infection, which produces a very sticky substance called a biofilm. The bacteria use this to protect and hide itself from your immune system. This infection is particularly prevalent in Lyme and Mold Illness.

MARCoNS reside deep in the nasal passage of those suffering from Biotoxin Illness and other chronic inflammatory illnesses, such as CIRS (Chronic Inflammatory Response Syndrome) and CFIDS (Chronic Fatigue and Immune Dysfunction Syndrome). This percentage increases when the person has also been treated with antibiotics for a month or more.

Once they have taken up residence, MARCoNS will lower your Melanocyte-Stimulating Hormone, increase cytokines, and lower T-reg cells. This results in chronic fatigue symptoms of body aches and debilitating exhaustion.

Interestingly, MARCoNS is not an infection, but a commensal colonization that can become an infection. These bacteria send chemicals into the blood (exotoxins A and B), that increase inflammation. By cleaving MSH, it causes a further decrease in MSH levels, which in turn creates more inflammation. Considering what you've read in this chapter it should be evident that CIRS can be a core complication in many neurological cases. The benefits of melatonin are obvious, and it makes perfect sense that it would support someone suffering from CIRS (Chronic Viral/Chronic Lyme/ Mold Illness).

Conclusion

Your brain is fairly important and protecting it should be a priority. Based on the information in this chapter you might consider melatonin supplements to improve your chances of living longer and keeping your brain sharper!

Melatonin improves detox through the lymphatics keeping your brain clean of heavy metals and other chemicals, as well as proteins that can build up. It further offers antioxidant protection during high energy demand and helps to keep your brain free of infection. Although doses in 1-20 mg can help, supra-physiological dosing of melatonin make more sense.

Melatonin should be used as a complementary therapy along with other strategies based on complicating factors leading to the inflammatory process in each person. This can be unique and as Dr. Dale Bredesen in his book *The End to Alzheimer's* brought attention to is that there are usually several factors that cause early aging of the brain as well as degenerative neurological diseases. Bredesen describes three subtypes of Alzheimer's disease: (1) Inflammatory (hot) (2) Atrophic (cold), and (3) Toxic (exposure to chemicals and infections). Using labs, as we do at Advanced Rejuvenation, doctors can now figure out the underlying cause of neurological challenges and work towards answers to correct those problems.

Besides melatonin for a healthy brain, you might consider activating autophagy and mitophagy to break down and recycle weak and dysfunctional cells and mitochondria through fasting and time-restricted feeding. mTOR is a gene you want to inhibit to gain better autophagy and mitophagy. Refeeding is also important as this is where you repair and grow new cells.

For further information on mTOR see Mito Fast and read my article on using fasting to improve brain function and mitochondrial health. Senescent cells as mentioned above can be harmful, and strategies to activate clearing of them are a good idea in any brain-based protocol. Using fasting as well as senolytics to help clear senescent cells can help greatly in neurological conditions.

Poor sleep can make all the following worse or even cause them:

- CIRS & Biotoxin illness due to chronic infections and mold.
- Gut Imbalances: Dysbiosis, Leaky Gut & inflammatory bowel disease. *Read in chapter 11.*
- Toxic accumulation of chemicals & heavy metals or fluoride causing calcification of the pineal.
- Poor Glymphatics: Toxic accumulation of immune-mediated proteins like beta-amyloid, alpha-synuclein, and tau.
- Immune Dysregulation: Poor NK cell production and healthy strong immune cells.
- Mitochondrial Function: Energy levels become critically low worsening brain function.
- Poor Autophagy & Mitophagy leading to a build-up of dysfunctional mitochondria and senescent cells.
- Poor Immune function causing chronic sinus infections or vice versa. (MARCoNs)

These above complications lead to the development and worsening of many neurological conditions. Testing and then addressing them as they are needed is the multifactorial and comprehensive approach that is needed!

What came first, the chicken or the egg? This saying rings true for most of the above-listed complications. Did one or more of the above cause the cascade of inflammation that led to the diagnosis of a neurological disease? Maybe the complication developed after the disease process was well on its way due to the weakened state of the central system and immune system keeping things in order?

Regardless of this answer, addressing sleep has the most "bang for the buck" out of all considerations. Moreover, addressing it with melatonin covers more bases than any other!

Reference

1. Wallace DM, Wohlgemuth WK, Trotti LM, Amara AW, Malaty IA, Factor SA, Nallu S, Wittine L, Hauser RA. Practical Evaluation and Management of Insomnia in Parkinson's Disease: A Review. Mov Disord Clin Pract. 2020 Feb 3;7(3):250-266. doi: 10.1002/mdc3.12899. PMID: 32258222; PMCID: PMC7111581.

2. Dominguez-Rodriguez A, Abreu-Gonzalez P, de la Torre-Hernandez JM, Consuegra-Sanchez L, Piccolo R, Gonzalez-Gonzalez J, Garcia-Camarero T, Del Mar Garcia-Saiz M, Aldea-Perona A, Reiter RJ; MARIA Investigators. Usefulness of Early Treatment With Melatonin to Reduce Infarct Size in Patients With ST-Segment Elevation Myocardial Infarction Receiving Percutaneous Coronary Intervention (From the Melatonin Adjunct in the Acute Myocardial

Infarction Treated With Angioplasty Trial). Am J Cardiol. 2017 Aug 15;120(4):522-526. doi: 10.1016/j.amjcard.2017.05.018. Epub 2017 May 30. PMID: 28645475.

3. Alghamdi B. S. (2018). The neuroprotective role of melatonin in neurological disorders. *Journal of neuroscience research*, *96*(7), 1136–1149. https://doi.org/10.1002/jnr.24220

4. Pandi-Perumal, Seithikurippu R. & Bahammam, Ahmed & Brown, Gregory & Spence, D. & Bharti, Dr. Vijay & Kaur, Charanjit & Hardeland, Rüdiger & Cardinali, Daniel. (2013). Melatonin Antioxidative Defense: Therapeutical Implications for Aging and Neurodegenerative Processes. Neurotoxicity research. 23. 267-300. 10.1007/s12640-012-9337-4.

5. Bondy SC, Lahiri DK, Perreau VM, Sharman KZ, Campbell A, Zhou J, Sharman EH. Retardation of brain aging by chronic treatment with melatonin. Ann N Y Acad Sci. 2004 Dec;1035:197-215. doi: 10.1196/annals.1332.013. PMID: 15681809.

6. Feng Z, Qin C, Chang Y, Zhang JT. Early melatonin supplementation alleviates oxidative stress in a transgenic mouse model of Alzheimer's disease. Free Radic Biol Med. 2006 Jan 1;40(1):101-9. doi: 10.1016/j.freeradbiomed.2005.08.014. Epub 2005 Sep 7. PMID: 16337883.

7. Gong, C. X., & Iqbal, K. (2008). Hyperphosphorylation of microtubule-associated protein tau: a promising therapeutic target for Alzheimer disease. *Current medicinal chemistry*, *15*(23), 2321–2328. https://doi.org/10.2174/092986708785909111

8. Gong, C. X., & Iqbal, K. (2008). Hyperphosphorylation of microtubule-associated protein tau: a promising therapeutic target for Alzheimer disease. *Current medicinal chemistry*, *15*(23), 2321–2328. https://doi.org/10.2174/092986708785909111

9. Rong-Yu Liu, Jiang-Ning Zhou, Joop van Heerikhuize, Michel A. Hofman, Dick F. Swaab, Decreased Melatonin Levels in Postmortem Cerebrospinal Fluid in Relation to Aging, Alzheimer's Disease, and Apolipoprotein E-ε4/4 Genotype, *The Journal of Clinical Endocrinology & Metabolism*, Volume 84, Issue 1, 1 January 1999, Pages 323–327, https://doi.org/10.1210/jcem.84.1.5394

10. Rong-Yu Liu, Jiang-Ning Zhou, Joop van Heerikhuize, Michel A. Hofman, Dick F. Swaab, Decreased Melatonin Levels in Postmortem Cerebrospinal Fluid in Relation to Aging, Alzheimer's Disease, and Apolipoprotein E-ε4/4 Genotype, *The Journal of Clinical Endocrinology & Metabolism*, Volume 84, Issue 1, 1 January 1999, Pages 323–327, https://doi.org/10.1210/jcem.84.1.5394

11. Glenna A. Dowling, Judith Mastick, Eric Colling, Julie H. Carter, Clifford M. Singer, Michael J. Aminoff, Melatonin for sleep disturbances in Parkinson's disease, Sleep Medicine,Volume 6, Issue 5,2005,Pages 459-466, ISSN 1389-9457, https://doi.org/10.1016/j.sleep.2005.04.004. https://www.sciencedirect.com/science/article/pii/S1389945705000961)

12. Capitelli C, Sereniki A, Lima MM, Reksidler AB, Tufik S, Vital MA. Melatonin attenuates tyrosine hydroxylase loss and hypolocomotion in MPTP-lesioned rats. Eur J Pharmacol. 2008 Oct 10;594(1-3):101-8. doi: 10.1016/j.ejphar.2008.07.022. Epub 2008 Jul 17. PMID: 18674531.

13. Ono K, Mochizuki H, Ikeda T, Nihira T, Takasaki J, Teplow DB, Yamada M. Effect of melatonin on α-synuclein self-assembly and cytotoxicity. Neurobiol Aging. 2012 Sep;33(9):2172-85. doi: 10.1016/j.neurobiolaging.2011.10.015. Epub 2011 Nov 25. PMID: 22118903.

14. Sae-ung, Kwankanit & Uéda, Kenji & Govitrapong, Piyarat & Phansuwan-Pujito, Pansiri. (2011). Melatonin reduces the expression of alpha-synuclein in the dopamine containing neuronal regions of amphetamine-treated postnatal rats. Journal of pineal research. 52. 128-37. 10.1111/j.1600-079X.2011.00927.x.

15. Atanassova PA, Terzieva DD, Dimitrov BD. Impaired nocturnal melatonin in acute phase of ischaemic stroke: cross-sectional matched case-control analysis. J Neuroendocrinol. 2009 Jul;21(7):657-63. doi: 10.1111/j.1365-2826.2009.01881.x. PMID: 19453822.

16. Kitkhuandee A, Sawanyawisuth K, Johns NP, Kanpittaya J, Johns J. Pineal calcification is associated with symptomatic cerebral infarction. J Stroke Cerebrovasc Dis. 2014 Feb;23(2):249-53. doi: 10.1016/j.jstrokecerebrovasdis.2013.01.009. Epub 2013 Feb 21. PMID: 23434443.

17. Mares J, Nohejlova K, Stopka P, Rokyta R. Direct measurement of free radical levels in the brain after cortical ischemia induced by photothrombosis. Physiol Res. 2016 Nov 23;65(5):853-860. doi: 10.33549/physiolres.933124. Epub 2016 Jul 15. PMID: 27429112.

18. Sewerynek E. Melatonin and the cardiovascular system. Neuro Endocrinol Lett. 2002 Apr;23 Suppl 1:79-83. PMID: 12019357.

19. Chen HY, Hung YC, Chen TY, Huang SY, Wang YH, Lee WT, Wu TS, Lee EJ. Melatonin improves presynaptic protein, SNAP-25, expression and dendritic spine density and enhances functional and electrophysiological recovery following transient focal cerebral ischemia in rats. J Pineal Res. 2009 Oct;47(3):260-70. doi: 10.1111/j.1600-079X.2009.00709.x. Epub 2009 Aug 26. PMID: 19709397.

20. Lin YW, Chen TY, Hung CY, Tai SH, Huang SY, Chang CC, Hung HY, Lee EJ. Melatonin protects brain against ischemia/reperfusion injury by attenuating endoplasmic reticulum stress. Int J Mol Med. 2018 Jul;42(1):182-192. doi: 10.3892/ijmm.2018.3607. Epub 2018 Mar 30. PMID: 29620280; PMCID: PMC5979830.

21. Curious molecule that makes mice smart leads to Breakthrough Prize (statnews.com)

22. Huang S. (2013). Inhibition of PI3K/Akt/mTOR signaling by natural products. *Anti-cancer agents in medicinal chemistry, 13*(7), 967–970. https://doi.org/10.2174/1871520611313070001

23. Huang S. (2013). Inhibition of PI3K/Akt/mTOR signaling by natural products. *Anti-cancer agents in medicinal chemistry, 13*(7), 967–970. https://doi.org/10.2174/1871520611313070001

24. Huang S. (2013). Inhibition of PI3K/Akt/mTOR signaling by natural products. *Anti-cancer agents in medicinal chemistry, 13*(7), 967–970. https://doi.org/10.2174/1871520611313070001

25. Huang S. (2013). Inhibition of PI3K/Akt/mTOR signaling by natural products. *Anti-cancer agents in medicinal chemistry, 13*(7), 967–970. https://doi.org/10.2174/1871520611313070001

26. Huang S. (2013). Inhibition of PI3K/Akt/mTOR signaling by natural products. *Anti-cancer agents in medicinal chemistry, 13*(7), 967–970. https://doi.org/10.2174/1871520611313070001

27. Huang S. (2013). Inhibition of PI3K/Akt/mTOR signaling by natural products. *Anti-cancer agents in medicinal chemistry*, *13*(7), 967–970. https://doi.org/10.2174/1871520611313070001

28. Huang S. (2013). Inhibition of PI3K/Akt/mTOR signaling by natural products. *Anti-cancer agents in medicinal chemistry*, *13*(7), 967–970. https://doi.org/10.2174/1871520611313070001

29. Huang S. (2013). Inhibition of PI3K/Akt/mTOR signaling by natural products. *Anti-cancer agents in medicinal chemistry*, *13*(7), 967–970. https://doi.org/10.2174/1871520611313070001

30. Huang S. (2013). Inhibition of PI3K/Akt/mTOR signaling by natural products. *Anti-cancer agents in medicinal chemistry*, *13*(7), 967–970. https://doi.org/10.2174/1871520611313070001

31. Huang S. (2013). Inhibition of PI3K/Akt/mTOR signaling by natural products. *Anti-cancer agents in medicinal chemistry*, *13*(7), 967–970. https://doi.org/10.2174/1871520611313070001

32. Valentina Gallo, Paolo Vineis, Mariagrazia Cancellieri, Paolo Chiodini, Roger A Barker, Carol Brayne, Neil Pearce, Roel Vermeulen, Salvatore Panico, Bas Bueno-de-Mesquita, Nicola Vanacore, Lars Forsgren, Silvia Ramat, Eva Ardanaz, Larraitz Arriola, Jesper Peterson, Oskar Hansson, Diana Gavrila, Carlotta Sacerdote, Sabina Sieri, Tilman Kühn, Verena A Katzke, Yvonne T van der Schouw, Andreas Kyrozis, Giovanna Masala, Amalia Mattiello, Robert Perneczky, Lefkos Middleton, Rodolfo Saracci, Elio Riboli, Exploring causality of the association between smoking and Parkinson's disease, *International Journal of Epidemiology*, Volume 48, Issue 3, June 2019, Pages 912–925, https://doi.org/10.1093/ije/dyy230

33. Valentina Gallo, Paolo Vineis, Mariagrazia Cancellieri, Paolo Chiodini, Roger A Barker, Carol Brayne, Neil Pearce, Roel Vermeulen, Salvatore Panico, Bas Bueno-de-Mesquita, Nicola Vanacore, Lars Forsgren, Silvia Ramat, Eva Ardanaz, Larraitz Arriola, Jesper Peterson, Oskar Hansson, Diana Gavrila, Carlotta Sacerdote, Sabina Sieri, Tilman Kühn, Verena A Katzke, Yvonne T van der Schouw, Andreas Kyrozis, Giovanna Masala, Amalia Mattiello, Robert Perneczky, Lefkos Middleton, Rodolfo Saracci, Elio Riboli, Exploring causality of the association between smoking and Parkinson's disease, *International Journal of Epidemiology*, Volume 48, Issue 3, June 2019, Pages 912–925, https://doi.org/10.1093/ije/dyy230

34. Nicotine Safety and Toxicity - Neal L. Benowitz - Oxford University Press (oup.com)

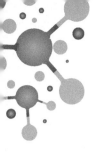

MELATONIN & GUT

Support, digestion & microbiome

"There is nearly 400x more melatonin in our digestive system than in the nervous system."

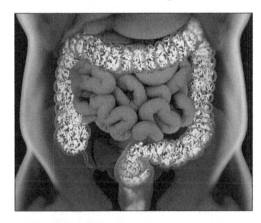

A robust, functional digestive tract is one of our most vital bodily functions. It's well-known that when one's gut is unwell, it affects the entire body's wellbeing. Yet, I find that very few traditionally trained medical practitioners have a proper under-standing of normal gut function.

Digestion starts during chewing when enzymes are released in your mouth. The contents then travel down into your stomach, where a strong acid further breaks down the food and converts pepsin into pepsinogen, which you need to break down your proteins. In the absence of strong stomach acid, there will be an inadequate breakdown of food, and your pancreas will fail to release a buffer once the food comes out of the stomach.

This buffer is critical to neutralize the acid contents moving into the small intestines and ultimately helps your small intestines from the irritation caused by acid. Without the strong acid from the stomach, this buffer will not be released, leading to lower-gut problems.

Without getting too deep in the woods about digestion, it is easy to see that there is much work going on along the digestive tract. Work from tissues and cells comes with a price: oxidative stress. Our miracle molecule is the premier antioxidant that neutralizes oxidative stress, thus keeping your gut healthy and working properly. Keep in mind that your gut has a massive turnover of cells, where new cells and tissues are constantly being formed along the entire digestive tract. In fact, the lining of your stomach turns over every 5 minutes!

Here as much or more than anywhere, there is a need to protect this process so that it works smoothly and the new cells have antioxidant protection, quality DNA, and strong mitochondria to keep up with this incredible demand. Melatonin can help keep your gut healthy and can even reverse the damage. Melatonin is an antioxidant molecule that can help with various digestive diseases caused by inflammation, poor flora, lack of circadian rhythm influence leading to poor sleep, and excessive oxidative stress.

Furthermore, melatonin can also help relieve symptoms of SIBO, leaky gut syndrome, and poor digestion. By reducing inflammation and improving the gut flora, melatonin comes to the rescue, particularly when used in higher doses. Of course, this comes as no surprise by now, as I have been suggesting much higher dosing than what many health-care providers typically recommend for sleep. I advocate super-physiologic dosing with melatonin, especially when there are health considerations, other than improving sleep. Research clearly shows that melatonin combats stress, is anti-aging, and also protects against runaway cytokine storms from infections through inflammasomes. Moreover, it can also repair cells in the body, including those in the brain, heart, and yes, even your GUT!

The role of endogenous circadian rhythmicity in gut health

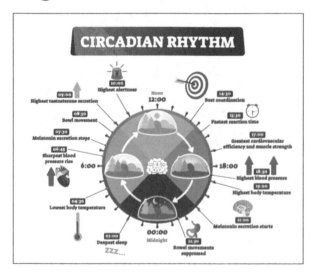

One research study, 'Human Gut Bacteria Are Sensitive to Melatonin and Express Endogenous Circadian Rhythmicity', published in the PLoS One in 2016, stated that "melatonin specifically increases the magnitude of swarming in cultures of E. aerogenes, but not in Escherichia coli or Klebsiella pneumoniae."

This study focused on assessing the impact of the body's circadian rhythms on gut health. Circadian rhythm is the fundamental property of most eukaryotes, including humans, animals, plants, and even fungi. However, the evidence that biological clocks can drive these rhythms in prokaryotes like blue-green algae, E. coli, and mycoplasma has been limited to Cyanobacteria.[1]

In invertebrates such as humans, the digestive system expresses a strong circadian pattern dependent on gene expression, which means it could be genetically linked. The motility of the bowels and secretion of different digesting enzymes and juices also depend on the circadian rhythm.

Recent studies suggest that the gut flora, which is composed of trillions of healthy bacteria, is regulated primarily by the circadian clock of the body. The circadian rhythm, in turn, is regulated by the amount and frequency of melatonin secretion in the body.

Healthy gut flora is an indication of a good and efficient digestive system, and it's also what your body needs in order to digest foods, absorb, and assimilate nutrients. By regulating the circadian rhythm, melatonin could play a critical role in improving gut flora and avoiding major digestive issues linked to the intestine's weak microbiota.

This study specifically demonstrated that at least one species of bacterium from the gastrointestinal system is sensitive to the effect of the neurohormone melatonin. This species is Enterobacter aerogenes. The findings of this study have revealed that, by expressing the circadian pattern of motility and swarming, the activities of Enterobacter aerogenes would be modified by melatonin secreted into the intestinal lumen.

Melatonin has been shown to specifically increase the magnitude of swarming in the

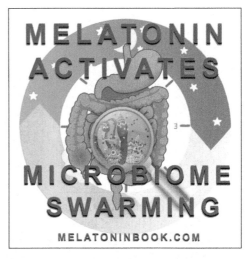

cultures of E. aerogenes, though not in other species such as in Klebsiella pneumoniae and Escherichia coli. The swarming appeared to occur on a daily basis and caused the transformation of E. aerogenes found to be temperature-compensated by the body's circadian rhythm synchronized perfectly in the presence of melatonin. Moreover, this data demonstrated the circadian clock in the non-cyanobacterial prokaryote and suggested that the human circadian system might regulate its microbiome by bringing about the entrainment of the bacterial clocks with the help of its own melatonin molecules.

In short, what this study demonstrates is that using melatonin to maintain your body's circadian rhythm is what your digestive system needs to function optimally. A regular circadian rhythm would create a favorable internal environment within the stomach and intestine, meaning that both digestion and gut flora are improved.

A separate study, 'Human Gut Bacteria Are Sensitive to Melatonin and Express Endogenous Circadian Rhythmicity', published in PLoS One in 2016, hypothesized that one human signal potentially affecting gut microbiota could be the secretion of melatonin into the lumen of the intestine.[2]

Although melatonin is regarded primarily as the *pineal* and *retinal neuromodulator* for the *circadian rhythm and photoperiodic functions*, it's present throughout the digestive system. While a part of this comes from the pineal secretion, there is evidence showing the presence of melatonin *biosynthetic enzymes* in the *biliary cholangiocytes* (liver and gallbladder), *intestinal mucosa* (gut lining), and *enterochromaffin cells* (also gut lining).

It's complicated but the evidence is clear that the gut is hard wired to your melatonin!

What is a biosynthetic enzyme?

Biosynthesis is an enzyme-catalyzed process where substrates are converted into more complex products in living organisms. This means melatonin is used for many critical chemical processes that occur inside your gut.

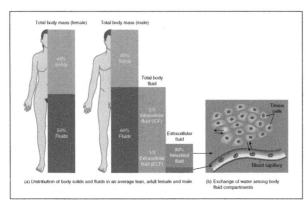

The study, 'Extrapineal melatonin: sources, regulation, and potential functions', published in Cellular and Molecular Life Sciences in 2014, revealed that melatonin is found in essentially all of the biological fluids, including bile, cerebrospinal fluid, synovial fluid, saliva, amniotic fluid, and even breast milk.

In some of these fluids, the melatonin concentration exceeds that of the blood. The continued availability of melatonin in these tissues and fluids at the cellular level is considered critical for all organs and systems' physiological regulation and maintaining optimum homeostasis. This explains why the presence of melatonin in bile and other digestive juices is essential for maintaining optimum gut health. All this information makes a good argument to use a much higher dosing of melatonin to achieve positive changes in a diseased or stressed gut. I have found this to be the case in virtually all of my cases, and I'll share my gut protocol with you later.[3]

According to a research study, 'Gastrointestinal melatonin: localization, function, and clinical relevance' published in the Digestive Diseases and Sciences in 2002, the gastrointestinal tract of humans is a rich source of pineal and extrapineal melatonin. The concentrations of melatonin in the gastrointestinal organs and tissues would surpass the blood levels by nearly 10 to 100 times, and there is nearly 400x more melatonin in our digestive system than in the pineal gland.[4]

Moreover, the gastrointestinal tract can contribute significantly to the circulating concentration of melatonin, especially during the daytime when melatonin might serve as an endocrine, pancreatic, and autocrine hormone to influence the regeneration of the epithelial lining of the stomach and intestine.

Your gut has an estimated composition of 100 trillion cells! That outnumbers your entire body's cells by a factor of 10. Besides outnumbering your own cells, they also express genes 10 times more so than your own cells.[5]

These complex communities of microbes that include bacteria, fungi, viruses, and other microbial and eukaryotic species, provide a tremendous enzymatic capability, and play a fundamental role in controlling most aspects of host physiology.[6]

> *This paper discusses the importance of your microbiome, immune health, and inflammation 'Role of the Microbiota in Immunity and inflammation' published in 2014. In this paper, the author states "The states of health or disease are the expressions of the success or failure experienced by the organism in its efforts to respond adaptively to environmental challenges".*

> *Melatonin release can have a direct effect on several gastrointestinal tissues and the digestive functions such as we have discussed: Support through circadian rhythm effect for the microbiome, bile & liver function and other gut functions, protection from oxidation, support gut regeneration through autocrine and endocrine influence, downregulate inflammation in the gut, balancing effect through the central nervous system via sympathetic and parasympathetic nerves.*

All of this means that ultimately you are your microbiome! Your health is intrinsically linked to how strong your microbiome is. Your microbiome creates messenger molecules, and t messenger molecules are produced based on your diet, activity levels, toxic exposures, mental and emotional signaling. The microbiome takes in this signaling to dictate your emotions, thoughts, and behaviors as well as the vitality of your immune system.

Through this endocrine influence, melatonin can also reduce unnecessary spasms or contractions of the gastrointestinal muscles.

This study has also stated that a portion of the melatonin found in the digestive tract could be of pineal origin. The production of melatonin in the pineal gland is regulated in a photo-periodical manner, based on the exposure through your eyes to the bright blue and green light or darkness. The release of gastrointestinal melatonin, on the other hand, seems to be linked more to our food intake. Food intake, and paradoxically, even long-term food deprivation or fasting, might increase the blood plasma and tissue concentrations of melatonin in the stomach and intestine.

This study has further stated that melatonin might prevent ulceration in the gastrointestinal mucosa by acting as an antioxidant, reducing the secretion of hydrochloric acid in the stomach (*makes sense as there is no need for hydrochloric acid while we sleep*), and stimulating the immune system.

We have already covered how it can support epithelial regeneration, which can be of great importance considering the massive damaging processes in the gut such as gastric ulcers or ulcerative colitis.

> *Why isn't this on the news like Tums and Prilosec? One word: "Patent". Without a patent, there is zero economic motivation for any company to pay for educating the public. You are being brainwashed through commercials to think of pharmaceuticals as the solution to your healthcare because this makes money for the machine called Big Pharma.*

> *The most common cause of heartburn is an infection and not due to too much acid! In fact, heartburn is usually due to too little acid being produced by your stomach. If not enough acid is produced, insufficient buffers will be released to neutralize it before it flows down the small intestines. The stomach contents become rancid ("sour stomach"), and they come back up. I use hydrochloric acid for my heartburn patients, and I address the chronic H. Pylori infection most have, plus put them on high doses of melatonin. This is called treating the cause and not chasing symptoms. Since you need the effect that acid gives you, which is killing harmful microbes in the food we eat, breaking down food, converting enzymes, and activating the buffer to protect the small intestines, we would not want to take a long-term acid blocker. Even the instructions on all the acid-blocking drugs say short-term use, but doctors commonly place patients on them for years or even lifetimes, as if the acid in the stomach is harmful.*

Yet, a critical point in the study was melatonin's ability to increase microcirculation in the gut. And lastly, a third crucial aspect of healing and repair is the ability to "*bring in the groceries and take out the garbage*" or blood supply. These unique properties make melatonin a must in the treatment of a wide range of digestive issues, including gastritis, colorectal cancer, gastric ulcers, ulcerative colitis, irritable bowel syndrome, and colic.

When we sleep our gut heals

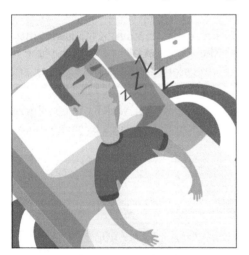

Melatonin inhibits the activities of unhealthy or harmful bacteria, thus allowing the healthy bacteria to survive and even thrive within the digestive system. This effect is hard linked to the circadian rhythm activating a robust microbiome growth phase called "swarming". Your microbiome is a complex and dynamic ecosystem of your gut and entire body.

There are some fascinating connections as well as shared influences between your sleep and gut flora. Scientists who have been investigating the relationship between sleep and gut flora have found that this ecosystem can affect sleep and sleep-related functions in many ways, possibly by shifting the circadian rhythms, modifying the body's sleep-wake cycle, and altering the hormones that control sleep and wakefulness such as melatonin. Sleep, in turn, may affect the diversity and health of the human microbiome.

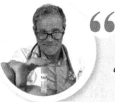

> *"What role does sleep play in maintaining the health of the gut microbiome, and how it contributes to our health so significantly?"*

The microbial life in our body is in perpetual flux, which means the microbes are being generated and dying constantly. Some of this form of decay or renewal occurs naturally during sleep. This brings us to an important question,

There are some critical signs of this significant connection: We have already seen that there are several studies demonstrating that circadian rhythm disruptions could have a negative effect on the gut microbiome. But what about sleep's connection? Well, there's an interesting study to note.[7]

This study highlights the important role of sleep is, 'Circadian Disorganization Alters Intestinal Microbiota' published in the Plos One in 2014. Researchers found that intestinal dysbiosis and disruptions in the circadian rhythm are associated with the risk of similar diseases such as obesity, inflammatory bowel disease, and metabolic syndrome. The overlap between the risks associated with dysbiosis and circadian disorganization is a strong indication of how your sleep is determined by your melatonin levels and linked to gut health, and how these influence each other.

Melatonin to the gut microbiome is like honey to the bee

The gut microbiome plays a key role in supporting the process of digestion and absorption of nutrients we consume. As mentioned previously, the microbiome helps in the breakdown, absorption, and assimilation of foods. Healthy gut flora is vital for ensuring all the nutrients from foods are efficiently absorbed into the blood. Meaning that a lack of healthy and diverse gut flora can affect digestive pro-

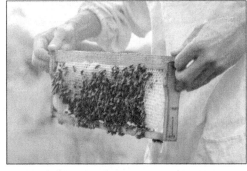

cesses, leaving some people with deficiencies in B vitamins, folic acid, calcium, iron, vitamin C, and other micronutrients.

Furthermore, healthy gut flora is also essential for supporting the activities of the immune cells. Patients with poor gut microbiota are more likely to develop symptoms of allergies, autoimmune disorders, and repeated infections due to the lack of efficient defense processes.

Studies have shown that melatonin might have the potential to improve the microbiota, especially in colitis. This study, 'Melatonin controls microbiota in colitis by goblet cell differentiation and antimicrobial peptide production through Toll-like receptor 4 signaling', was published in Scientific Reports in 2020. The results of this study are based on the concept that microbial dysbiosis could be associated with the pathogenesis of IBD (inflammatory bowel disease). The study proposed that the anti-colitic effect of melatonin could be related to this sleep hormone's ability to improve gut flora. It showed that melatonin supplementation helped improve the symptoms of colitis induced by DSS (dextran sulfate sodium) by reversing microbial dysbiosis.

The improvement in the gut flora was also followed by the induction of healthy goblet cells. Goblet cells are types of mucosal epithelial cells lining the intestinal walls. These cells serve as the primary site for the digestion of nutrients and their absorption through the mucosal lining. Goblet cells also secrete mucus to protect the intestinal lining against damage by the food traveling through the GI tract, which often holds enzymes, abrasive surfaces, and various harmful agents such as toxins and pro-inflammatory substances.

Melatonin treatment of the intestinal epithelial cells also improved mucous production and stimulated wound healing while inhibiting the growth of Escherichia coli. This means melatonin may also help protect the gut flora by encouraging the healing of the mucosal lining and preventing damage by infection-causing bacteria.

Earlier, we discussed the swarming effects melatonin activates with the good bacteria in the gut, causing them to increase in number. Yet these studies ultimately conclude that melatonin also holds significance in the management of IBD through its ability to improve gut microbiota.

Melatonin and Leaky Gut Syndrome

"Leaky gut" is a condition associated with an unhealthy gut lining, where the gut becomes permeable to larger food items due to stressors. This is what leads to many food sensitivities, such as IgG food sensitivities. We regularly test for these in my practice, and it is not a matter of "if"; it's a matter of how many foods you are sensitive to. These sensitivities can be delayed up to 4 days, and therefore, it can be notoriously difficult to gauge this reaction directly without lab testing. Due to the constant activation of the immune system, this problem fuels many situations, including chronic inflammation. The activation of chronic inflammation is one of the leading causes of most diseases in the body, and autoimmune conditions are an excellent example of a condition created by a leaky gut. For example, studies have shown a direct relationship to leaky gut in autoimmune conditions such as Hashimoto's disease, and multiple sclerosis.[8]

This is why I typically test for these intolerances as soon as possible and remove these foods to reduce the inflammatory burden. See more on this at Ultimatecellularreset.com

The next study, 'The gut-brain axis: The role of melatonin in linking psychiatric, inflammatory and neurodegenerative conditions' published in the Advances in Integrative Medicine in 2015, has further explored the link between lower melatonin secretion and the increased risk of leaky gut syndrome. It showed that melatonin has the potential to restore the lining of the intestine. This study further highlighted the importance of using melatonin to manage various disorders by regulating immune-inflammatory processes, neuroregulatory stressor tryptophan catabolites (TRYCATs), and oxidative and nitric oxide stressors called nitrosative stress (O&NS).

It identifies impaired gut permeability and lack of diversity in the gut microbiome as the etiology and course of several diseases, including mental health issues such as depression. Increased gut permeability would be evident in several medical conditions. Moreover, it can contribute to the higher immune-inflammatory cytokines, TRYCATs, and O&NS. By regulating the pathways that control the secretion of immune-inflammatory cytokines, TRYCATs, and O&NS. Meaning, that melatonin could provide a solution to the disorders that have leaky gut syndrome as a root cause.

This study has also assessed the role of reduced melatonin in gut permeability, primarily through the regulation of inflammasomes. Inflammasomes have been found to have serious consequences across a range of medical conditions, including fatty liver disease, Alzheimer's disease, fibromyalgia, obesity, and alcoholism. Simply put, by regulating the activities of inflammasomes, melatonin might restore normal gut permeability and minimize the implications of leaky gut syndrome, thereby reducing the risk of these diseases.[9]

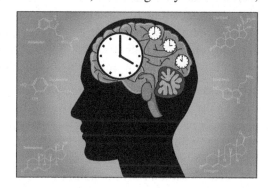

How often do medications provide both symptomatic relief and cure? Not often, but melatonin can do just this!

Does melatonin work for colitis?

Ulcerative colitis is a common inflammatory bowel disease characterized by recurrent bouts of loose stools, constipation, abdominal pain, and blood in stools. If not appropriately managed, ulceration in the colon may become deeper, eroding the intestinal lining. In some cases, the ulcerated tissues may turn cancerous, thus increasing the risk of colorectal cancer.

Studies aimed at assessing the role of melatonin in the management of ulcerative colitis have shown encouraging results. Let's take a look!

According to one study, 'Melatonin improves experimental colitis with sleep deprivation', published in the International Journal of Molecular Medicine in 2015, melatonin supplementation might help control the signs of colitis. This study has recognized sleep deprivation as an epidemic phenomenon and an aggravating factor responsible for triggering the development of inflammatory bowel disease.

Melatonin could help to control the symptoms of this disease by acting as an antioxidant and anti-inflammatory agent. It would reduce oxidative stress on the intestine's delicate mucosal lining and protect these tissues against damage by free radicals, thereby reducing the risk of ulceration. This is another excellent example of how melatonin comes to the rescue when we are under stress.

The study further focused on the measurable effect of sleep deprivation on experimental colitis and whether melatonin's protective effect could be effective in minimizing these changes. The participants were divided into four experimental groups as follows: the first group included participants with colitis; the second was composed of those with colitis and sleep deprivation; the third group had participants with colitis and sleep deprivation and treated with melatonin, while the fourth was the control group.

Colitis in the first three groups was induced artificially by the administration of 5% DSS (dextran sulfate sodium) in their drinking water for about six days. The participants were later sleep-deprived for three days, and subsequently, the changes in the histological analysis of colon tissues, body weight, and the levels of genes and pro-inflammatory cytokines were evaluated.

The results of this study showed that sleep deprivation causes worsening of the inflammation in the colon, as was evident in the histopathological analysis of the tissues. It was also found that the group of participants that were treated with melatonin had favorable results. The inflammatory changes in the tissues caused due to sleep deprivation were reversed by melatonin. Additionally, even the weight loss caused due to colitis was reduced significantly by melatonin treatment, and it also led to an improvement in the survival rates.

There was a rise in the levels of proinflammatory cytokines, including interleukins, interferon-γ, and tumor necrosis factor-α in the serum of the sleep-deprived group. However, the levels of these proinflammatory substances were reduced remarkably following the treatment with melatonin. Furthermore, gene analysis showed that the expression of some inflammatory markers was initially increased due to sleep deprivation and later reduced following treatment with melatonin.

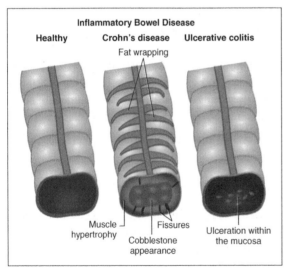

Inflammatory Bowel Disease

Healthy   Crohn's disease   Ulcerative colitis

Fat wrapping

Muscle hypertrophy   Fissures   Cobblestone appearance   Ulceration within the mucosa

The results of this study have provided a remarkable breakthrough in the management of colitis. It has shown that melatonin holds great potential as an anti-inflammatory agent and could reverse the effect of sleep deprivation risk of ulceration and inflammation in the colon.

I suggest that anyone under stress would benefit from melatonin supplementation - and who isn't these days? Lack of sleep is one of the worst stressors there is, perhaps worse than poor nutrition and lack of exercise.[10]

Melatonin in the management of colorectal cancer

Melatonin has been found to play a role in inhibiting the abnormal proliferation of cells responsible for triggering the development of many cancers, including colorectal cancer.

Colorectal cancer is the third most commonly detected cancer. It's also a significant cause of cancer-related deaths around the world. Multiple factors are associated with the development of colorectal cancer, including poor sleep, poor gut function, general aging, dietary habits, inadequate physical activities, and smoking.

At their root, all cancers are related to the poor function of your mitochondria. Melatonin might help reduce the chances of developing this cancer by supporting mitochondria as a primary antioxidant. Through this mechanism of supporting and protecting your mitochondria, melatonin also protects against colorectal cancer as an anti-inflammatory agent, creating immune modulation and activating anti-oncogenic and oncostatin actions. All these work to inhibit the progress of many cancers, including colorectal cancer.

Given that melatonin is produced in the gastrointestinal tract, it produces a direct local effect on the cancer-causing agents the colon and rectum are exposed to, thereby preventing the growth and spread of abnormal cells.

Moreover, the secretion of melatonin in the digestive tract holds particular importance here as the total levels of melatonin are nearly 400 times more than that produced in the pineal gland. This has been proven in a study, 'Thirty-four years since the discovery of gastrointestinal melatonin', published in the Journal of Physiology and Pharmacology in 2008.[11]

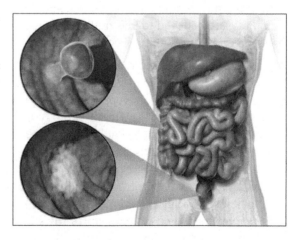

Another study, 'Therapeutic Opportunities in Colorectal Cancer: Focus on Melatonin Antioncogenic Action' published in the Biomed Research International in 2019, showed that the antitumor functions of melatonin, coupled with the ability of this hormone to regulate the body's circadian rhythm, would help people avoid the risk of colorectal cancer.[12]

Problems in the circadian rhythm were observed in patients with colorectal cancer and reduced melatonin production, indicating the possible involvement of melatonin deficiency as a possible cause for this condition.

Another study confirms that melatonin has the potential to block colon carcinogenesis. 'Melatonin suppresses AOM/DSS-induced large bowel oncogenesis in rats' published in the chemical-biological Interactions in 2009 has supported these findings.

The study assessed the inhibitory effect of exogenous melatonin on the cancerous changes occurring in the colon. It showed that the administration of melatonin helped to inhibit the development of colonic adenocarcinoma. Moreover, exposure of the colon to exogenous melatonin also modified the process of mitosis (a form of cell division) and apoptosis (programmed cell death in cancer tissues), thereby indicating the efficacy of melatonin as an anticarcinogenic agent. By regulating mitosis, melatonin might inhibit the abnormal proliferation of cancer cells, limiting the growth and spread of cancer. This means melatonin might also help support the division or regeneration of new and healthy cells in the tissues affected due to cancer, thereby supporting faster repair and healing. The improvement in apoptosis brought about by melatonin would encourage programmed cell death, enabling the body to selectively attack and destroy cancer cells, ultimately limiting the extent of cancer mass.

Also noted in the study, was the possibility that melatonin might control the secretion of inflammatory substances in patients with colonic adenocarcinomas, minimizing damage to the tissues. These results indicate the beneficial effects of exogenous melatonin on colon carcinogenesis, particularly related to the inflammation in the colon, suggesting the potential application of this hormone for inhibiting the development of colorectal cancer. [13]

Altogether, these results suggest that melatonin might inhibit the development and progression of colorectal cancer in humans. Which are extremely interesting findings, that could make waves in the prevention and treatment of specific types of cancer.

There is a cross-link between melatonin deficiency and the higher occurrence of colorectal cancer. The lack of adequate levels of this hormone might prevent the body from fighting cancer naturally. Several potential mechanisms, including autophagy, suppression of cancer cell proliferation, angiogenesis, and the activation of apoptosis and cancer-related immunity, are believed to be stimulated by melatonin while limiting the development and progression of the colorectal colon.

Moreover, there is experimental evidence showing that melatonin might act through the membrane and nuclear receptors. One research study, 'Possible involvement of the nuclear RZR/ROR-alpha receptor in the antitumor action of melatonin on murine Colon 38 cancer' published in the Tumor Biology in 2002 proposed that the nuclear melatonin receptors are identical to the nuclear orphan receptors, suggesting that the antitumor effect of melatonin also depends on nuclear signaling. This means melatonin may produce an oncostatin effect on colon cancer cells by regulating nuclear signaling mechanisms and reducing the excessive proliferation of tumor cell nuclei. Once the proliferation of tumor cell nuclei is prevented, it would automatically cause inhibition of cellular proliferation. This demonstrates one of melatonin's roles in the body: to stop the growth of colorectal cancer by creating an inhibitory effect on the division of the nuclei of cells.[14]

The main takeaway from this chapter is that melatonin is a gut-protective agent that helps enhance the immune functions of the gut flora, reduce peristalsis, alter the intestinal microbiome diversity, and restore healthy functions of the stomach and intestine.

Conclusion

The high concentration of melatonin within the gut (400x's) compared to the melatonin produced by the pineal gland demonstrates how important it is in gut health. The protective effect of melatonin on the gastrointestinal tract has been proven with a variety of studies. Melatonin further supports the beneficial bacteria through a robust circadian rhythm signaling which causes the good bacteria to "swarm", and has a negative effect on the bad bacteria, thereby improving the microbiome in your gut.

The microbiome should primarily live in your large intestines and not so much in the small intestines. Using a suppository or enema implant with probiotics and butyrate can be helpful. Especially when a post-fast protocol to improve the health of your microbiome is desired. A 24 hour or even 3-5 day fast followed with a supra-physiologic melatonin dose to support a strong microbiome swarming effect is effective. Fasting is a positive stress to the microbiome, and refeeding after the fast is how the microbiome comes back with stronger health.

You can support your gut by restoring melatonin levels through supplementation. Once melatonin levels increase, the circadian rhythm would be restored, and the gut functions would be regulated, thereby preventing mechanisms responsible for poor gut health.

When deciding how much melatonin to supplement for gut support, consider that the level of melatonin in your gut is four hundred times higher than the levels associated with the pineal gland. I believe that the typical 3-20mg prescribed by most doctors falls short of the optimal dosage, where one can receive the most benefit from the miracle molecule.

Reference

1. Reconstitution of an intact clock reveals mechanisms of circadian timekeeping (science.org)

2. Paulose, J. K., Wright, J. M., Patel, A. G., & Cassone, V. M. (2016). Human Gut Bacteria Are Sensitive to Melatonin and Express Endogenous Circadian Rhythmicity. *PloS one, 11*(1), e0146643. https://doi.org/10.1371/journal.pone.0146643

3. Acuña-Castroviejo D, Escames G, Venegas C, Díaz-Casado ME, Lima-Cabello E, López LC, Rosales-Corral S, Tan DX, Reiter RJ. Extrapineal melatonin: sources, regulation, and potential functions. Cell Mol Life Sci. 2014 Aug;71(16):2997-3025. doi: 10.1007/s00018-014-1579-2. Epub 2014 Feb 20. PMID: 24554058.

4. Bubenik GA. Gastrointestinal melatonin: localization, function, and clinical relevance. Dig Dis Sci. 2002 Oct;47(10):2336-48. doi: 10.1023/a:1020107915919. PMID: 12395907.

5. Belkaid, Y., & Hand, T. W. (2014). Role of the microbiota in immunity and inflammation. *Cell, 157*(1), 121–141. https://doi.org/10.1016/j.cell.2014.03.011

6. Belkaid, Y., & Hand, T. W. (2014). Role of the microbiota in immunity and inflammation. *Cell, 157*(1), 121–141. https://doi.org/10.1016/j.cell.2014.03.011

7. Smith, R. P., Easson, C., Lyle, S. M., Kapoor, R., Donnelly, C. P., Davidson, E. J., Parikh, E., Lopez, J. V., & Tartar, J. L. (2019). Gut microbiome diversity is associated with sleep physiology in humans. *PloS one, 14*(10), e0222394. https://doi.org/10.1371/journal.pone.0222394

8. Melatonin and the thyroid — BOOST Thyroid: Hashimoto's and Hypothyroid App

9. Advances in Integrative Medicine,Volume 2, Issue 1,2015,Pages 31-37,ISSN 2212-9588,https://doi.org/10.1016/j.aimed.2014.12.007.https://www.sciencedirect.com/science/article/pii/S2212962614000819

10. Park, Y., Chung, S., Lee, S., Kim, J., Kim, J., Kim, T. ... Baik, H. (2015). Melatonin improves experimental colitis with sleep deprivation. International Journal of Molecular Medicine, 35, 979-986. https://doi.org/10.3892/ijmm.2015.2080

11. Bubenik GA. Thirty four years since the discovery of gastrointestinal melatonin. J Physiol Pharmacol. 2008 Aug;59 Suppl 2:33-51. PMID: 18812627.

12. Hucong Wu, Jiaqi Liu, Yi Yin, Dong Zhang, Pengpeng Xia, Guoqiang Zhu, "Therapeutic Opportunities in Colorectal Cancer: Focus on Melatonin Antioncogenic Action", *BioMed Research International*, vol. 2019, Article ID 9740568, 6 pages, 2019. https://doi.org/10.1155/2019/9740568

13. Tanaka T, Yasui Y, Tanaka M, Tanaka T, Oyama T, Rahman KM. Melatonin suppresses AOM/DSS-induced large bowel oncogenesis in rats. Chem Biol Interact. 2009 Jan 27;177(2):128-36. doi: 10.1016/j.cbi.2008.10.047. Epub 2008 Nov 5. PMID: 19028472.

14. Winczyk K, Pawlikowski M, Guerrero JM, Karasek M. Possible involvement of the nuclear RZR/ROR-alpha receptor in the antitumor action of melatonin on murine Colon 38 cancer. Tumour Biol. 2002 Sep-Oct;23(5):298-302. doi: 10.1159/000068569. PMID: 12595746.

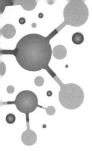

12

MELATONIN FOR JET LAG & DISRUPTED SLEEP-WAKE CYCLE IN SHIFT WORKERS

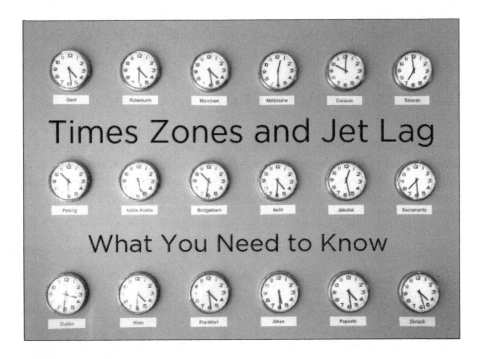

What's more important than nutrition and exercise? Sleep is the answer! Sleep is so important that it is now illegal to run research on sleep deprivation due to the extreme harm it can do to us.

I recently traveled for a weekend spiritual retreat and my flight was so early I had to set my alarm at 3:30am. I was so concerned I wouldn't wake up that I didn't trust going to sleep at a deep level and played in bed half asleep until 3:30am when I pulled myself out of bed and dragged myself to the airport feeling horrible. This was a rare occasion, but the after-effect was my hands were shaking and I was unsteady on my feet all day. I was unable to recall many simple words, and ideas were difficult to express in conversation. All due to a poor night's sleep. It hit me like a brick wall and what's amazing to me is that there are so many individuals out there that deal with this night after night. It has become completely normal.

Sleep is an active process. It takes an extremely specific release of chemicals, and of course melatonin.

Many people experience difficulties falling asleep due to anxiety like I did a few nights back. Sleep deprivation or the lack of adequate sleep could work as a dangerous precursor to the decline in brain and physical function, plus life and work productivity, and performance.

Sleep does things for us that reach into every aspect of our health and we will be diving into this subject a little further in this chapter, as well as how we can leverage the use of melatonin to improve this. I will also be covering ways to maximize sleep besides melatonin, so for those that have sleep difficulties, this chapter is perfect for you!

We will also be looking at how traveling through time zones causes jet lag and whether this hormone could be used to avoid the symptoms of jet lag for frequent travelers or the adverse effect of changing sleep-wake patterns in people working shifts, such as in the ER or security guards.

What does melatonin do?

Melatonin plays a vital role in improving the duration and quality of your sleep. The secretion of this hormone in the pineal gland varies at different times throughout the day. Melatonin production depends on the amount of light or brightness your body is exposed to. Some other factors including your daily schedule, seasons, and emotional health can also influence the secretion of melatonin in the pineal gland, thereby creating a positive or negative effect on your sleep-wake cycle.

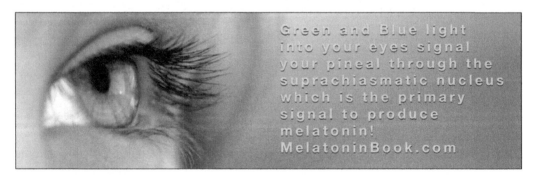

Green and Blue light into your eyes signal your pineal through the suprachiasmatic nucleus which is the primary signal to produce melatonin!
MelatoninBook.com

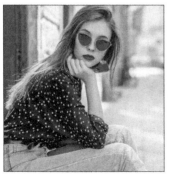

For example, during evening hours, as darkness approaches, the body begins to prepare itself for sleep by releasing the secretion of melatonin. On the other hand, as daytime approaches, the body is exposed to bright sunlight. So, during the early morning hours, the secretion of melatonin begins to reduce to prepare your body for wakefulness. Cortisol is an opposing hormone to melatonin and when melatonin decreases in the morning hours cortisol increases, and vice versa in the evening.

These changes in melatonin production are regulated by exposure to bright light and governed primarily by the suprachiasmatic nucleus which is hard wired to your eyes. It's a part of the brain that is responsible for sending signals to the pineal gland to produce and release melatonin at night and then, suppress its production and release it during the daytime.

The increased level of melatonin during night hours is meant to help you sleep, meanwhile the reduced level of melatonin along with elevated cortisol during the daytime keeps you alert and awake.

Melatonin could be beneficial for those who are producing less due to sleep stress factors. These include lack of sunlight exposure to eyes, poor bedroom hygiene such as too hot or lack of total darkness, too much exposure to green and blue light after sunset, meals too late in the evening, and high physical, mental or emotional stress. Melatonin may also be useful for managing the symptoms of jet lag which frequent travelers often experience.

Melatonin supplementation taken at specific times based on the difference in the time zones of your origin and destination would reduce the impact of jet lag symptoms. Trust me, I grew up in Hawaii and currently live in Florida, so I fly back often to visit friends and family which is a 5–6-hour time difference and I know jet lag well. I have figured out how to beat this with something I call the "Travel Hacker Kit" which includes a very high-dose melatonin product called Sandman. This protocol has been a complete game changer and I am able to get right into the fun when I arrive at my destination the first day. Incidentally, I'm actually writing this chapter while on a flight to Hawaii at this very moment. I'm flying over the Pacific Ocean right now headed to Hawaii for x-mas!

These strategies can be used by frequent travelers to feel fresh and reset their body's circadian rhythm according to the day and night times of the destination. This will happen naturally over time, but we want to get right into the swing of things when we arrive so speeding this up is desirable. Achieving a shorter acclimation duration using melatonin and even more impactful the Travel Hacker Kit method is a big advantage. Therefore, it is important to explore the right ways melatonin supplementation can be used in your travel plans to be able to avoid the impact of jet lag. Luckily, we will outline my special hack later in this chapter.

The dual role of melatonin during the night and daytime also holds importance for people who work in shifts. The lack of regular working schedules and changing sleep-wake cycles prevents the body from creating its own biological clock. This lack of regular routine ultimately disrupts the body's circadian rhythm. The dysregulation of the circadian rhythm, in these cases, would not just affect the ability of the person to sleep well, but also cause a decline in productivity during working hours.

Above all, the disruptions in the rhythmic activities of the body would create an adverse effect on all functions that are regulated by the sleep wake cycle including repair and healing mechanisms, inflammation, and the defense activities of the immune system. The overall impact of these changes could be severely harmful.

Melatonin supplementation might provide a solution to the health issues linked to shift working and enable people to have healthy sleep-wake cycles while avoiding acute and chronic diseases linked to the distorted circadian rhythm.

We have already discussed what melatonin means and how it affects sleep in earlier chapters. But, in this chapter, we will specifically look at the role of melatonin supplementation for reducing jet lag and the effect it can have for those working in shifts.

What is it about the sunlight and melatonin secretion?

One of the best ways to stimulate the pineal gland and cells to produce melatonin is to get some sun every day. Exposure to sun rays for at least 10 to 15 minutes every day could support optimum secretion of this hormone in the body. During the daytime, when the sun rays fall onto the retina, they stimulate the optic nerve, which, in turn, sends a message to the brain about the presence of bright sunlight outside. Once the brain knows it is daytime, it sends a message to the pineal gland to stop releasing melatonin to prevent sleepiness and promote mental and physical alertness which is essential for us to perform our daytime activities.

Exposure to the sun in the morning hours would also regulate the production of melatonin in the pineal gland such that when you go to sleep, the melatonin levels are at the peak allowing you to have quality sleep.[1]

Melatonin is also secreted in the fluid in your eyes. So, it makes sense to set aside your sunglasses in the morning hours while traveling. Not wearing sunglasses will allow the sun rays to enter your eyes and promote the synthesis of melatonin in the intraocular fluid. If you're a shift worker you might consider investing in one of the hats or sunglasses products that puts out green and blue light, or if you're traveling you should get out in the sun in the morning and ditch those sunglasses.[2][3][4]

Whether you're traveling or not you might consider removing your sunglasses before 11 am and after 3-4 pm. This would be an effective way to ensure adequate signaling of the circadian rhythm and production of melatonin in the pineal gland.[5]

Support your pineal gland

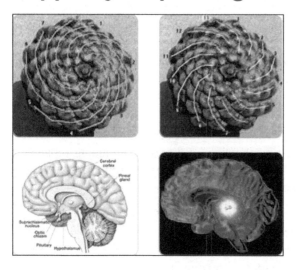

Pineal calcification is calcium deposition in the pineal gland, which has long been reported in humans. The occurrence of pineal calcification depends on environmental factors, such as sunlight exposure, toxins like fluoride, and increased metabolic activity. This calcification is seen in many chronic conditions.

Studies have found that the more metabolically active the pineal gland is, the more likely it is to form calcium deposits. Furthermore, researchers have conducted animal studies where gerbils who were exposed to less light than others had higher amounts of pineal gland calcifications. darkness strongly influences the pineal to release melatonin. If the pineal gland has to produce larger amounts of melatonin due to less sunlight exposure, calcification can occur. Do certain chronic medical conditions increase the likelihood of pineal gland calcifications or is pineal calcification lowering melatonin, therefore, these conditions appear? Examples of these medical conditions include Alzheimer's disease, migraine headaches, kidney disease, and schizophrenia.

Fluoride & your pineal gland?

Researchers have studied a potential connection between increased fluoride exposure and pineal gland calcifications. Fluoride is a naturally occurring mineral that some areas add to their water supply to reduce tooth decay. The mineral is present in most toothpaste because it helps to strengthen tooth enamel. Yet, fluoride is naturally attracted to calcium, and some researchers believe increased fluoridation leads to increased pineal gland calcification.

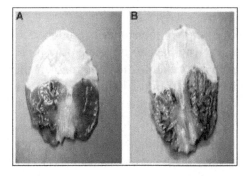

A study in 2019 in rats found those who were placed on a fluoride-free diet for 4 to 8 weeks experienced a greater increase in the number of pineal gland cells compared with those who consumed fluoridated food and drinking water. See the chapter on pineal for more details on this subject.

Can you decalcify your pineal gland?

It's pretty simple really, stop consuming fluoridated water. If you're on a public water system, you can request support from your water supplier, which will contain information about fluoride and chlorine, which is another mineral that may contribute to calcifications. As an alternative, some people will either filter their water or drink bottled water. Avoid using toothpaste that contains fluoride. Fluoride is also used in pesticides and some chemicals used to create non-stick compounds for pots and pans. Eat organic foods and avoid processed foods to reduce fluoride consumption. Calcium supplementation consumed in excess could be problematic. Especially if you're low in vitamin D and

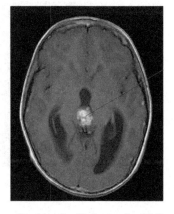

K-2. Or you may be taking too much vitamin D and not enough vitamin K-2, as the K-2 is needed to prevent the calcium from depositing into your tissues.

Either way, to answer the question: Yes, it is possible to decalcify the pineal gland.

The importance of using melatonin supplements for sleep

Besides melatonin being a sleep-inducing hormone, it plays a major role in regulating the body's internal biological clock. It basically works by regulating the sleep-wake pattern and helps to improve the quality and duration of sleep. But let's not forget that it also works on your body and brain in so many other ways as you have read throughout this book. Dialing in the circadian rhythm can be as important as an exercise or nutrition program. This becomes even more important when traveling and in shift workers due to the stress both these situations place on your body.

Even though melatonin is produced in the body naturally, people who work in shifts or those who have to travel across different time zones frequently, are unable to derive the potential benefits of this hormone, simply because the specific conditions needed for the time-dependent or light-dependent secretion of melatonin by the pineal glands are not adequate under these stressful situations.

Neither the shift workers nor frequent travelers get an opportunity to set their body's rhythm so that it gets a similar amount of exposure to sunlight at fixed times of the day or night. And this is the reason they need to depend on melatonin in the form of supplements to be able to enjoy the therapeutic benefits of the miracle molecule.

How to use melatonin supplements for sleep?

Since melatonin is a sleep-wake cycle regulating hormone, it's important that you use it at the right time to suit your routine, keeping in mind the time you need to sleep against the time you need to be awake and productive.

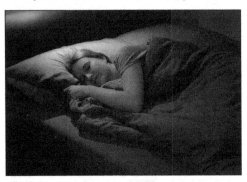

If you struggle to fall asleep often due to jet lag or working in shifts, you should take melatonin supplements about 30 minutes before bedtime. The other option is spending several hours trying to fall asleep. I know which one I prefer! Moreover, some research suggests when taking smaller doses of melatonin such as 3-20mg may be better for sleep latency, but these doses should be taken 3-4 hours before bed, such as after dinner. This principle does not seem to be true for the supra-physiological dosing of melatonin, such as 100-200mg.

You need to consider your sleeping habits when you start using melatonin for improving your sleep quality. This is true irrespective of whether you're an early bird or a night owl. These are the basic chronotypes that determine the rhythmic activities your body follows to allow you to perform and maintain various functions.

Night owls are basically the people who tend to stay awake until the late hours of the night. So, they also tend to get up later. Early birds, on the other hand, are those who get to sleep early like by 9 or 10 pm and are early to rise.

Therefore, depending on whether you are an early bird or a night owl, you need to time the doses of your melatonin supplements so that it matches your current sleep-wake cycle. You also need to consider your expected sleep-wake schedule. This means if you plan to change your bedtime routine or the time you wake up, you'll also need to change the time you take melatonin supplements to derive optimum benefits.

If you are an early bird, it's advisable to take melatonin in a slow-release delivery format so that the melatonin is provided throughout the evening. Oral routes generally have a short half-life and fast absorption, versus a suppository which can release slowly over 5-7 hours. Liposomal versions can also be time-released, nevertheless, I have found the suppository to be the most effective. Also, keep in mind studies show oral melatonin is only 2.5% absorbable, so a Liposomal or suppository might be best all around.

In the case of early birds who often wake up too early in the morning, say at 3 or 4 am, using a melatonin supplement might be helpful for you to signal a stronger sleep cycle through your circadian rhythm. Melatonin will extend the sleep duration allowing you to sleep for the extra 2 hours, meaning that you would wake up at 5 or 6 am. Tracking your sleep is a great way to know for certain the quality and exact duration of rest you're getting each night. Oura rings are what I use as they have been studied to be one of the best products on the market, but there are also several options to choose from.

Most people believe that going to bed early and waking up early is a good habit. However, while it's true that sleeping and getting up early is good for health, the total duration of sleep should still be 8 hours. If you sleep early but wake up too early, you may not get adequate sleep. Your total sleep time would be shortened by a few hours. This might deprive your body of the multiple benefits of having a sound sleep, and it may also hamper the biological processes like memory storage, and healing that occur more efficiently while sleeping.

This is the reason why even early birds may need to take melatonin supplements to extend their sleep duration. Proper dosing of melatonin taken at the right time could help early birds get the correct amount of sleep and prevent their risk of diseases linked to poor immunity, inflammation, oxidative stress, and degeneration all of which are connected to sleep insufficiency.

Should night owls try and return to the natural rhythms of the earth?

The need to use melatonin supplements is more important in night owls than it is for the early birds. This is because the night owls are more likely to already be suffering from health issues linked to poor sleep habits. They are out of sync with the earth's natural rhythms!

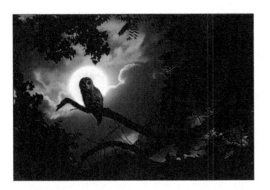

Staying awake until late hours and then subsequently waking up late in the morning can disrupt the body's circadian rhythm, which is regulated by the amount of exposure to sunlight. If your actual sleep-wake cycle is not in sync with the night-time and daytime, your brain would fail to be in sync with various mechanisms that depend on the circadian rhythm to function efficiently.

Your brain will be left confused about whether to follow the signals received through exposure to darkness and sunlight based on external conditions or whether to follow the signals provided by you with your out-of-sync sleep-wake schedule.

This might create huge disturbances in the overall functioning of all organs and systems putting you at risk of several diseases. For instance, it could cause disruptions in your immune system, your heart rate, body's healing mechanisms, natural antioxidant defenses, and much more. So, the only way to restore health here is to reset your sleep-wake cycle so that it is attuned to the actual day and night cycles of the earth.

Melatonin supplements along with some lifestyle factors can be effective tools to rebalance your sleep-wake cycles. Night owls can start taking melatonin supplements approximately 2 hours prior to their normal bedtime in order to fall asleep early and bring your body's circadian rhythm closer to that of the sun's rhythm. This would advance your sleep-wake schedule and sync your body's circadian rhythm.

How much melatonin should one take for these situations? I feel 10-20mg can be a good place to start. Although we've discussed supplementing with much higher doses, where sleep is concerned these are unnecessary. Lower doses can be tried and if they work well then higher doses could be used occasionally for a "Melatonin Reset", which is something we will discuss a little later in this chapter.

Jet lag & time zone acclimation

What is jet lag?

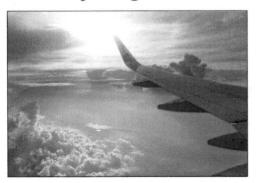

Jet lag refers to a physiological state that is characterized by the disruption in the sleep-wake cycles of a person due to the rapid traveling across multiple time zones leading to imbalances in the circadian rhythm.

The circadian rhythm, as we already know, is the internal biological clock your body is accustomed to following in order to determine the time to sleep and stay awake, eat meals, bowel movements, and so on.

When you travel through more than two time zones in a short period, say in 5 to 6 hours, it does not provide adequate time for your body to adjust to the new day-night cycle of the destination.

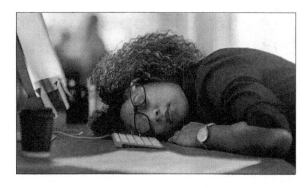

As a result, you may experience an inability to sleep during the night and stay awake during the day once at your new destination, resulting in what we call jet lag. In simple words, it means your body is lagging in terms of the time zone you jet traveled from causing you to be out of tune with the time zone you are currently in.

What about people who have to put up with frequent changes in their sleep-wake cycles due to the need to travel across multiple time zones? Working professionals and businessmen often have to travel from one country to another to attend meetings, give presentations, and so on. They often have to jet set from one location to another across time zones throwing a monkey wrench in their circadian rhythm.

In cases like these, if the difference in the time zone of their place of origin and the destination is approximately a 5/6-hour difference, as is the case from Florida to Hawaii, then the body's sleep cycle gets disrupted.

What are the common signs of jet lag?

It's surprising to note that in spite of using the words, jet lag, repeatedly, most travelers are not aware of the specific symptoms they may develop. Most of the time people say they have jet lag just to describe the fatigue caused due to the lack of proper sleep after having traveled to a different time zone.

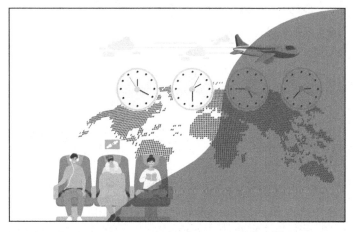

However, unbeknown to most, jet lag does not only involve loss of sleep or fatigue.

It's important to be aware of the specific symptoms of jet lag so that you know the long-term implications this problem may cause if you choose to ignore it. Jet lag is characterized by several symptoms that can disturb your routine schedule significantly.

Here are the top 3 common signs and symptoms that frequent travelers often develop due to jet lag:

1. Disturbed sleep and daytime fatigue

A research study 'Jet Lag: Current and Potential Therapies' published in the Pharmacy and Therapeutics in 2011 has shown that patients may develop extreme daytime fatigue for the first few days after arriving at the destination. This may occur due to the inability to sleep well at night.[6]

It has been found that the loss of sleep after travel is linked to the disturbances in the production of melatonin, the primary function of which is to regulate your sleep-wake cycle.

Most people find it too difficult to get enough sleep because the new time zone they have arrived at has a different schedule than what their body's circadian rhythm is used to.

As a result, when nightfall arrives at the new destination, they cannot sleep, or experience fragmented or disturbed sleep. This might affect their daytime productivity and make them feel tired and drowsy while performing tasks.

This indicates why it's important for frequent travelers to not ignore jet lag and use melatonin to be able to avoid these symptoms. This is especially important if they need to attend meetings or events that hold high importance in their life or career. Feeling tired with low motivation while performing such tasks might negate the very purpose of traveling to the destination and lead to unpleasant consequences.

2. Lowers cognitive skills

Frequent jet lag may affect your cognitive skills by reducing your sleep duration and quality.

A research study, 'How To Travel the World Without Jet lag' published in the Sleep Medicine Clinic in 2010 showed that jet lag may also reduce your concentration and prevent you from focusing on tasks.[7]

As a result, your ability to make quick decisions and your sense of judgment can be negatively affected.

3. Irritability

Lastly, one of the more notable symptoms of jet lag is irritability. might experience severe irritability and anger issues during the period in which your body is trying to adjust to the day-night cycle of the new time zone.

A research study, 'Associations Between Jet Lag and Cortisol Diurnal Rhythms After Domestic Travel' published in Health Psychology in 2011 showed that jet lag could disrupt the production of cortisol in the brain. As a result, you may develop irritability and poor mood.[8]

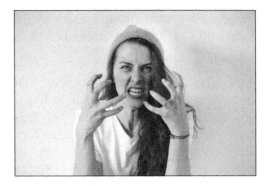

Most of these symptoms of jet lag are related to the changes in the production of melatonin within the pineal gland. Ultimately, travelers should leverage the use of melatonin supplements to restore their body's circadian rhythm and avoid jet lag caused by hopping across different time zones. Moreover, melatonin taken even before the trip can be helpful, for instance dosing a day or two before your trip around the approximate bedtime of the destination you're traveling to. I usually suggest a dose of 20-60mg in this case. It is advisable that you understand how a daytime melatonin dose affects you prior to doing this so you don't have any disruption in your travel plans.

I find this advice difficult going to time zones where it is earlier where you would be dosing the melatonin in the middle of the night. I feel getting good rest according to the cycle you're in at this point is more important. However, heading to later time zones as with a Hawaii to Florida trip is a different story.

When it comes to folks that travel frequently, say more than once every month or so, their bodies ultimately never get adequate time to adjust to any time zone. As a result, their circadian rhythm remains disrupted month after month and they are largely deprived of the benefits of having a well-regulated body clock. This happens because, by the time they get adjusted to the day-night cycle of one time zone, it's the time to pack their bags and head off on another trip.

But fear not! If you're a frequent traveler and have to hop across different time zones several times in a year, I'm sure you'll want to know how you can avoid the effect of jet lag and hack your body clock as quickly and efficiently as possible. In this next section, "Melatonin Reset" I'll highlight exactly how to effectively reset the body's circadian rhythm.

Melatonin Reset

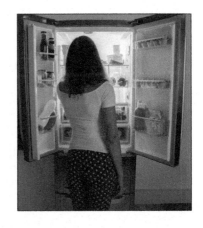

If you're wanting to really reset your circadian rhythm this method is for you. It's what I will do tonight on my first evening in Hawaii.

First of all, I'll take advantage of as much sunlight as I can this afternoon to make the most of as much natural signaling as I can. I won't wear sunglasses, which I rarely do these days for the same reason anyway.

Secondly, I will try and get some physical exercise as well by going for a short hike to build up sleep stress.

Thirdly, I'll use caffeine this afternoon to keep me alert as it can be quite difficult to stay awake till 9 or 10pm the first night without some form of energy beverage.

Ok so here is the real magic…

For the melatonin reset ill dose 200mg of melatonin in the form of a suppository at 9/10pm this evening. And if you've been reading through other chapters in this book, you're probably already more than familiar with the safety and efficacy of using melatonin in these high doses. It's nontoxic at very high levels, does not shut down your natural production with any negative feedback loop, and it works quite well for this utility. However, if you're an executive or travel for business, let me forewarn you that the first time or two you take this much melatonin you could be a little groggy the next morning.

Melatonin also detoxifies heavy metals from the brain so you won't want to be detoxing while on vacation, and while 90% of people will do just fine doing 200mg of melatonin right out of the gate, however there is a small percentage of individuals who might need a few days to acclimate themselves to that dosage.

Eating late & melatonin

This information is from chapter 7 yet it's worth mentioning here again, as traveling can oftentimes throw our mealtimes out of whack.

In your pancreas, you have MT1 & MT2 receptors for melatonin. These are called "G-coded melatonin receptors". This means that there is a direct link between your pancreas, insulin, and melatonin. When you go to sleep, these receptors are activated by melatonin. And subsequently, insulin is lowered, and glucose is increased, via these MT1&2 receptors.

These receptors have a direct action through cAMP and cGMP which is an important signal to your metabolism. This activation and signaling enables you to have more glucose which ultimately helps make repairs needed within the body while you sleep.

The point I'm trying to make is although eating late might increase serotonin, which helps to increase building blocks for melatonin, it might not be best for your health long term. Especially if you're leaning towards Type 2 diabetes. Therefore, this is something to be extremely mindful of if you're a frequent traveler.

Travel hacker kit

I find traveling daily stressful and before I discovered the protocol, I'm going to share with you now I always needed a few days to feel "normal" after any trip.

My personal challenges were partly due to time zone changes, yet there are other factors that I struggled with, especially when using air travel. Nevertheless, I suspect that air travel might be better now that the airlines have been somewhat forced to use better air filtration systems due to the COVID pandemic.

I say this because I was diagnosed with severe mold illness, therefore my tolerance for poor air quality is low.

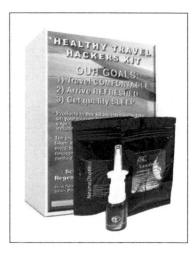

Another reason many of us feel quite tired after a long flight is the EMF exposure from the engines, plane, and altitude. I find a very high CBD dose to be immensely helpful to combat the EMF exposure, which I prefer in a suppository form. I take a product called NeuroDiol 300mg which offers a neuroprotective and inflammatory effect while flying.

I also enjoy using a nice natural antimicrobial nasal spray a few times while on the plane to keep my sinus clear and prevent picking up any unwanted nasties on the flight as well.

I've been using the travel hack kit for a while now and it's never let me down. It's well worth it, especially if you're someone who's either sensitive to EMFs, air quality, and environmental changes such as time zones.

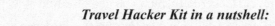

Travel Hacker Kit in a nutshell:

300 mg CBD suppository upon take-off and redose 5 hours into the flight if it's a long-haul flight.

Antimicrobial nasal spray each hour or so while flying, I like GlutaStat Nasal Spray.

Take 100-200mg melatonin in suppository or liposomal form the night of and for several nights into my trip.

"I've also found NAD+ support to help during traveling using NAD+ Max."

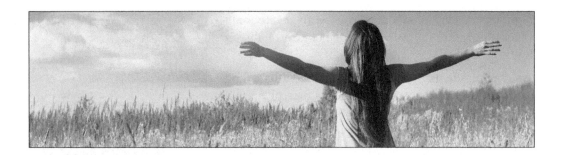

Conclusion

In this chapter we've seen how melatonin can be used when travelers wish to reset their circadian rhythm, and how it can further be leveraged by night owls in order to create healthier sleep-wake cycles that are more in tune with nature.

We also highlighted the use of melatonin for shift workers. And although melatonin can be applied successfully in these cases, it's also super important to sleep in complete darkness during the night and get out in the sunshine when possible. Shift workers could also use blue or green lights at night to mimic the sun's neurologic influence on the circadian rhythm. Moreover, nowadays there are even hats and glasses that are designed to shine these daylight mimicking colors into your eyes.

We further discussed the Travel Hacker Kit which you can also find at MitoZen.com.

In the various strategies covered in this chapter the melatonin dosages can vary from 10-200, yet it's definitely worth testing as there are numerous health challenges poor sleep leads to in the body, and correcting sleep-wake cycles can be an important factor in reaching optimal and balanced health.

Reference

1. Mead M. N. (2008). Benefits of sunlight: a bright spot for human health. *Environmental health perspectives*, *116*(4), A160–A167. https://doi.org/10.1289/ehp.116-a160

2. Choi, J. H., Lee, B., Lee, J. Y., Kim, C. H., Park, B., Kim, D. Y., Kim, H. J., & Park, D. Y. (2020). Relationship between Sleep Duration, Sun Exposure, and Serum 25-Hydroxyvitamin D Status: A Cross-sectional Study. *Scientific reports*, *10*(1), 4168. https://doi.org/10.1038/s41598-020-61061-8

3. Tosini, G., Baba, K., Hwang, C. K., & Iuvone, P. M. (2012). Melatonin: an underappreciated player in retinal physiology and pathophysiology. *Experimental eye research*, *103*, 82–89. https://doi.org/10.1016/j.exer.2012.08.009

4. Tosini, G., Ferguson, I., & Tsubota, K. (2016). Effects of blue light on the circadian system and eye physiology. *Molecular vision*, *22*, 61–72.

5. Lok R, van Koningsveld MJ, Gordijn MCM, Beersma DGM, Hut RA. Daytime melatonin and light independently affect human alertness and body temperature. J Pineal Res. 2019 Aug;67(1):e12583. doi: 10.1111/jpi.12583. Epub 2019 May 9. PMID: 31033013; PMCID: PMC6767594.

6. Choy, M., & Salbu, R. L. (2011). Jet lag: current and potential therapies. *P & T : a peer-reviewed journal for formulary management*, *36*(4), 221–231.

7. Eastman, C. I., & Burgess, H. J. (2009). How To Travel the World Without Jet lag. *Sleep medicine clinics*, *4*(2), 241–255. https://doi.org/10.1016/j.jsmc.2009.02.006

8. Doane, L. D., Kremen, W. S., Eaves, L. J., Eisen, S. A., Hauger, R., Hellhammer, D., Levine, S., Lupien, S., Lyons, M. J., Mendoza, S., Prom-Wormley, E., Xian, H., York, T. P., Franz, C. E., & Jacobson, K. C. (2010). Associations between jet lag and cortisol diurnal rhythms after domestic travel. *Health psychology : official journal of the Division of Health Psychology, American Psychological Association*, *29*(2), 117–123. https://doi.org/10.1037/a0017865

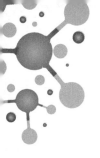

13

MELATONIN & SKIN

Skin Disease & Anti-aging strategy for skin

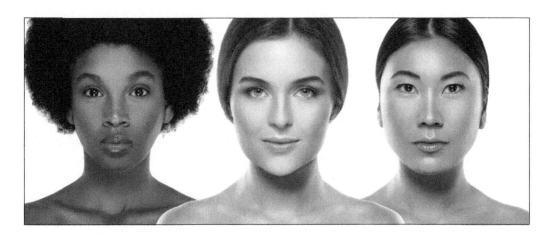

I started working with a woman who was dealing with cancer a while back and she asked me to connect with her holistic doctor to discuss using high-dose melatonin. Her doctor was super-open to adding melatonin to her program as she already had a good experience with using melatonin in the past. She was mainly applying it for her female patients for skin in a melatonin cream. She asked if we made any melatonin skin products and at that time, it was the first I had heard of melatonin used this way.

She stated that she was seeing dramatic skin results with a cream she was having made through a compound pharmacy. It made sense to me as the science behind this approach would work just like it does with many of the other conditions we have discussed in this book. As antioxidant and mitochondrial support, it could help your skin be healthier and more youthful.

So, I began making a facial serum and a body lotion with melatonin and, of course, I had to boost this with my own additions of resveratrol, apocynin, GHK peptide, methylene blue, and hyaluronic acid.

I found this to be an amazing combination for skincare. Besides the direct application of melatonin to the skin, there is also the quality of your sleep as "beauty sleep". Beauty or the health of your skin is dependent on the quality of your sleep. If you get consistent quality sleep every night, you will look fresh, and your complexion will glow with radiance.

But can melatonin, orally or in the forms of gels or creams, bring back the glow on your face? We will dive into this subject in this chapter.

Using melatonin for improving skin health

When we think of melatonin, the odds are that you will think of sleep. Yet, as we have discussed in prior chapters, melatonin is not just a sleep hormone that regulates our circadian rhythm and improves our sleep-wake cycle. Melatonin is also one of the most effective natural remedies to improve our skin health, as it's considered a natural anti-aging hormone. These "skin benefits" of melatonin are related to the ability of this hormone to improve your sleep pattern, protect your skin against oxidative damage through its antioxidant qualities, and the cellular energy it provides to your skin through the support of your mitochondria in cells.

How is this possible? It turns out that besides being produced in the brain by the pineal gland, melatonin is also produced in your skin cells. This makes your skin a site of local production and activity of melatonin. Melatonin has a somewhat wider range of action when it comes to the skin. For example, melatonin suppresses the UV-induced damage to the skin cells and works as the skin's own natural antioxidant, protecting cellular DNA against free-radical damage, delaying the aging signs like wrinkles, improving the thickness of the skin, and maintaining its tone.

Let's take a closer look at each of these melatonin benefits for your skin, and what has been revealed through research about the effect the miracle molecule can have on your skin and overall external beauty.

The anti-aging benefits of melatonin for skin

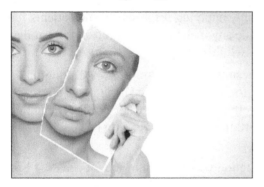

Do you know why those signs of aging appear on your skin? Those wrinkles and fine lines on your face give away your actual age. These signs are nothing but the effect of loss of collagen in your skin.

As you age, your skin begins to lose both collagen and elastin. These two are the most important components of the skin and primary contributors to its appearance. Collagen and elastin together form a strong matrix of skin tissues and provide a firm structure that supports your skin. Unless you do something to prevent the loss of your collagen and elastin, your youthful appearance can only last if you are young. Therefore, slowly, it begins to lose its elasticity like a rubber band that has lost its stretchable nature.

Now that we know why these wrinkles and fine lines appear, it's time to learn how we can influence the skin to produce more elastin and collagen. The best way to do this is to ensure your skin is supplied with a rich amount of melatonin.

According to a study, 'Protective Effects of Melatonin on the Skin: Future Perspectives' published in the International Journal of Molecular Sciences in 2019, melatonin has the potential to stimulate the production of collagen and elastin in the skin.[1] It might strengthen the skin matrix and prevent or slow down the degradation of the skin structure due to aging.

Melatonin may also be used to protect the skin against sun damage that is known to accelerate the signs of aging. Exposure of the skin to harsh ultraviolet rays in the sunlight can cause wrinkles and fine lines to appear at a younger age. The skin may look dry and dull and loses its natural glow due to excessive exposure to sunlight.

The damage to the superficial and deeper layers of the skin due to UV radiation can also lead to the appearance of age spots and dark patches, that can make you look older than your actual age. The effects of sun damage to your skin could be avoided by using melatonin. Moreover, this study shows the natural antioxidant potential of melatonin can minimize free radical damage in the skin and slow down the effect of sun exposure.

Melatonin may also stimulate mitochondrial functions locally within the layers of the skin, reduce inflammation, and modify the expression of some genes, thereby improving your skin tone and complexion. Consequently, melatonin has been shown to have an excellent anti-aging effect on the skin.

When used regularly, you will notice your skin looking firmer and more elastic. This would occur not just due to the increased collagen and elastin produced in the skin following melatonin supplementation, but also due to how this sleep hormone stimulates the healing processes throughout your body. Moreover, melatonin would accelerate the repair of the dead and damaged skin cells and stimulate the regeneration of new cells so that they can replace the old cells.

Exploring the Gut – Sleep – Skin axis

There is another mechanism through which melatonin can create a favorable response on your skin, and that mechanism works through the gut-sleep-skin axis.

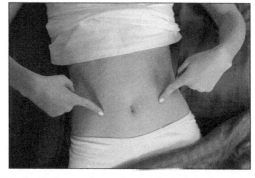

Your gut and skin are closely related. And the gut flora, in turn, is linked to your sleep. As we discussed in Chapter 11, your gut bacteria or the microbiome goes through a daily regenerative phase called swarming, which is primarily signaled through the circadian rhythm and the release of melatonin. This is different from the melatonin release in the brain and is called gut melatonin which is 400 times more elevated than the brain levels.

Melatonin for gut flora and swarming

Melatonin plays a key role in supporting the development of healthy gut flora. Moreover, healthy gut flora is essential not just for improving the functions of the digestive system but also for strengthening your immunity.

Healthy gut functions and a strong immune system, in turn, can have a remarkable and positive influence on your skin's health.

Let's dive deeper into how your skin is linked to your gut flora, sleep, and your immune system.

What forms the gut-sleep-skin axis?

The health of your skin at any given time can be the result of several factors. From hormones and genetics to your diet and nutrition, your skin is the reflection of what is happening inside your body.

There is no larger influence on your skin health-driven through internal conditions than the state of your gut. Besides improving skin health, there are a few common skin diseases driven through an unhealthy gut such as d, eczema, rosacea, psoriasis, severe skin redness, severe itching, severe rashes, and even acne eruptions are all reflections of a sick and inflamed gut with a poor microbiome. The gut-sleep-skin axis is so important that it can oftentimes lead to some of the worst skin conditions doctors see in their clinics.

According to the Human Microbiome Project by the National Institutes of Health (NIH), our body consists of trillions of microorganisms, including bacteria that outnumber human cells by a huge margin of 10 to 1. That gives you an idea of the number of microorganisms residing in your body. The largest number of these microbes are found in your gut flora located within your large intestines.[2]

As reported by the researchers at the Harvard School of Public Health, microorganisms in the gut flora support digestion, stimulate the immune functions, break down toxic compounds, and synthesize amino acids and vitamins like all your B vitamins which are critical to bodily functions.[3]

In the intestine, bacterial imbalances are associated with inflammatory conditions such as irritable bowel syndrome (IBS), and leaky gut syndrome. These gut issues can manifest in several other organs of the body, among which skin is the commonest. For example, the overgrowth of bacteria in your gut, due to a condition called small intestinal bacterial overgrowth (SIBO), is linked to the two most common skin conditions, namely acne, and rosacea.

Bottom line is that if you take good care of your gut, it will eventually have a positive impact on your skin's health and appearance. Moreover, in Chinese medicine, they call the skin the reflection of what is going on inside your gut. On the other hand, if you experience any gut issues, like inflammation, or leaky gut, your skin would likely be the first place where you'd notice problems.

Scientists have proven the direct as well as the indirect connection between gut flora and skin issues like eczema, psoriasis, dermatitis, rosacea, and acne. For example, one study, 'Allergic Disease Linked To Irritable Bowel Syndrome' sourced from the Rush University Medical Center has shown that inflammation in the gut may spread to the skin.

This might happen due to the involvement of the immune system in gut flora. The increased secretion of inflammatory substances by the immune system would cause damage to the gut tissues due to which may develop *into* digestive diseases like ulcerative colitis, colorectal cancer, leaky gut syndrome, or inflammatory bowel disease. The inflammatory substances would be carried to the skin through the blood due and thus you may notice redness, itching, rashes, acne eruptions, rosacea, and sunburns all of which are characterized by skin inflammation.

Now, this direct impact of gut diseases in your skin can be easily avoided if you take good care of your gut flora. Maintaining a healthy and diverse gut flora would improve the functions of your immune system so much so that it can calm down the excessive secretion of proinflammatory substances by the immune cells. The immediate effect of this would be evident first in your gut and then with your skin.

Ultimately, by healing your gut you'd further start to notice how you no longer develop skin rashes, itching, and redness. There may also be a reduced chance of frequent flare-ups of dermatitis, eczema, rosacea, psoriasis, and so on.

This is how strengthening your gut-sleep-skin axis would have a healthy influence on your skin and protect you against several skin diseases. If you don't have a skin condition you may find supporting your microbiome with melatonin orally and/or topically might greatly improve your *skin's* youthful appearance as well.

Skin Microbiome: how does it relate to your melatonin levels and immune health?

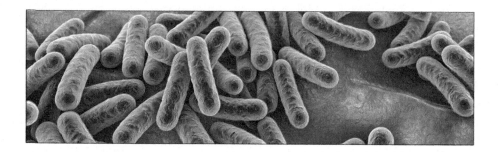

The skin microbiome is a vital parameter for assessing the ability of your skin to protect itself against infections and other disease-causing agents like inflammation, sun exposure, and oxidative stress. Interestingly enough, melatonin can get into the skin microbiome and help restore a diverse skin microbiota just like it does for the gut flora.

The skin microbiota is made of a number of microorganisms. Most cutaneous organisms can produce molecules that can inhibit the colonization or growth of other microorganisms and even alter their behaviors. Moreover, the skin microbiota in healthy adults remains stable and keeps them protected against the development of skin diseases like eczema, psoriasis, and sunburns. What is more interesting is these skin microorganisms also play an important role in training the adaptive and innate arms of the cutaneous immune system. This means having a healthy skin microbiota is vital for ensuring the immune cells in the skin are able to work efficiently.

The role of the skin microbiome in maintaining skin health

The interaction of the surface of the body with the external environment occurs through the skin that acts as a physical barrier and prevents the invasion of foreign bodies, including pathogens. The harsh physical landscape of the human skin, particularly in the nutrient-poor, desiccated, acidic environment, may contribute to the adversities that pathogens face while colonizing the human skin. Despite this, the skin is often colonized by diverse strains of microorganisms.[4]

The term skin flora, commonly called the skin microbiota, refers to the microorganisms residing on the skin. Furthermore, the skin's microbiota may also be composed of different strains of fungi that reside on the skin and cause diseases or symptoms like itching, rashes, and redness. These fungi are mainly found in different parts of the skin including the chest, forearm, ear canal, the back of the head, between the eyebrows, the heel, behind the ear, toenails, between the toes, back, groin, nostrils, and palms.

Skin flora is often non-pathogenic in nature. It is either commensal, which means not harmful to the host, or mutualistic, which means it might offer a benefit. The benefits that bacteria can offer to the skin and human body include the prevention of the colonization of the skin surface by the transient pathogenic organisms competing for vital nutrients, stimulating the immune system of the skin, and secreting chemicals against them. But resident microbes may also cause skin diseases or enter the bloodstream, creating life-threatening consequences, particularly in people with immunosuppressed states. So, it is considered important to adopt measures to restore a healthy skin microbiota so that it can provide benefits to your skin, or at least, not be harmful to the body.

I found some studies aimed at assessing the impact of melatonin on the skin microbiome and whether the effect of melatonin could help modify the risk of skin problems.

One study, 'Gut microbiota and nutrient interactions with skin in psoriasis: A comprehensive review of animal and human studies' published in the World Journal of Clinical Cases has revealed that the risk of psoriasis, a chronic systemic inflammatory disease, strongly associated with the interactions between genetic susceptibility, environmental triggers, and immune response could be modified by using melatonin.

Allergies and gut issues

The link between your gut is clearly visible in the research! If you suffer from skin issues, it's likely your gut is not in the best health. This leads to the development of allergies and inflammation throughout the body. Here is a study that showed people with rosacea and acne are 10 times more likely to have chronic gut issues. This study, 'Allergic Disease Linked To Irritable Bowel Syndrome' was conducted by researchers at the Rush University Medical Center and published in 2008.

Moreover, adults with allergy symptoms have a higher incidence of Irritable Bowel Syndrome (IBS), suggesting another link between allergic disorders and gut health. It showed that 34 percent of patients with irritable bowel syndrome have skin manifestations reiterating why you must consider the health of your gut health, especially when you are having skin problems. [5]

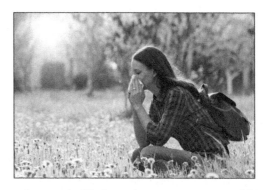

The Gut-Skin Axis is today a widely researched concept by researchers. It has been clinically proven that when the digestive balance is thrown off guard, -whether due to stress, poor sleep, issues with the microbiome, or lack of nutrients in your diet - the gut is likely to become overrun with harmful bacteria called dysbiosis. This also leads directly to skin-aggravating manifestations especially allergies and inflammation.

Getting enough sleep, having higher levels of melatonin, eating healthy fermented foods, and managing stress are some ways that could restore healthy and diverse gut flora and reverse these skin manifestations.

Melatonin and sun burns

We learned that melatonin supplementation, especially in the form of a liposomal or suppository could be just what you need to improve gut health. The benefits of melatonin to your skin have both a direct and indirect effect on your skin. The direct effect of melatonin is attributed to its anti-inflammatory and antioxidant effects. And the indirect effects could come from an improved microbiome, a stronger immune system, and better sleep, thus leading to more efficient repair processes.

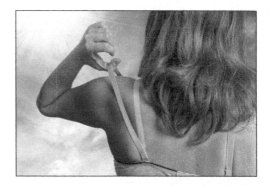

Speaking of repair processes, let's consider for a moment how prolonged sun exposure can play havoc with your skin and create oxidative stress that the body then subsequently needs to deal with

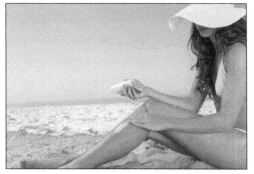

Prolonged skin exposure to the harsh sun rays causing sunburns can lead to redness, blisters, long-term dark or white patches, and wrinkles. In some cases, sun damage can be serious enough to trigger cancerous changes. This is one of the most common causes of a form of skin cancer called melanoma. You need to be careful but not too careful as you need UV exposure, we will discuss this later.

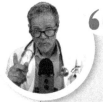

“

Here is what I recommended for supporting the microbiome:

Take a spore-based probiotic

Rotate probiotics as the diversity is as important as the quantity.

Eat plenty of fermented foods.

Take a spore-based probiotic.

Rotate probiotics as the diversity is as important as the quantity.

Eat plenty of fermented foods.

Cut down on simple carbohydrates as it supports the "bad"

bacteria in your gut.

Consider a carnivore diet and or a lectin-free diet to cut down on gut inflammation.

Consider a fast such as "Mito Fast" see MitoFast Fasting is "good" stress to the microbiome and supports healing of the gut lining. Taking high doses of melatonin post fast will greatly improve a strong bounce-back of the microbiome through swarming.

Do a food allergy panel like Doctors Data or Cyrex Labs and avoid IgG allergies for a month while doing a cleanse to support the gut lining to heal and strengthen.

Take a quality protein such as Collagen, Perfect Aminos, or Kion Amino's for building blocks to build healthy gut lining.

Do a parasite and candida cleanse by using broad-spectrum antimicrobial herbs for a month.

Do a sinus cleanse such as the one discussed on UltimatecellularReset.com/ sinuscleanse/ as the nasal passage (a filter) needs to be cleaned and serviced to prevent "bad" things from growing there. The bacteria that can colonize there can seed into your gut continuously and act as a primary source of gut issues.

Practice meditation and deep breathing to support vagal tone and your autonomics for improved nerve flow to your gut. Also, see Zen meditation mist at MitoZen.com for vagus nerve strengthening.

Do an extended fast such as with MitoFast for 3-5 days to stress the microbiome and activate a hermetic positive effect on your flora strains. Always follow this fast with a re-feeding strategy with melatonin, probiotics, and fermented foods.

Practice good sleep hygiene and supplement with melatonin to support swarming.

The Melatoninergic System

A study revealed that the melatoninergic system discovered in the epidermis could be a possible modulator for inflammation a nd healing. The cyclic nature of sunlight influences the activities of an area of the brain called the suprachiasmatic nucleus (central clock) which regulates melatonin production. Moreover, the peripheral tissues, such as the skin (peripheral clock), also contain this melatoninergic system.

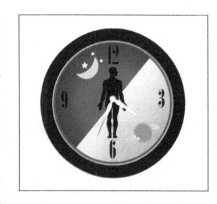

The shift in circadian rhythm caused due to the changes in the levels of melatonin during night and daytime is particularly evident in psoriatic patients. Interestingly, this study has also found that night-shift workers exhibit an increase in severity of the psoriatic flares, suggesting that the shift in the circadian rhythm linked to the lower levels of melatonin could be a risk factor for psoriasis. In such cases, sunlight, in the form of a narrow band UVB (Red Light Therapy) activating the melatoninergic system, might also be curative for the psoriatic skin! The melatoninergic system allows for the reprogramming of the body's central circadian clock through light exposure to the skin.[6]

The efficacy of Melatonin in the management of skin issues linked to sun exposure

One study 'Protective Effects of Melatonin on the Skin: Future Perspectives' published in the International Journal of Molecular Sciences in 2019 revealed that melatonin possesses the efficacy of fighting the damage to the delicate skin due to ultraviolet A and B rays in sunlight. This study showed that melatonin might suppress the production of reactive oxygen species in the skin and protect it against oxidative stress and inflammation. Let me explain how this action works and helps:[7]

The photoaging processes are initiated in the skin following excessive sun exposure by an increase in the production of reactive oxygen species (ROS). These reactive oxygen species, in turn, can lead to an activation of some pathways that trigger inflammation and

induce the activation of pro-inflammatory factors. This would worsen the inflammatory skin processes and cause activation of proteases like MMPs (matrix metalloproteinases), which can weaken the structure of your

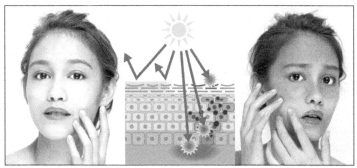

skin. Moreover, a gradual rise in the MMP expression is also proposed to be one of the mechanisms responsible for altering the elastic fiber network in the skin. Repetitive UV exposure can contribute to the activities of MMP due to which the elastic fiber network in your skin would be further hampered.

Melatonin could be highly effective in such cases for reversing these changes. This study showed that melatonin could suppress the production of ROS and consequently, reduce MMP-1 expression. It may also stimulate the repair processes in the skin allowing the skin to heal and regenerate faster.

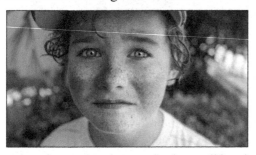

This is how melatonin could play a key role in protecting your skin against sun damage, by reversing oxidative stress and inflammation. This would also protect the skin against cancerous changes reducing your risk of melanoma.

But that's not all! The regenerative potential of the skin tissue also declines with aging due to the changes in the proliferation and differentiation of cells. So, when your age increases, your skin may no longer have the ability to repair and regenerate itself after sun exposure. This marks the importance of providing additional protection to your skin by using melatonin to support the natural repair processes.

Melatonin has also been shown to reduce water loss after UVB treatment. This just goes to show that melatonin might play a multitude of roles in protecting your skin against a wide range of effects of sun exposure including faster aging, cancer, and water loss. It could restore hydration of your skin keeping it soft and supple.[6]

Yes, we must take precautions to protect our skin against the sun by wearing long-sleeved clothes, using a wide-brimmed hat, and applying healthy sun protection, and at the same time get some exposure to our whole body and into our eyes, to be our healthiest! It's a catch 22, but similar to most things in life, balance is key.

Our skin makes vitamin D through sun exposure; therefore, total avoidance isn't a good idea. As long as you don't burn, you're ok to get sun without protection. In fact, 20-30 minutes of sun per day without any protection or sunglasses is a good idea. The best time to sunbathe would be before 11:00 am or after 3-4:00 pm so that you're avoiding the most intense sun's rays.

Ditch the shades and get out in the sun!

Believe it or not, when you wear your sunglasses, you're more likely to get burnt. This is because you trick your brain into not creating melanin, and melanin is what offers a protective action against the sun UV rays.

This concept has been proven during one study, 'The Protective Role of Melanin Against UV Damage in Human Skin' published in the Photochemistry and Photobiology in 2009. This study revealed that skin pigmentation brought about by melanin is the most important photoprotective factor. Melanin, besides acting as a broadband UV absorbent, also functions as an antioxidant and free radical scavenging agent.[8]

Melanin is primarily stimulated by the light that enters the eyes. This light is measured by the brain and tells your skin how much melanin to make based on the amount of light detected. It's a genius built-in sensor (supra the suprachiasmatic nucleus aka central clock) yet we make the mistake of always wearing sunglasses.

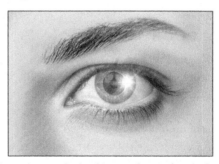

Try to avoid your sunglasses in the morning on your drive to work. Instead, allow the light to enter your eyes. If it feels too bright that's ok! It was like that for me when I first started doing this and it gets better once you retrain your eyes to deal with REAL light. I honestly never wear sunglasses while driving unless it's a long trip and try to not wear them most of the time. Not just for the melanin, but for more melatonin to get produced through the influences on the suprachiasmatic nucleus (central clock) regulates the melatonin production and light exposure to the peripheral tissues or skin (peripheral clock), in numerous ways.

Moreover, light exposure to the eyes strengthens the circadian rhythm, and it's made stronger when you're telling the brain its day and when it's night. It's about the natural rhythm that the light activates and making sure that it's supporting your healthy sleep and wake states. If you want to be more rested after a night's sleep, and more energetic, alert, and sharp during the day then you need to consider following these suggestions.

Melatonin might help kids with eczema to avoid sleep issues

Nowadays, we have kids on smartphones, tablets, and TVs for hours after the sun goes down. This paired with poor nutrition, EMF, and toxins in our environment is a headwind to the release of melatonin with our children. This is why, coincidentally, children with a skin condition called eczema often experience trouble sleeping.

A new study has suggested that melatonin might be helpful in such cases to boost their sleep. The study, 'Melatonin for Children with Eczema' was published in the online edition of the journal JAMA Pediatrics in 2016.[9]

Eczema, also referred to as atopic dermatitis, is characterized by recurring episodes of itching, redness of the skin, and rashes. It affects as many as 30% of children, more than half of whom develop sleep difficulties. These sleep problems could be more difficult to treat in children as compared to adults with similar problems because sleeping pills and anxiolytics are not safe in children.

Having said that it doesn't mean that the use of sedatives is a great idea for adults either. Yet with children, the risks of serious side effects and dependency are much higher than in adults, and in fact, most sedatives have contradictions for use in children.

What are better options for kids to help them sleep well?

Researchers have revealed that supplementation with melatonin could be a safer and more effective alternative for helping children with eczema to fall asleep faster and avoid other issues related to poor sleep hygiene such as academic performance and behavioral changes like irritability, impulsiveness, aggressiveness, and anger. Melatonin, being a natural human hormone without the risk of severe adverse effects, seemed like a good choice for children with eczema, which is what prompted researchers to study its effects in detail.

This study was conducted to assess the safety and efficacy of melatonin supplementation in 48 children between the ages of 22 months to 18 years. The children received melatonin treatment at bedtime for 4 weeks. The results showed that the children who took melatonin not only slept better but also experienced reduced severity of eczema symptoms. Moreover, it was also observed that the kids who were treated with melatonin fell asleep nearly 21 minutes earlier than the kids who were given a placebo. In fact, the total nightly sleep in the melatonin group increased by an average of 10 minutes, while it reduced by 20 minutes in kids who were treated with a placebo. This study ultimately provided greater insights into the safety and efficacy of melatonin not just for the management of sleep issues but also for chronic skin conditions like eczema.

While the study was primarily focused on checking whether melatonin supplementation could be advisable for kids with sleep issues, as an added benefit, it also opened the doors for assessing its use for relieving the signs of eczema. The research results indicated that melatonin could be useful for kids, as well as adults, who suffer from atopic dermatitis not just for improving their sleep but also for reducing annoying symptoms like itching, redness, and rashes.[10]

For patients with eczema, sleep disturbances are commonly known to affect the quality of life, and m has demonstrated powerful anti-inflammatory effects. To evaluate its efficacy in reducing the severity of eczema (and, the resulting sleep disturbances), researchers conducted one randomized study in patients who had at least 5 percent of their body surface affected by this condition, with subsequent documented sleep problems.

The study, 'Melatonin and Atopy: Role in Atopic Dermatitis and Asthma' was published in the International Journal of Molecular Sciences in 2014. It showed that the immuno-regulatory action of melatonin could be effective in the management of allergic diseases.

This study was based on the concept that the abnormal activation of the immune system in patients with eczema could lead to excessive free radical production, which might also be associated with reduced melatonin secretion and depressed activities of other antioxidant enzymes, as is the case in several other inflammatory diseases.

Several skin disorders, including eczema, are accompanied by the activation and infiltration of mast cells that release pro-inflammatory and vasoactive mediators. There is experimental data suggesting that melatonin supplementation might inhibit the development of atopic eczema by reducing the level of total IgE antibodies and proinflammatory mediators like interleukins. In these cases, melatonin would regulate and influence the immune response. This role of melatonin supplementation as an immunomodulatory agent could be effective in the management of atopic eczema and help patients derive significant relief from the symptoms in a safe and effective manner.[11]

Furthermore, the safety of melatonin, our miracle molecule, has been confirmed in asthmatic patients, and perhaps someday doctors might consider its routine use in bronchial asthma.

Melatonin may have important immunostimulatory actions in allergic diseases, in addition to its well-known antioxidant and cytoprotective effects in several inflammatory conditions. The activation of the immune system leads to free radical production, which is associated with decreased melatonin levels and depressed antioxidant enzyme activities in several inflammatory diseases. Many skin disorders, including atopic dermatitis, are accompanied by infiltration and activation of mast cells, which release vasoactive and proinflammatory mediators.

Allergic asthma is a condition characterized by bronchial hyperresponsiveness and the presence of IgE antibodies in response to inhaled allergens; often there are also enhanced total serum IgE levels. Melatonin could, however, act as a pro-inflammatory agent in asthma, leading to bronchial constriction. The safety of melatonin as a sleep-inducing agent has been confirmed in asthmatic subjects, but its routine use is not recommended in bronchial asthma.[12]

Can melatonin help to manage the symptoms of psoriasis?

Melatonin may affect the morbidities that lead to the development of psoriasis by producing an anti-inflammatory and immunomodulatory effect. Psoriasis is a common skin condition that causes the skin cells to build up and form white silvery scales. This condition is also marked by intense itchiness of the skin and dryness. This condition is believed to be an immune system problem. The common triggers include infections, mental stress, and cold exposure. While the most common symptom of Psoriasis is rashes on the skin, sometimes the rash may involve the joints and nails. This indicates that psoriasis could be linked to widespread internal disruptions in the body that affect tissues other than just the skin. From my experience, normally always a gut connection in these cases.

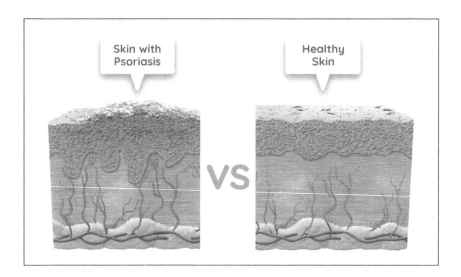

This is why treatment needs to be on a deeper and more comprehensive level. Working on the body at the cellular level so that the underlying anomalies affecting the immune system and sleep issues are corrected. Yet, the immunoregulatory properties of melatonin have been found to be effective in this regard.

One study has revealed how melatonin acts when administered to patients with immunological diseases affecting the skin like psoriasis. This study, 'Exploring the Physiological Link between Psoriasis and Mood Disorders' published in the Dermatology Research And Practices in 2015 revealed that the anti-inflammatory properties of melatonin could play a key role in reversing the pathologies responsible for causing Psoriasis.

This study is based on the concept that inflammatory cytokines are not the only biomarkers that link depression and psoriasis. Depression may also be associated with the disruption in the secretion of melatonin. By reducing the levels of pro-inflammatory substances like TNF-, IL-8, and IL-6, melatonin might attenuate the severity of inflammatory disorders like psoriasis. This study further noted that melatonin dysregulation is common in patients with Psoriasis Vulgaris.

The disruptions in the cyclic secretion of melatonin would contribute to the skin inflammation observed in patients with Psoriasis. Moreover, nighttime melatonin levels are also found to be significantly lower in people with psoriasis.

It's also interesting to note that in patients with depression, reduced melatonin levels coupled with the dysfunctional circadian rhythm might affect the secretion of the melanocyte-stimulating hormone that is linked to a high risk of seborrhea and psoriasis. We also see this with cases with CIRS due to mold exposure and these conditions are typically linked.

This suggests that supplementing with this miracle molecule might provide patients with adequate relief from the symptoms of psoriasis by addressing the underlying problem and not just treating symptoms.

Deep sleep and regeneration of tissues and skin health

Deep sleep is linked to faster and more efficient regeneration of the body's tissues. Remember we discussed earlier, that as you age, your skin loses its elasticity? It is because the production of collagen and elastin reduces as age increases. Now with aging, even the skin cells begin to degenerate at a faster rate than new cells can regenerate. And this is why, despite the body's best efforts, the skin starts looking 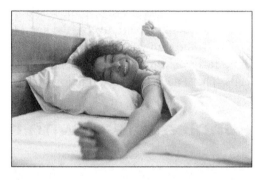 older and older. I also told you earlier that one of the best ways to boost your skin health and achieve that vibrant glow, even during older age, is to use melatonin. Why?

Because melatonin has the potential to act both directly and indirectly on your skin and stimulate the regeneration of new cells as well as new collagen and elastin.

I came across one research study that shows melatonin can support regeneration in the skin and several other tissues of the body. The study, 'Tissue regeneration: Impact of sleep on stem cell regenerative capacity' was published in the Life Sciences un in 2018. It showed that the circadian rhythm of the body orchestrates several cellular functions, including metabolism, cell division, cell migration, and intracellular biological processes through how much melatonin the cells receive. The physiological changes occurring in your body during sleep are believed to promote the perfect microenvironment suitable for the proliferation, migration, and differentiation of the stem cells.

While we slumber, our body repairs tissues, cleans out metabolic wastes, and heals DNA that has suffered inflammation and oxidative stress. Every cell in our body is repaired and restored in some way while we are sleeping. Also, new cells and tissues are created from stem cells and these cells are then used as a scaffolding for forming new tissue that can replace the old skin damaged by aging and all the stresses from the preceding days and weeks.

These effects are mediated directly by the circadian clock genes, as well as indirectly by hormones like melatonin and cortisol. For instance, when your body is exposed to darkness in the late evening hours, the melatonin secretion would be enhanced allowing the stem cells to be activated to replace all necessary cells.

A new study, 'Circadian Rhythm, and the Skin: A Review of the Literature' published in the Journal of Clinical and Aesthetic Dermatology in 2019 demonstrated how sleep can promote tissue repair and a regenerative process. That mechanism works primarily through melatonin. Before we fall asleep, our body begins producing a high level of melatonin, which signals the production of messenger molecules that can activate circadian genes promoting tissue regeneration. That's not all, melatonin also lowers our body temperature, which in turn, causes our metabolic activity to become slower to allow more of the available energy to be channelized into the repair processes.[13]

This correlation between melatonin and the circadian rhythm, and its effects on tissue regeneration in the skin matrix could provide us answers to how we can slow down or at least reverse some of the effects of aging.

What these studies suggest, is that the ability of melatonin to promote sleep and reset the circadian rhythm could reverse the age clock of your skin by stimulating it to regenerate new cells through your own stem cells. So, if you sleep well, your skin is going to regenerate faster and produce new cells that can replace the dead, damaged, or degenerated cells. These new cells would help your skin look younger, firmer, and more youthful.

Supplementing with melatonin for gut health

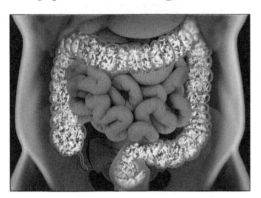

Can improving your skin by taking melatonin really be that simple? And how much melatonin should you take for good signaling and gut health?

I would offer that the melatonin necessary for sleep is much lower than levels needed for gut health. In fact, I often tell my patients that we are not giving you melatonin just for sleep with the super physiological dosing. Seeing as gut melatonin is 400 times higher than the amount released in the brain through the pineal gland, it makes sense to use much higher levels than what we use for sleep. Also, consider the large intestines as the primary location for your microbiome, and that unless you have SIBO, you should have zero bacteria growing in your small intestines. That means the melatonin within the large intestines or colon is what can move the needle most on a healthy microbiome.

This is what brings us to suppositories and the benefit of administering melatonin directly to this area. Keep in mind studies show oral melatonin dosing is only 2.5% absorbed, so using it in an alternative route of delivery can be more beneficial for this reason.

Next, I feel liposomal delivery can be a great route for those who would prefer an oral option. We have had some cases where we used both due to the delivery to both the upper and lower GI tract. Dosing of 100-200 mg and even higher can be both safe and effective for improving the gut-sleep-skin axis. It may not be necessary to do this high-level dosing for long periods and can be alternated for days, weeks, or months at a time to create a positive internal change that can improve even the worst of skin conditions.

Melatonin can also be applied directly to the skin in a cream. This can be done before bedtime or throughout the day. Even though some melatonin will be absorbed systemically through the transdermal route, melatonin used while in the presence of natural light will not generally lead to tiredness. I have found using a melatonin-based cream on my face and body to be one of the most effective strategies I've encountered both personally, as well as with many patients. Nevertheless, for individuals with poor gut health, high-level dosing with liposomal and/or suppositories should be the primary options.

Conclusion

It is clear that melatonin can be incredibly helpful for skin health.

When one takes care of their inner health it is expressed in the outer layers of health as well. That's why melatonin works so well because it supports so many aspects of inner health and vitality, which ultimately show with improved skin. Moreover, melatonin also serves to protect the skin from oxidative stress.

There is also a benefit to applying melatonin as a cream directly to the skin's surface. MitoZen.com will be introducing a product called Mitoskin in the near future, which's going to be a combination of some of the most powerful antioxidants as well as absorbable melatonin.

I have been personally utilizing this on my own skin and trialing on close friends and family with spectacular results. I've also found that supplementing with melatonin has prevented me from burning and instead manage to acquire a nice tan. All my life I have gotten terrible burns, even after being in the sun for 30 or 45 minutes. Now, I can be out in the sun virtually all day and still not burn due to melatonin's protecting abilities. Please see MitoZen.com for our face cream called MitoSkin which is a melatonin, peptide, apocynin based face cream.

Reference

1.   Rusanova I, Martínez-Ruiz L, Florido J, Rodríguez-Santana C, Guerra-Librero A, Acuña-Castroviejo D, Escames G. Protective Effects of Melatonin on the Skin: Future Perspectives. Int J Mol Sci. 2019 Oct 8;20(19):4948. doi: 10.3390/ijms20194948. PMID: 31597233; PMCID: PMC6802208.

2.   NIH Human Microbiome Project defines normal bacterial makeup of the body | National Institutes of Health (NIH)

3.   The Microbiome | The Nutrition Source | Harvard T.H. Chan School of Public Health

4.   Byrd, A., Belkaid, Y. & Segre, J. The human skin microbiome. *Nat Rev Microbiol* **16**, 143–155 (2018). https://doi.org/10.1038/nrmicro.2017.157

5.   Rush University Medical Center. "Allergic Disease Linked To Irritable Bowel Syndrome." ScienceDaily. ScienceDaily, 31 January 2008. <www.sciencedaily.com/releases/2008/01/080130170325.htm>.

6.   Damiani, G., Bragazzi, N. L., McCormick, T. S., Pigatto, P., Leone, S., Pacifico, A., Tiodorovic, D., Di Franco, S., Alfieri, A., & Fiore, M. (2020). Gut microbiota and nutrient interactions with skin in psoriasis: A comprehensive review of animal and human studies. *World journal of clinical cases*, 8(6), 1002–1012. https://doi.org/10.12998/wjcc.v8.i6.1002

7.   Rusanova I, Martínez-Ruiz L, Florido J, Rodríguez-Santana C, Guerra-Librero A, Acuña-Castroviejo D, Escames G. Protective Effects of Melatonin on the Skin: Future Perspectives. Int J Mol Sci. 2019 Oct 8;20(19):4948. doi: 10.3390/ijms20194948. PMID: 31597233; PMCID: PMC6802208.

8.   Brenner, M., & Hearing, V. J. (2008). The protective role of melanin against UV damage in human skin. *Photochemistry and photobiology*, *84*(3), 539–549. https://doi.org/10.1111/j.1751-1097.2007.00226.x

9.   Melatonin for Children with Eczema (jwatch.org)

10. Yung-Sen Chang, M.D., M.P.H., attending physician, department of pediatrics, Taipei City Hospital Renai Branch, Taiwan; Lawrence Eichenfield, M.D., chief and professor, pediatric and adolescent dermatology, University of California, San Diego and Rady Children's Hospital, San Diego; Nov. 16, 2015, *JAMA Pediatrics*, online

11. Marseglia, L., D'Angelo, G., Manti, S., Salpietro, C., Arrigo, T., Barberi, I., Reiter, R. J., & Gitto, E. (2014). Melatonin and atopy: role in atopic dermatitis and asthma. *International journal of molecular sciences*, *15*(8), 13482–13493. https://doi.org/10.3390/ijms150813482

12. Marseglia, L., D'Angelo, G., Manti, S., Salpietro, C., Arrigo, T., Barberi, I., Reiter, R. J., & Gitto, E. (2014). Melatonin and atopy: role in atopic dermatitis and asthma. *International journal of molecular sciences*, *15*(8), 13482–13493. https://doi.org/10.3390/ijms150813482

13. Lyons, A. B., Moy, L., Moy, R., & Tung, R. (2019). Circadian Rhythm and the Skin: A Review of the Literature. *The Journal of clinical and aesthetic dermatology*, *12*(9), 42–45.

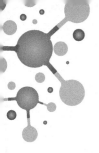

14

MELATONIN, EMF & MELATONIN DISRUPTORS

EMF, Light Pollution & Drugs That Deplete Melatonin

Melatonin is just as useful for our body as it is vulnerable to the effect of adverse factors like EMF, "melatonin toxic" substances, and light pollution. When vitality and overcoming disease are the priority of your life, it becomes equally important for you to protect your melatonin.

Melatonin is produced in your pineal gland, the cells in your gut, and each and every cell in your body to deal with stress, and therefore it's important to consider a method to protect it against "Melatonin Toxic Factors". These melatonin toxic factors are known to cause immense damage to your health simply by depleting your melatonin and robbing you of your primary stress protection and restorative sleep.

Let's take a deep dive into "Melatonin Toxic Factors" and explore what they are and how we can make changes in our lives to improve melatonin, vitality, life span, and overcome diseases.

What are melatonin toxic factors?

If you have trouble with sleep or find yourself at the receiving end of infections just too frequently or are suffering from one of many diseases linked to inflammation or oxidative stress, you might consider melatonin as a supplement. Melatonin is secreted in the pineal gland and all cells of the body in adequate amounts. This is the body's own natural way of enhancing its stress defense mechanisms. But, this melatonin, though produced in adequate amounts, may simply get depleted, used up, or destroyed if you are not careful enough.

Sometimes, your pineal gland just may not produce enough melatonin. This can occur if your lifestyle and habits do not allow this gland to function optimally. In short, it all

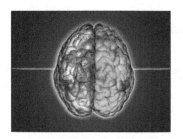

depends on how you work toward improving the melatonin levels and preventing the depletion linked to reduced secretion and increased usage.

Meaning that you need to be aware of these factors first so that you can adopt measures to protect yourself against them. Here are some of the main toxic factors that we'll be discussing throughout this chapter:

- Light pollution (avoiding blue and green lights after sunset)
- EMF (Electromagnetic Pollution)
- Drugs (melatonin Toxic drugs)
- Food and Nutrients (natural substances that are Melatonin toxic)
- Sleep habits and environment (body temp, bed, pillow.
- Dietary and Dinner time factors (foods that are melatonin toxic & eating too late)
- Sleep Drugs that prevent deep and REM

Too much artificial light can reduce melatonin secretion

We are in a new era where we have multiple artificial light sources bombarding our retinas 24/7 that simulate the effects of natural light and influence an active "wake" response, thus decreasing your production of melatonin in the same way natural sunlight would do. Natural sunlight in the morning and during the day is the most powerful signal to building up melatonin, and darkness is the primary signal to releasing this molecule so that it can exercise its function by helping you with cellular stress, chronic infections, cancer, toxins like heavy metals, regeneration of your body, and a healthy brain and nervous system. For instance, if you have typical lights in your bedroom, you're getting lots of blue and green within that white light. This will confuse your nervous system into thinking that it is still the daytime, and it will release hormones such as cortisol that will ramp up your wakefulness. Your eyes can't tell the difference between artificial lights and natural lights.

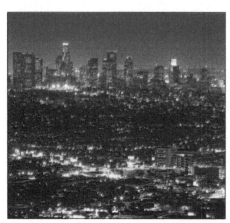

Therefore, if the lighting arrangement in your house is too bright, the rays entering the eyes will send signals to your brain indicating it is still daytime, when, in reality, it is nighttime. This would disrupt the circadian rhythm and melatonin secretion

Exposure to these lights creates a sense of alertness in the brain, encouraging it to modify the body's functions and hormonal signaling in a way that's favorable for you during the daytime, however, this is catastrophic toward sleep and melatonin release.

Modifying the lighting arrangement in your house, especially in the areas where you spend time during the evening becomes an especially important melatonin enhancing strategy. For example, I would advise you to have red lights in your bedroom so that when you go to bed, your brain would be signaled to get ready for sleep according to the reduced exposure to the blue and green light spectrum, thus signaling the secretion of melatonin to be normally released as it would ideally happen during the nighttime.

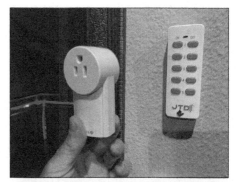

Another "melatonin must" may be to place dimmer switches around the house, so that you can dim the lights during evening hours when you're not doing any form of activity that requires brightness. Companies also make Bluetooth-enabled lights that you can control from your phone! How convenient right?

The dimmers are not the best alternative though, red-light lamps are, as I have found for my own home. What I have done is purchased cheap remote control plug outlets adaptors. You can get these online at Amazon.com for $20-30. While you're online get yourself some red-light bulbs as well to go into your lamps. Lamo are easy to find at Lowes or home depot. See the images here of my own home and how I set my home up for nighttime lighting. See the red rope light that I have attached with plastic ties to the railings both inside and outside of my house, so I don't have to be exposed to bright light after the sun goes down. This protects my circadian rhythm and natural melatonin production

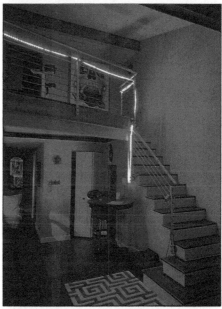

If your bedroom lights are too bright, when you go to sleep, these light rays would enter your eyes and reach the retina where signals will be sent to the brain to shut down the melatonin production. Once melatonin production declines, you will find yourself feeling more alert without any feeling of sleepiness. Without adequate levels of melatonin secreted in your brain, you

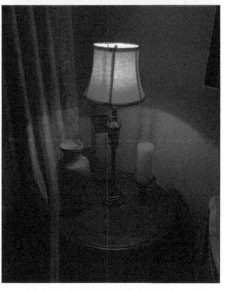

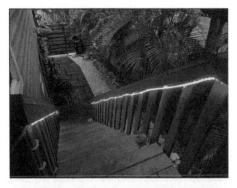

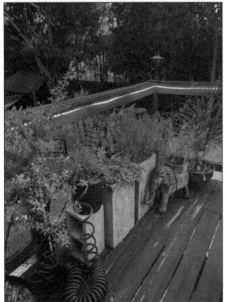

will have difficulty falling asleep. This high-lights the remarkable effects the bright lights vs dim lights create on the melatonin levels in your body

Now, let's talk about technology and how it affects your melatonin.

Technology Pollution:

Although technology is supposed to be helpful, and in many ways is, it is also dangerous. This is more so the case when it comes to the latest technologically advanced. that allow us to have access to a whole entire world of information, right at our fingertips. I'm talking about smart-phones, computers, laptops, smart TVs, and everything else in between. These technologies or commodities have revolutionized our lives in so many ways, but they've most definitely caught our health and priorities off guard.

These gadgets are harmful primarily due to the blue light they emit. This blue light can do much more damage to your melatonin levels. If you haven't heard of blue light, let me first introduce you to what it is and how it affects your melatonin and sleep.

I came across research that was published in Molecular Vision in 2016 which highlights the effects of blue light quite well. This study, 'Effects of blue light on the circadian system and eye physiology' was aimed at assessing the impact of light-emitting diodes (LEDs) on sleep and melatonin secretion. This study also analyzed the effect of blue light on the body's internal biological clock called the circadian rhythm by interfering with the phys-iology of the eyes.

Ultimately, the study concluded that LEDs that have been commonly used to provide illumination in domestic, commercial, and industrial environments can hamper melatonin secretion significantly. LEDs are also used in computers, televisions, smartphones, lap-tops, and tablets. The light emitted by these LEDs often appears white to us, yet, the truth is that LEDs have a peak emission range of blue light (400 to 490 nm), and this is the reason why they are called blue light.

The accumulating evidence has indicated that the exposure of the body to blue light can affect several physiologic functions, by inducing photoreceptor damage. This is the rea-son why it is important to consider and analyze the spectral output of the LED-based light sources to avoid the dangers associated with blue light exposure.

This study demonstrated that blue light from smartphones, television screens, and laptops emitted in the range of 460 to 480 nm can do significant damage to our sleep pattern by reducing melatonin secretion and causing disruption in the circadian rhythm.

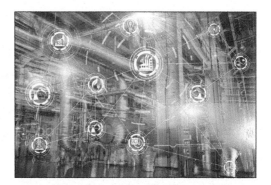

As I mentioned earlier the exposure to bright lights in your living room and bedroom during late evening hours could prevent you from sleeping well. These light rays can enter the eyes and suppress melatonin secretion by signaling the brain that it is daytime.

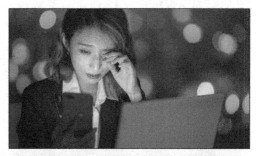

But the impact of blue light from electronic gadgets like smartphones is much higher than the effects of these bright lights. It's not uncommon for adult men and women and even children to stay glued to their smartphones for different purposes during the evening hours. Some of you may be using smartphones to check out the latest news and some might be just watching videos and movies on the OTT platforms. In children, it is commonly observed that they spend a lot of time playing games on smartphones, laptops, or tablets before bedtime. Whereas teenagers are likely to spend their

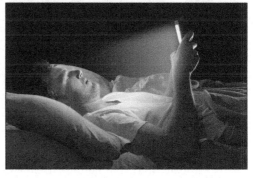

time catching up with friends and chatting with them on social media platforms. These activities can increase your exposure to blue light at a time of the day when you should ideally be shutting down your exposure to ANY form of screen-based technology.

These habits can cause a sharp decline in the production of melatonin in the pineal gland as it is primarily determined by the amount of exposure to light and affected by the day-night cycle of the earth. As a result, you will not only have trouble sleeping but also be deprived of the natural antioxidant, anti-inflammatory, and immunity-boosting benefits of this sleep hormone.

Consistent with these results, it was also found that in older people, acute or short-term exposure to blue light could significantly decrease their alertness and suppress their sleep and melatonin production more severely as compared to the younger people.

The decline in melatonin secretion in elderly individuals might worsen inflammation and oxidative stress in the brain tissues putting them at risk of degenerative diseases like Alzheimer's and Parkinson's. This also explains why they might experience a lower level of alertness when they use smartphones during nighttime. The blue light from these devices can reduce the efficiency of brain functions and trigger faster cognitive decline due to which their memory, attention span, focus, and ability to stay alert are affected. This is another very important reason why everyone, including older people, should minimize the use of devices that release blue light.[1]

Let me reveal a few more ways by which blue light can affect your health and increase your risk of diseases.

Top health risks of blue light:

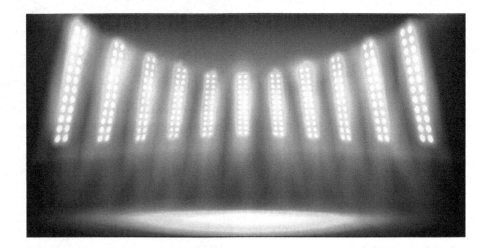

- **Insomnia**

  I already told you that blue light exposure, especially at night, can lower the secretion of melatonin, which controls your sleep-wake cycles. The brighter the light and the longer the time of exposure, the lesser would be the melatonin secreted in your brain. Needless to say, the lowered production of melatonin would contribute to the risk of insomnia because of which you will find yourself staying awake for several hours even after you have switched off your smartphones, ultimately feeling sleep deprived and unrefreshed!

- **Stress and depression**

  This duo of mental health diseases could be right around the corner waiting for you if you're not careful and take steps to minimize your exposure to blue light in the evening and at night. The exposure to blue lights could lower melatonin levels causing stimulation of the release of the stress hormone called cortisol in the nervous system. This hormone is already infamous for making us feel stressed out even without any apparent reason. Cortisol would make you prone to anxiety disorders and even depression. So, it could be more mental health issues for you if you're not serious about reducing your exposure to blue light!

- **Weight gain**

  If you're trying to lose weight, blue light could create obstacles for you. I say this because I recently came across an interesting study, 'Night shift work at specific age ranges and chronic disease risk factors' that has specifically shown how blue light contributes to obesity and prevents weight loss.[2]

  Exposure to blue light could reduce melatonin secretion in your brain and create imbalances in the levels of hunger hormones, such as ghrelin and leptin, thus enabling unwanted weight gain. The decline in melatonin production and the disruptions in the levels of ghrelin and leptin could increase your hunger, slow down fat burning, and reduce calorie use by your body. As a result, you could find losing weight much harder, or nearly impossible. Additionally, exposure to blue light may also increase your BMI, waist circumference, and height ratios.

- **Increases diabetes risk**

  Exposure to blue light could further worsen your risk of diabetes and diabetic complications, both directly and indirectly. Blue light could raise your risk of diabetes by affecting carbohydrate metabolism. It might further prevent the efficient utilization of sugars from foods and keep your blood glucose levels higher making you more dependent on insulin injections and oral anti-diabetes drugs.

  Blue light may also create disturbances in your blood sugar levels by preventing the optimum secretion of melatonin. The reduced melatonin levels could affect the synthesis of insulin in the pancreas. At the same time, it may also worsen insulin resistance. Both effects could cause you to have persistently elevated blood sugar levels putting you at risk of diabetes and more serious complications of this disease.

- **Affects cardiac functions**

  Blue light might even affect the functions of vital organs like the heart and brain. Blue light could disrupt your sleep affecting the internal biological clock of your body. This could put muscle cells of the heart out of sync increasing your risk of cardiac diseases, such as myocardial infarction (heart attacks), and cardiomyopathies (enlargement of the walls of the heart).

  The cardiac functions would also be hampered due to the loss of melatonin. The reduced melatonin secretion following blue light exposure would result in the decline in the amount of energy received by the cardiac muscles making them less efficient. This would reduce the efficiency of the heart and prevent it from pumping out enough blood during each contraction. This effect of reduced melatonin on the heart functions can affect the health of your heart, as well as other vital organs like the brain, kidneys, and gut leading to serious implications. This could be easily avoided by protecting your melatonin by reducing your use of smartphones and laptops at night.

- **Affect your eyesight**

  Exposure to blue light, specifically at night might contribute to vision loss, by triggering the development of macular degeneration. It may bring about the destruction of cells in the retina. The blue light entering your eyes may also trigger inflammation of the delicate retina. The retina is the surface or a mirror on which the image of what is there in front of you is formed. The damage to retinal tissues could affect your eyesight and increase your risk of macular degeneration.

  The reduced melatonin level caused due to exposure to blue light may also increase your risk of another eye disorder called glaucoma. In patients with glaucoma, the functional cells in the retina tend to become susceptible to the damage caused by blue light causing a faster worsening of the condition.

  Moreover, if you have had cataract surgery recently, you have one more reason to protect your melatonin levels against the effect of blue light. Watching television and using smartphones should be strictly avoided for a few days or weeks after cataract surgery, to enable the tissues of the eyes to heal completely. Exposure to blue light from electronic gadgets might slow down recovery after cataract surgery, putting you at the risk of postoperative complications.

  These are just some of the many negative health effects of blue light. You can protect your melatonin levels by minimizing your use of these gadgets, especially after evening hours and at night.

How to protect your melatonin from the harmful effect of blue light?

Now that you have realized how dangerous blue light can be, you must be worried thinking about how to keep yourself safe and protected from it. Here are some tips that would help you safeguard your melatonin from exposure to blue light:

- Avoid extended exposure to artificial lights after evening hours and sunset by closing the curtains and shades to block the streetlights.
- Use dimmer lights or set up red light lamps throughout your house after dinner to lower the light exposure.
- 'Power Down' and avoid the use of electronic gadgets at least 2 hours before bedtime, and that includes your smartphones and laptops too.

How does the electromagnetic field interfere with melatonin secretion?

Electromagnetic field or EMF is another culprit responsible for causing depletion in the levels of melatonin secreted in your body. The dangers of EMFS are just as severe as those caused by blue light emission from electronic gadgets. But before we jump into the negative effects of EMFs, let us first find out what exactly EMF means.

What are electromagnetic fields?

Electromagnetic fields refer to the combination of invisible magnetic and electric fields of forces that exist in our surrounding atmosphere. These forces are generated by natural phenomena such as the Earth's magnetic field and also by human activities, primarily through the use of electricity. Power lines, mobile phones, and computer screens are some examples of equipment that generate and emit electromagnetic fields.

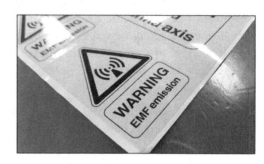

Some of the man-made electromagnetic fields can reverse their directions at a regular interval of time. The frequencies of these fields may range from extremely high radio frequencies, as in the case of mobile phones, intermediate frequencies from computer screens, or extremely low frequencies that are generated by power lines

The term static is used to refer to the fields whose frequencies do not alter with time. They usually have an incredibly low frequency. Static magnetic fields are commonly used in medical imaging tests and are generated by appliances that use a direct current. This information goes on to indicate how difficult it is for us to avoid exposure to electromagnetic fields and can therefore develop related complications due to continual bombardment.

After an in-depth review of various scientific reports, it is obvious that there exists a close link between exposure to electromagnetic fields and the risk of adverse health effects.

Let's take a look at how EMFs could affect your melatonin levels and why it is necessary to protect yourself against these invisible forces:

A comparative study, 'Pineal melatonin level disruption in humans due to electromagnetic fields and ICNIRP limits' published in the Radiation Protection Dosimetry in 2013 has revealed that the exposure to EMF could be highly counterproductive for the melatonin levels secreted in the pineal gland.[3]

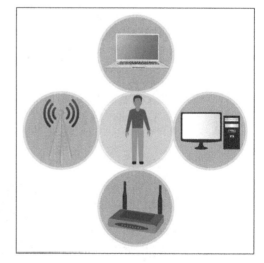

This study recognized the classification of electromagnetic fields as possibly carcinogenic agents for humans by the IARC (International Agency for Research on Cancer). IARC issued a warning indicating the potential of EMFs to transform normal cells into cancerous cells. Also, owing to the higher utilization of electricity in our day-to-day life, exposure to EMF with a power frequency in the range of 50 to 60 Hz could be unavoidable.

This study was aimed at assessing whether exposure to EMF could affect melatonin levels and worsen the likelihood of developing cancers further. The finding of this research concluded that man-made EMFs might influence the functions of the pineal gland. The pineal gland is likely to sense or perceive the EMFs as light, and consequently, it may be encouraged to stop melatonin production. This incorrect perception of EMFs by the pineal gland is considered to be a major factor responsible for the decline in the production of melatonin.

In this review, more than 100 experimental data points from animal and human studies assessing the changes in the melatonin levels following exposure to the power-frequency magnetic and electric fields were analyzed. The results were compared with the maximum limit recommended by the ICNIRP (International Committee of Non-Ionizing Radiation Protection). Moreover, a comparison of the results was made with the findings of existing experimental studies to assess the biological effects of magnetic fields to quantify the severity of complications.

The results have drawn attention to the importance of limiting exposure to EMFs. The observations made by this study were consistent with that of earlier research conducted to evaluate the effects of EMF on cancer risk and melatonin production.

It was further confirmed at a later date that varying degrees of disruptions in melatonin secretion may occur due to the exposure to EMFs of weak frequencies. And this may possibly lead to more severe long-term health effects in humans.[3]

Look at the penetration of EMF into the brain when one uses a cell phone. The penetration is well within the range to be affecting the pineal gland. This can have detrimental effects on melatonin which affects the overall circadian rhythm. It seems children are more susceptible to this than older adults.

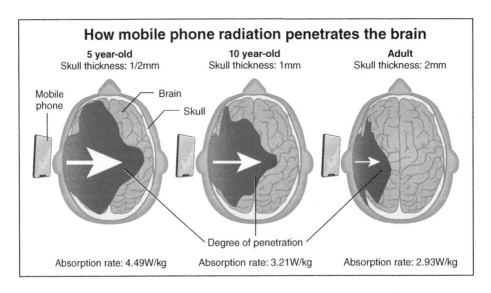

How mobile phone radiation penetrates the brain

5 year-old
Skull thickness: 1/2mm

10 year-old
Skull thickness: 1mm

Adult
Skull thickness: 2mm

Mobile phone — Brain

— Skull

Degree of penetration

Absorption rate: 4.49W/kg   Absorption rate: 3.21W/kg   Absorption rate: 2.93W/kg

Protecting yourself at night while you sleep form EMF

Using a carbon-based paint in your bedroom is one option to minimize the EMF exposure while you sleep which could protect your melatonin as well as other harmful effects of EMF exposure. I painted my bedroom while we were remodeling it whereas even before the flooring went in the carbon paint was coated around all of the walls and floors. I find it hard to get a good signal in my bedroom which is sometimes inconvenient, but it is an inconvenience I am willing to live with knowing how harmful EMFs are to our health. Keep in mind if you do this that you want to minimize the use of your cell phone within the space as the radiation coming off of your phone or ricochet and bounce around the room a bit more than typical. I still occasionally use my phone in my bedroom however I am putting it on airplane mode before bed every night. Like many people I use my cell phone as my alarm clock, so it sits next to my bed. Putting your phone on airplane mode at night is important of course unless there is some sort of need for you to be communicated with. For instance, some people need to leave their phone on in case their children might call late in the evening if there was some emergency. Outside of that I think the phone should be turned off.

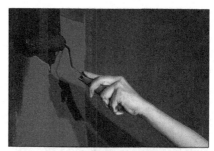

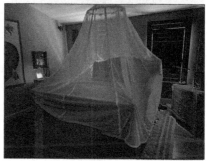

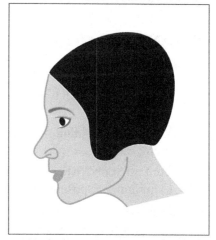

There are companies that make clothing that protects and shields from EMF. They also produce cabs that might be important to shield your brain and pineal gland in particular. This might be a viable option for some people especially at night. If you were exposed to a lot of EMS during the day, then these could be something to consider as well but I feel that nighttime is probably the most important where we should be shielding and protecting ourselves from these harmful microwaves.

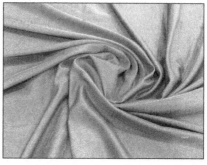

How to properly set up your bedroom for maximum melatonin and sleep quality.

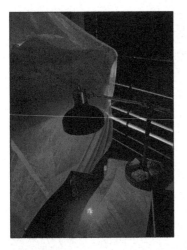

Look at the image here of my bedroom showing a lamp with a red-light bulb and remote control are located where I can reach it from in my bed. The remote controls all the lights in the bedroom and down my stairs to the living room. find the remote controls to be helpful so I can simply lean over and turn them off when I'm ready to go to sleep. Also, the red lamp that I could reach from my bed is nice so that I could turn it on and off by hand and see my way to the bathroom late at night. This way I don't have to turn on any bright lights containing blue or green colors which will tell my brain that it is morning which will interrupt my sleep and melatonin production.

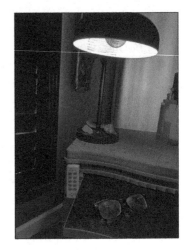

Important points to consider for EMF protection at night.

- If you use your cell phone as an alarm clock, then turn it on airplane mode at night.
- I'm sort of shielding such as a carbon-based paint for your bedroom or a silver lining canopy.
- Turn off your Wi-Fi router at night. Consider the placement of your Wi-Fi router to minimize exposure as well.
- Be careful of electronics that might be around your bed that he met a Wi-Fi signal. An example is CPAP machines or other electronic gadgets now have Wi-Fi continuously being admitted.
- Don't wear any EMF admitting wearable devices such as the new watches from Apple. If possible, turn them on airplane mode if you're using them for tracking sleep.
- Consider EMF shielding clothing and caps that will protect at night while you're sleeping.

Should you avoid sunlight completely to protect your melatonin?

So far, we've discussed how you can avoid exposure to bright lights in order to protect your melatonin levels. But protecting your melatonin is a bit tricky. It is not as simple as just avoiding exposure to bright lights or EMFs. The negative effect of bright light on melatonin production is limited to the late evening hours or nighttime. So, it would be very wrong to assume that you need to avoid sunlight completely. In fact, 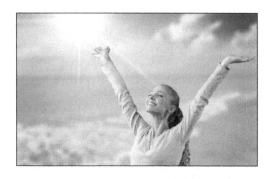 doing so might put you at a risk for other health issues like vitamin D deficiency. So, ultimately this all comes down to how to regulate your exposure to sunlight so that it is neither too high nor too low.

To increase your melatonin naturally, your body requires a certain amount of sunlight. This is because sunlight can stimulate the secretion of another hormone called serotonin, which is a precursor of melatonin. After sunset, the leftover serotonin could be converted into melatonin, which is why you need to have ample exposure to sunlight during the day-time to make sure enough serotonin is created to support the production of melatonin later.

Sunlight exposure may also stimulate the secretion of cortisol that could keep you awake during the daytime so that by the time night approaches, your body would circle back to the phase of sleep and start stimulating melatonin once again.

All these mechanisms involved in the secretion of melatonin, serotonin, and cortisol occur in a cyclical manner depending on the day-night phases created by the earth's rotation. Let me explain this with the help of a study that has beautifully described the importance of sunlight for maintaining health.

This study, "Benefits of Sunlight: A Bright Spot for Human Health' was published in the Environmental Health Perspectives in 2008. The purpose of this study was to establish the importance of exposure to sunlight for maintaining bodily functions and bust the common misconception that sun rays are harmful to our health. Moreover, this study was also focused on revealing both the sides of sunlight exposure - the advantages as well as the disadvantages - so that people can make the right decisions about how much exposure to sunlight is necessary. This approach is expected to help us derive the benefits of sun exposure without experiencing any adverse complications like sunburns and skin cancers.

This study is based on the fact that humans are diurnal creatures, programmed to be outdoors when the sun is shining and at home in bed during the night. This is the reason why melatonin production begins when it becomes dark and stops upon the optic exposure to the bright daylight. This pineal hormone is considered the key pacesetter for most of the body's activities related to the circadian rhythm. Furthermore, the same study also confirmed that the diurnal variation in the levels of melatonin also plays a key role in countering cancer, inflammation, infections, and auto-immunity.

When our body is exposed to sunlight or bright artificial lights in the morning, the nocturnal melatonin production in the evening tends to occur a bit sooner. This can allow us to enter into a deep phase of sleep more easily once we hit the bed.

Melatonin secretion also shows seasonal variations that could be relative to the availability of sunlight, with the hormone being produced for a longer duration of time in the winter months as compared to that in the summer. The melatonin secretion phase advancement caused by the exposure to bright sunlight in the morning could be effective against insomnia, seasonal affective disorder (SAD), and premenstrual syndrome.

The secretion of serotonin, which is a melatonin precursor, is also affected by the exposure to daylight. Serotonin is normally produced during the daytime and is converted to melatonin later when it becomes dark. High melatonin levels usually correspond to longer nights and shorter days, while a high serotonin level in the presence of melatonin usually reflects shorter nights and longer days indicating longer exposure to UV radiation. Also, moderately high levels of serotonin might lead to an improvement in moods allowing you to stay calm yet focused.

Therefore; seasonal affective disorder is commonly linked to lower serotonin levels during the daytime as well as with the phase delay in the melatonin production during the nighttime.

The study concluded that our skin can also produce serotonin and convert it into melatonin and that several types of skin cells have receptors for both melatonin and serotonin. This suggests exposure to sunlight is essential for the production of serotonin.

Our modern-day penchant for indoor activities and staying up past dusk could reduce nocturnal melatonin production, taking our sleep-wake cycle far away from being healthy and robust. Also, the sunlight our body can receive from being outside on summer days is much brighter than what we are likely to experience by being indoors. For this reason, it's important for people working indoors to get outside periodically. This can have a major positive impact on the melatonin rhythms and result in improvements in sleep pattern, mood, energy, and overall sleep quality.

Moreover, people in jobs that prevent them from having adequate sunlight exposure can use full-spectrum lighting to stimulate serotonin secretion. Going shades-free while in the sunlight, even for just 10 to 15 minutes, could confer significant health benefits.[4]

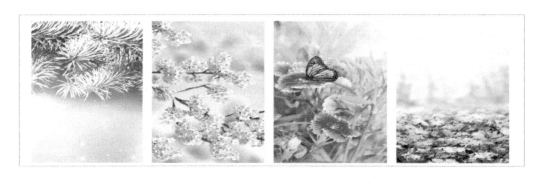

Seasonal changes & melatonin

Seasonal change is another factor that can affect your melatonin levels. During the fall and winter, there is less light. So, your body will naturally produce a high level of melatonin.

At some point or another, you must have experienced how hard it is to get out of bed during the cold winter months. Don't worry, we've all had those days!

But, interestingly enough, it's not just the cold that makes you feel like staying in bed for longer. This is where melatonin comes into the picture. The increased secretion of melatonin makes you feel sleepy causing you to curl up in bed until late in the morning hours. Now you can explain away those lazy days without feeling guilty, right? But, as the season changes, your body might have a harder time adjusting to the change in the levels of sunlight exposure. For example, as spring and summer approach, you might find yourself staying awake for several hours at night without any desire to sleep. This may happen due to the decline in the secretion of melatonin during the bright spring and summer days.

The increase in your body's exposure to sunlight, which is not only brighter but also shines for longer, would dip your melatonin levels sharply. As it is bright and sunny outside until late in the evening, your brain won't send signals to the pineal gland to start secreting melatonin. As a result, the time of the secretion of melatonin would also be delayed. So, instead of, say at 4 pm or 5 pm on winter days, your body will start secreting melatonin at about 6 pm to 7 pm on summer days.

Our bodies will need time to adjust to the new routine based on the reduced sunlight exposure during the daytime of this season. So, even after the winter or fall begins, you'll notice how you're unable to sleep well, at least for a few days. Later, as your body gets attuned to the reduced exposure to the brightness during the daytime or the reduced duration of the daylight availability, it will start producing more melatonin. Studies aimed at checking the impact of different seasons and their effect on melatonin levels have confirmed these findings. One study, 'Melatonin and seasonal rhythms' published in the Journal of Biological Rhythms in 1997 has helped to analyze the change in the secretion of melatonin in the pineal gland due to seasonal variations.

According to this study, the seasonal changes in the lengths of the nightfall (scotoperiod) can induce a parallel or proportional change in the duration of the secretion of melatonin. This study has shown that when the duration of nighttime increases, as happens during winters and fall, there is also a rise in the duration for which melatonin is secreted in the pineal gland. The increased duration for which the body is exposed to the darkness due to the late sunrise and early sunset during these seasons allows the body to secrete more melatonin.

These variations in the duration of nocturnal melatonin secretions, in turn, might trigger a seasonal change in your behavior. It is primarily found to affect your sleep-wake cycle.

Moreover, this study confirmed that the response of the RHP (retinohypothalamic-pineal) axis to bright light is highly conserved in our bodies. So, in a human body, the secretion of melatonin is interrupted when we are exposed to lights during the nocturnal phase of its secretion. This means in most individuals, the RHP axis can detect the change in the length of the nighttime, allowing the body to make a proportional adjustment in the duration of the nocturnal secretion of melatonin. This is why you will find each person responding to the change of season in a different manner. While one person may find it too difficult to fall asleep during the initial days of the summer months, some people may be able to adjust to the change of season with ease.

This variation in the response could be attributed to the body's ability to improve the duration and amount of melatonin secretion in spite of a limited or reduced amount of darkness the body is exposed to. So, even when the sunlight is bright, the body can regulate the response of the RHP axis so that the secretion of melatonin in the pineal gland is restored. This can allow the person to sleep well even during the summer months.

Moreover, the RHP axis also helps to regulate the production of the type of melatonin messages that the body can use to trigger the seasonal change in behavior of a person in terms of the circadian rhythm. This has been shown in naturalistic research, in which the melatonin profiles of a group of participants were compared in winter and summer, and even in experimental research in which the melatonin profile was compared after long-term exposure to the varying duration of artificial "nights".

These studies revealed that individuals living in a modern urban environment tend to differ in the degree or extent to which the intrinsic duration of the secretion of melatonin can respond to the seasonal change in the duration of the solar night. The duration was measured based on the exposure of the body to constant dim light. It was found that the change in the intrinsic duration of the production of melatonin that is induced by the change in the scotoperiod can be significantly correlated with the change in the intrinsic timing of the offset of the secretion of this hormone in the morning and is weakly correlated with the change in the intrinsic timing of the onset of its secretion in the evening.

This finding has suggested that the differences in the ways in which an individual is exposed to the morning light in different seasons could affect his responsiveness to the change in the duration of experimental or natural scotoperiods. So, as the duration of the nighttime or darkness changes when the season transitions from the summer to the winter or vice versa, the body would modify the secretion of melatonin both in the morning and evening to adjust to the reduced or increased duration of the nighttime.

Nevertheless, the response of everyone to the change in the melatonin secretion and the subsequent response to adjust the melatonin levels may be different.

This indicates that the human RHP axis is clearly capable of detecting the change in the length of the nighttime. But the body may take a variable time to adjust to the change in the season, and until it's attuned to the new season, the person may continue to experience the same sleep-wake cycle that he was used to before the transition into the new season.[5]

The point here is the melatonin levels are bound to change - both increase or decrease - each time the weather changes. But your body will take its own time to adjust to the change in the amount of exposure. Meaning, it might take you about a week or two to start getting better sleep as your body starts producing more melatonin when the season changes from summer to winter.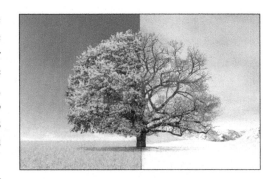

The problem here is that it isn't possible for us to avoid the change of season. If you are struggling with sleep issues or want to have your melatonin levels improved to enhance your body's ability to fight inflammation or oxidative stress, there is little you can do to stop the seasons from changing. If this is something that's bothering you, then the answer is simple. You may not be able to change the weather, but you can definitely trick your body into believing it's the winter season by simply reducing your sunlight exposure after the late evening hours. If you suffer from insomnia, my advice is to avoid going outdoors in the evening hours. It's best for you to stay indoors after evening hours as this is where you can manage the lighting arrangements so that your body is not exposed to bright lights. Moreover, I normally advise my patients to use dark shades for their windows. That way, after say, 5 or 6 pm, you can pull down the shades so that the bright light from outside, whether sunlight or streetlights, doesn't enter your house.

The reduced exposure to lights, even when there is bright sunlight outside, will help your body produce good amounts of melatonin. So, when you hit the bed, your pineal gland would have secreted enough melatonin allowing you to rest peacefully. Lastly, there's one more thing you can do in the summer months to protect your melatonin levels, and that is to minimize your use of smartphones and laptops. We already discussed the reasons why these gadgets are not good for your melatonin production. The blue light from these gadgets can prevent your brain from sending signals to the pineal gland to start secreting melatonin. This effect could be more severe in the summer months. Therefore, as the season changes from winter to summer, it's time for you to further minimize your use of smartphones, laptops, and similar tech that has bright screens.

To sum things up:

Seasonal changes require you to switch up your routine so that the effect of change in light exposure does not have any adverse impact on the melatonin secreted in your pineal gland. You may find it difficult to follow the tips laid out in this chapter in the beginning. But, once you get a hang of it, you'll know exactly what you need to do for a smooth seasonal transition.

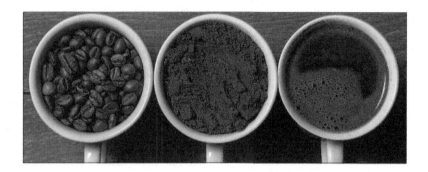

Too Much Caffeine

This probably will not come as a surprise to most of you because we already know that caffeine is a stimulant, and it can prevent us from sleeping well. You've most likely heard doctors advising patients to limit their intake of coffee to ensure they can get some sound sleep.

Not only does it provide a wake-promoting effect that we crave, but also makes us feel more alert and awake. This is why; coffee shops have become a place for business meetings and social gatherings making the beverage easily available for us at any time. Unfortunately, the easy availability of coffee has also made today's generation of young men and women sleep-deprived. In fact, the survey conducted by the National Coffee Association of the U.S.A. has found that nearly 83% of Americans drink coffee several times a day.

Moreover, an average cup of coffee contains anywhere from 50 to 560 mg of caffeine. And the grand-size cup of coffee often contains more than 300 mg of caffeine. The caffeine in coffee is quickly absorbed into the bloodstream. Coffee's half-life is about 3.5 to 5 hours as discovered by the sleep medicine researchers and in a study published in the journal of Sleep Medicine. Also, caffeine can start to affect our bodies quite quickly, in fact, it can reach the peak level in your blood in just 30 to 60 minutes of consumption.

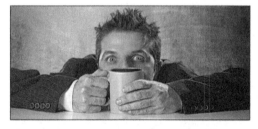

After drinking a cup of coffee, you can expect to stay wide awake for at least 5 hours or even more. This clearly means even if you have a cup of coffee at say 5 pm or 6 pm, you'll still experience difficulty sleeping if you go to bed around 9 or 10 pm.

But what most people don't know is that caffeine can also suppress melatonin secretion, which is actually why it can help people to stay awake up. Drinking coffee to refresh yourself in the morning or after a stressful meeting is fine. But, to drink a cup of coffee in the evening just to feel better is a strict no.

The mechanism of action of caffeine is the antagonism or inhibition of the activity of adenosine receptors in the central nervous system. Adenosine is a kind of sleep promoter.

It works by increasing melatonin secretion in the pineal gland. When you drink a cup of coffee, the caffeine in it blocks adenosine from binding to its receptor promoting wake-fulness. It is clear that this effect of caffeine could cause you to remain alert for several hours, and thus the overall quality and duration of your sleep would be affected.

Because even a cup of coffee would be enough to reduce your melatonin secretion. And this would not just keep you wide awake, but also prevent you from experiencing any of the other long lists of benefits that this sleep hormone has to offer. If you're curious to know what happens to your melatonin when you drink coffee, just read the next research example.

The study, 'The effects of coffee consumption on sleep and melatonin secretion' published in Sleep Medicine in 2002, specifically exam-ined the effects of caffeinated beverages on the quality of sleep, based primarily on how it affects melatonin secretion.

Melatonin secretion is regulated by neu-rotransmitters, which can be affected by the excessive consumption of caffeine. In the first part of this study, 6 volunteers were asked to drink either regular coffee or decaffein-ated in a double-blind manner. This idea was to not get influenced or prejudiced due to being aware of what they drank.

Later, after 7 days, they were asked to drink the alternate beverage. The sleep parameters of these participants were assessed with the help of actigraphy. The urine samples of these participants were assessed every 3 hours for the quantitation of 6-SMT (6-sulfatoxymel-atonin), which is the main metabolite of melatonin passed in the urine. In the 2nd part of the research, it was found that the subjects, who drank either regular coffee or decaffein-ated beverage, had differences in the amounts of 6-SMT in the urine.

The results of this study indicated that drinking caffeinated coffee caused a sharp decline in the total duration of sleep and the quality of sleep, compared to drinking the decaffein-ated beverage. There was also an increase in the duration of sleep induction in participants who drank coffee, as compared to those who drank decaffeinated coffee. The caffeinated drink caused a decline in the excretion of 6-SMT in the urine throughout the next night.

These results have confirmed the widely held belief that the consumption of coffee can interfere with the quantity and quality of sleep. In addition, it was also found that the intake of caffeine can decrease the 6-SMT excretion. This suggests that people who suffer from sleep issues should strictly avoid caffeinated beverages during the evening hours.

Conclusion

Melatonin plays an important role in the protection of the pineal gland and the chemistry involved in melatonin release.

I think some of the easiest lifestyle changes to make are the ones described in this chap-ter, such as setting your house up with red light lamps and remote controls and using blue-blocking sunglasses when the sun goes down while you're watching TV or looking at your cellphone or computer screen. Turning the brightness down on your computer and cell phone screen is also important in addition to the blue glasses. I only wish we could turn the brightness down on our television sets, but it does not seem like this technology has caught up with our health needs quite yet.

Try to minimize the EMFs at your home office by using old fashion wires to connect and keep your cell phone away from you and off of your body, especially when you're not using it. Another easy thing to consider is turning off your Wi-Fi router at night. Moreover, there are lots of exciting new products being brought to market, such as carbon-based paint as well as silver-lined canopies that can be used to protect you from harmful EMFs while you sleep.

Most importantly, go out and get sun during the daytime without sunglasses and avoid artificial light at night to improve your circadian rhythm and melatonin release. We live in such a stressful high-tech environment which includes light and EMF pollution, among other stressors, that have negative effects on our melatonin production.

Even with all the lifestyle changes described in this chapter, it is obvious that supplementing with melatonin makes sense, as just the aging process itself and having birthdays is enough to produce massive declines in melatonin. When you stack those natural age declines on top of all of these other subsequent stressors you start to set the stage for a lot of the diseases we are seeing in our technologically advanced and industrialized world.

Reference

1. Tosini, G., Ferguson, I., & Tsubota, K. (2016). Effects of blue light on the circadian system and eye physiology. *Molecular vision*, *22*, 61–72.

2. Ramin, C., Devore, E. E., Wang, W., Pierre-Paul, J., Wegrzyn, L. R., & Schernhammer, E. S. (2015). Night shift work at specific age ranges and chronic disease risk factors. *Occupational and environmental medicine*, *72*(2), 100–107. https://doi.org/10.1136/oemed-2014-102292

3. Malka N. Halgamuge, Pineal melatonin level disruption in humans due to electromagnetic fields and ICNIRP limits, *Radiation Protection Dosimetry*, Volume 154, Issue 4, May 2013, Pages 405–416, https://doi.org/10.1093/rpd/ncs255

4. Mead M. N. (2008). Benefits of sunlight: a bright spot for human health. *Environmental health perspectives*, *116*(4), A160–A167. https://doi.org/10.1289/ehp.116-a160

5. Wehr TA. Melatonin and seasonal rhythms. J Biol Rhythms. 1997 Dec;12(6):518-27. doi: 10.1177/074873049701200605. PMID: 9406025.

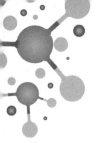

15

MELATONIN FOR CHILDREN

Autism, ADHD, Infections & Behavior

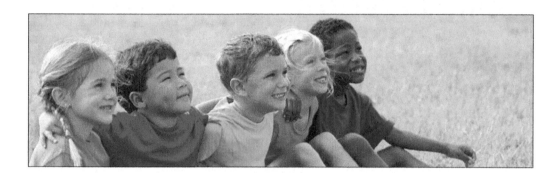

My own "Pain to Purpose" story.

I have a special connection with this chapter as I feel if melatonin were given to me as a child, it would have been beneficial in more than one way.

After being expelled from two schools I was placed into special education classes and diagnosed with ADHD and dyslexia. I remember my mother crying while speaking with the administrator as we both sat around the conference table as they told her there were no other options available for me. We lived in Hawaii at the time and little did I know I was about to be placed into classes with kids much worse off than I was.

I endured these special education classes until I was taken out by my parents just before high school. The system still wanted me in these classes, but I had plenty enough of being teased and looked down upon by the other kids in the "normal' classes.

Obviously, things worked out well for me over time and I believe those challenges lead me to become the person I am today. They say strong winds lead to strong timber. My strong winds were not the ADHD, nor the dyslexia…really. My problems would be revealed to me over time as 2 main contributing factors. Both issues I now feel melatonin would have helped. These two factors were in fact, severe food allergies and exposure to neurotoxins.

When I was in my 20's I found out that I was allergic to gluten and dairy, and when I stopped consuming them it was like a miracle for me and my brain. Over the years voiding them has improved my energy and ability to focus greatly. Now when I consume either of these food's I go into a zombie state with severe brain fog. Most likely this was why I couldn't sit still and learn when I was younger. No wonder I had ADHD! Food sensitivities are considered "inflammatory stresses" as the immune system is seeing gluten and dairy as a foreign invader, like an infection. This inflammation is due to a bad gut (leaky gut and poor microbiome) which causes the immune reaction. The allergen would have then caused inflammation throughout my body, and in particular, to the brain, leading to enhancement of the ADHD challenges.

Refer back to chapters 5 & 11 for how this works and how melatonin can support the gut, allergies, and immune system.

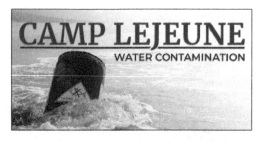

Besides the allergies, I also was born and raised for my first 2 years of life on Camp Lejeune in the early 70's, which at the time was the epicenter of the worst environmental toxic water contamination in US history. The contamination primarily included perchloroethylene (PCE), trichloroethylene (TCE), dichloroethylene (DCE), vinyl chloride, and benzene. Very nasty chemicals that settled into my central nervous system.

Much has now been learned about how these chemicals can cause cancer as well as challenge the developing nervous system. My father has recently been diagnosed with Leukemia, my mother has developed debilitating arthritis, and both parents have auto-immune thyroid conditions. It's difficult to say how much this exposure has affected my own nervous system, but hard to rule out the possibility that it contributed to my ADHD and Dyslexia. It could have been that the effects to my nervous system led to the poor gut function, and then that subsequently led to the food allergies. You see it's not the symptom that is usually the problem, it's usually deeper and involves an underlying breakdown in the proper function of the body.

Although I've done lots to clear these toxins from my system over the years, I now know that I would have greatly benefited from melatonin during this toxic exposure. You see melatonin has been shown in studies to protect the brain during various toxic exposures, such as heavy metals and harmful drugs like amphetamines. If only my parents knew about the miracle molecule when I was growing up, maybe things would have been much different for us all?

If you're a parent and you have kids with these challenges you now have this powerful knowledge. I feel like my past challenges or my *"Pain to Purpose"* story has led me to discover answers to these problems that I am passing on to you so that you and your children won't have to suffer the same way I did.

So how do we gain our circadian rhythm in utero and as babies?

When we are young, we rely on our mother to provide the signaling to our circadian rhythm through the hormones in her breast milk or even placental transfer. This important function of entrainment to the light/dark cycle becomes fully functional by 3 months of age. [1] Entrainment may also be important for development, seeing as a mother whose sleep is not disturbed by a baby on a different circadian rhythm will improve her caregiving

and low melatonin production in mothers of some autistic children.[2]

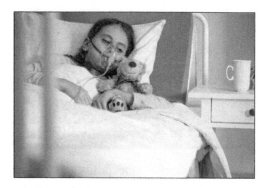

The benefits of melatonin are certainly not limited to adults. Many people are surprised to hear melatonin supplementation can also be of benefit for children, as there are times when various stresses can have adverse effects neurologically and cause a decline in their melatonin levels. There are also times when pulsing higher doses of melatonin can support things like the immune system during an infection, heavy metal toxicity, mold exposure, respiratory diseases, and any child who might suffer from sleep disorders or learning and behavioral disorders due to the reduced melatonin levels.

Melatonin can be effective for the management of health issues in children and there are a few conditions that have been scientifically studied, which we'll be diving further into throughout this chapter.

Severe respiratory distress syndrome

Studies have revealed that melatonin could be effective for relieving the symptoms of severe respiratory distress syndrome in premature infants. The ability of melatonin to support immunomodulation, along with its anti-oxidation action would reduce swelling and inflammation in the respiratory passages. This can help to improve breathing in infants.

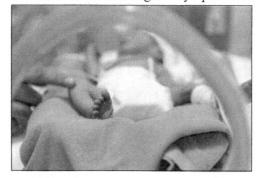

Additionally, the inhibition of the pro-inflammatory mediators or cytokines through the melatonin mechanisms (discussed in chapter 5 & 6) can be of benefit to severe respiratory distress syndrome, especially in premature infants.

I came across one study, 'Melatonin in bacterial and viral infections with a focus on sepsis: a review' published in Recent Patents on Endocrine, Metabolic, and Immune Drug Discovery in 2012. This study shows that melatonin could be effective in fighting various viral and bacterial infections in the respiratory system in children. The administration of melatonin supplements has been shown to control chlamydial infections, and the infective conditions induced by Mycobacterium tuberculosis.

The specific mechanisms of the antimicrobial action of melatonin are discussed in detail in chapter 5 and 6, so if you need to review, please do that now. But if you want the short version here it is:

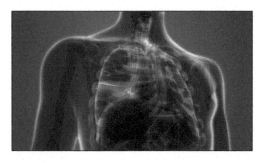

Inflammation runs wild due to out-of-control oxidation. Melatonin has a powerful antioxidant or inhibitory effect on free radical formation. This molecule is normally produced in the energy-producing units in each cell, yet mitochondria and infections can shunt this energy to 10% of what is normally created from oxygen and glucose. This lack of energy to the immune cells causes it to decrease the ability to fight the infection which then causes the inflammation to run wild. This is called a cytokine storm. It goes even deeper in the lungs as melatonin can also slow the duplication of bacteria and viruses, thereby, preventing faster growth and multiplication of microorganisms within the respiratory tissue. Meaning, that it would render the bacteria and viruses unable to survive thus causing the infection to clear within a shorter period.

Besides, melatonin may also be effective in the management of sepsis in newborns and premature infants. This effect has been demonstrated in several animal models, showing the action of melatonin supplementation in septic shock. The protective action of melatonin against sepsis has been attributed to its antioxidant and immunomodulating properties, as well as its inhibitory effect against the activation and production of pro-inflammatory mediators. Basically, this means that melatonin helps to calm down the cytokine storm and allows the immune cells to work harder.

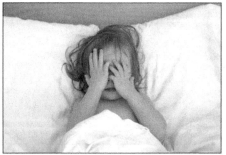

The results of this study have provided evidence linking the use of melatonin to faster improvement in premature infants diagnosed with severe respiratory distress syndrome or septic shock. Furthermore, melatonin also offers great therapeutic potential in the treatment of multi-organ failure associated with septic shock in critically ill patients.[3]

This research clearly demonstrates that melatonin can be beneficial for children and infants born prematurely. Why then is melatonin not used regularly for these conditions? And why has the public not been informed about it while lives are being lost due to the massive stressors, we now deal with that suppress melatonin?

ADHD & Autism related sleep disorders

Other pediatric conditions that have benefited from melatonin supplementation include sleep disorders of various origins, autism spectrum disorders, and epilepsy, including febrile seizures. One study, 'Clinical uses of melatonin in pediatrics' published in the International Journal of Pediatrics in 2011 revealed some amazing results in the use case of melatonin when administered to children.

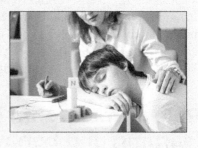

> ## Dr John's Comment:
>
> *My suggestion would be to give kids, who suffer from an inability to fall asleep, lower doses such as 3-20 mg about 2-4 hours before their bedtime. Disturbed sleep at night might also be helped with melatonin in this same dosing schedule or even higher such as 20-60 mg. Of course, this is meant to be only a guide and not a substitute for medical advice, as you should always consult your doctor before starting any supplement*

This study has analyzed the results of several clinical trials aimed at assessing the effects of melatonin supplementation in children, focused mostly on a variety of kinds of sleep disorders.

Melatonin was found to be beneficial for the treatment of dyssomnias, particularly delayed sleep phase syndrome. This means children who suffer from different forms of sleep problems, such as inability to fall asleep and disturbed sleep at night, would be able to enjoy a sound and undisturbed sleep routine following melatonin supplementation. It would also prevent the delayed sleep phase syndrome, which means melatonin would help them fall asleep within a much shorter period once they hit the bed.

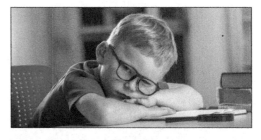

The benefits of melatonin are found to be pronounced in children who suffer from learning and behavioral disorders, like I did, such as attention-deficit hyperactivity (ADHD), and even autism spectrum disorders. The sleep disturbances associated with these conditions are linked to the imbalances in the psychological, emotional, and neurological disturbances. Melatonin could support the health and functions of the nervous system. Moreover, melatonin can further have a positive impact on the brain due to how metabolically sensitive it is. Kids have an incredible energy requirement as they are in growth and on top of that they also have many of the same stressors we have as adults. Melatonin can restore the normal functions of the brain by protecting the energy it needs.

Febrile seizures and epilepsy have also been found to be susceptible to treatment with melatonin. These supplements can be used alone or in combination with conventional anti-epileptic drugs. Melatonin would prevent the progression of brain damage in children with epilepsy and seizures, thus improving the quality of their life.

In newborns, particularly in those who are delivered preterm, supplementation with melatonin would reduce oxidative stress linked with asphyxia, sepsis, respiratory distress, and surgical distress. Moreover, the administration of melatonin to infants would help them adapt to the sleep-wake cycles of adults. It would improve their nocturnal sleep allowing them to set their circadian rhythm to that of adults, including their parents. This effect of melatonin could be of great relief to parents, especially first-time moms, and dads, who struggle to adapt to the sleep-wake cycle of the newborn baby, which is often not in sync with the day-night cycle of the earth.[4]

Role of melatonin in the management of learning and behavioral disorders

In recent years there has been a sharp spike in the incidence of learning and behavioral disorders like Autism and ADHD (Attention deficit hyperactivity disorders). We spoke earlier about entrainment which is an extremely important aspect of the development of the baby's circadian rhythm. A mother whose sleep is disturbed by a baby on a different circadian rhythm can cause issues to her ability to pass along the signaling for the development of the pineal gland and melatonin receptors being formed which create the baby's circadian rhythm. Supplementing the mother with melatonin might solve this issue. Most importantly, giving the mother melatonin during the third and fourth trimesters when the neonate's melatonin receptors begin to function.[5]

Studies aimed at assessing the therapeutic role of melatonin in the management of these conditions have exciting and amazing results.

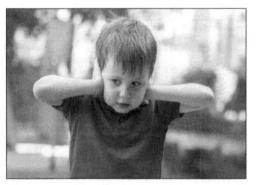

One study, 'Updated View on the Relation of the Pineal Gland to Autism Spectrum Disorders' published in the Frontiers in Endocrinol in 2019 has provided evidence linking the use of melatonin supplementation with improved performance of children with autism and ADHD.

This study is primarily focused on evaluating how the higher risk of autism could be associated with pineal gland malfunctioning. It is believed that the abnormal functioning of the pineal gland can result in the lower production of melatonin, due to which the development of autism could be triggered. This hypothesis is supported by observations revealing a low concentration of melatonin in children with autism. It was found that nearly 65% of children with autism have less than 50% of the average value of melatonin.

Also, sleeplessness has a higher prevalence of nearly 50 to 80% in autistic children, as compared to just 9 to 50% in normal children of the same age.

Moreover, studies have shown that exogenous supplementation with melatonin could be highly beneficial for reducing the time until the onset of sleep and improving sleep duration.

This means the treatment of autistic children with melatonin could enhance the quality and duration of their sleep while also reducing the time taken to fall asleep. This benefit of melatonin may also be effective in the management of other behavioral disorders like ADHD, which is marked by hyperactive and impulsive behaviors. The reduced sleep onset latency period brought about with the help of melatonin supplements could reduce the hyperactive behaviors of ADHD children and even improve their focus and attention span.

There is a strong genetic link to explain the benefits of melatonin in children with autism or ADHD. Genetically, the autism-linked mutations are usually found in the genes that encode the key enzymes for melatonin synthesis, such as AANAT (Arylalkylamine N-acetyltransferase), and ASMT (Acetylserotonin O-methyltransferase). The reduced expression of the genes encoding AANAT is also a characteristic finding in children with autism. These genetic abnormalities have been found even in the genes encoding the 2 melatonin receptors called MT1 and MT2.

This suggests that the higher incidence of autism in children with melatonin dysfunctions could be genetic in origin. One of the best ways to reverse the effects of these mutations is to improve melatonin levels in the brain, which could be achieved easily through the use of melatonin supplementation. It is advisable that parents speak to their health care providers about melatonin supplementation for children with learning and behavioral disorders.

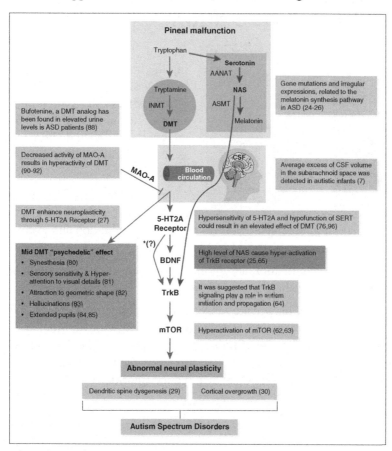

Besides, there is also the need to explore the link between melatonin, DMT, and autism. Because researchers have begun speculating on the possibility of the abnormal metabolism of N-dimethyltryptamine (DMT), from the pineal gland, causing aberrant neuroplasticity or abnormalities related to the neural connectivity in autistic patients. It has been previously suggested that the abnormal neural plasticity-like cortical overgrowth and dendritic spine dysgenesis are common neurological symptoms in children with autism. The abnormal activation of the mTOR (mammalian target of rapamycin) is proposed as the primary cause for the abnormal neurological development linked to autism. Fasting to inhibit mTOR might be worth considering in addition to melatonin. Moreover, it was also suggested that the disruptions in the activities of the BDNF (brain-derived neurotrophic factor) through TrkB (tyrosine kinase B) signaling pathways may play a role in the initiation and propagation of autism.

Interestingly, the disruptions in the synthesis of melatonin in children with autism have been found to be associated with a rise in the secretion of melatonin precursors, N-acetylserotonin (NAS), and serotonin. NAS works as an agonist for the TrkB receptors and so, in conjunction with serotonin, it can contribute to the abnormal plasticity of the neurons in autism.

The pineal gland can become non-functional and calcified due to fluoride in children

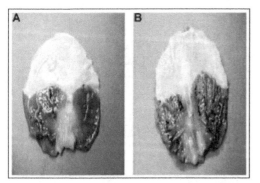

One of the defense mechanisms protecting the body against the effects of fluoride toxicity seems to be its deposition in calcified tissues. The symptoms of excessive fluoride accumulation in bones and teeth are known and well documented, classified as skeletal fluorosis and dental fluorosis, respectively

Calcium deposition into the pineal gland is like that found in bones. The process of calcium accumulation in the pineal gland is initiated in childhood and even in newborns.

Calcification is accompanied by a reduction in melatonin synthesis. Hence, the conclusion that pineal gland calcification has an indirect effect on the production and secretion of this hormone. The image here shows the severe calcification of the pineal.

Considering this science, it may make sense to limit fluoride intake by avoiding drinking most municipal water sources, which have been fortified with fluoride, as well as many conventional kinds of toothpastes. Furthermore, fluoride is also used in pesticides and some chemicals used to create non-stick compounds for pots and pans. Eating organic foods and avoiding processed foods can also reduce fluoride consumption.

> **Dr John's Comment:**
>
> I can't overstress the importance of pineal gland health, and the impact fluoride and calcification can have on melatonin production, especially in children. In fact, I've dedicated an entire chapter of this book (chapter 17) to the pineal gland because I firmly believe that this gland plays a vital role in our wellbeing and overall health.

Conclusion

Using melatonin supplementation with children might at first surprise many people, as it is unnecessary. Children require lots of melatonin, maybe much more than adults do as they are going through very high metabolic activities with growth.

There are multiple headwinds to kids producing their own melatonin to keep up with the demand the body requires to buffer stress. Some of these stressors include toxins, like when I was exposed to toxins in Camp Lejeune, our kids are now exposed to mercury in seafood and vaccines, pesticides, aluminum, and many other industrial chemicals and solvents. Melatonin would work to protect this delicate developing nervous system in this toxic world we live in.

Another big stressor to consider is light pollution. Kids are on their iPhones and iPads after the sunsets, which are preventing them from the normal sleep-wake cycle which will ultimately suppress melatonin production. Moreover, the electromagnetic stresses that we have today are much greater than at any other time in our history. It is unknown how severe the health risks will be with 5G, and yet our kids are bombarded with an onslaught of these potentially melatonin-killing invisible EMF stressors. Also consider the general stress level of many mothers in today's world, and how they are not training their kids for a normal circadian rhythm because they don't have a strong signal of their own to transfer. On top of all that, there are also genetic considerations.

What is the bottom-line regarding melatonin for children?

There probably was not a need for melatonin 50 or 100 years ago, however, in today's world it might be a necessary tool for parents, pediatricians, and alternative healthcare practitioners that work with children to consider.

One of my close colleagues and friend Dr. Dan Pompa works closely with children and performs detox protocols with them using products he's developed. We are collaborating with various protocols to safely detox many harmful substances from the nervous system in particular.

By using various binders and chelating agents, many afflictions we see with children can be improved by including some of these detox protocols. A multi-modal approach needs to be used with many conditions we see, specifically developmental and neurological problems with children.

These are some of my bullet points to consider:

- *Food Sensitivities and Gut Health.*
- *Chronic Infections (EBV, Lyme Mold)*
- *Environmental Toxins and Biotoxin Illness*
- *Poor Sleep Hygiene (light pollution)*
- *Lack of Proper Physical Activity and Brain Activation for brain development (See Disconnected Kids by Dr. Robert Melillo)*
- *EMF Exposure*
- *Cranial Bone Issues (See Functionalcranialrelease.com)*

I hope this chapter opens the eyes of parents to the incredibly long list of benefits that melatonin has to offer. I also really hope that this chapter helps kids to avoid the challenges I went through personally. My journey would have been much different if I were given melatonin as a child, but as I said earlier, my pain might have led to my purpose to learn what I can about health through my own personal journey. Melatonin has been a big part of my healing, even though it was somewhat "late to the party".

Reference

1. Lewy A. (2010). Clinical implications of the melatonin phase response curve. *The Journal of clinical endocrinology and metabolism*, *95*(7), 3158–3160. https://doi.org/10.1210/jc.2010-1031

2. Lewy A. (2010). Clinical implications of the melatonin phase response curve. *The Journal of clinical endocrinology and metabolism*, *95*(7), 3158–3160. https://doi.org/10.1210/jc.2010-1031

3. Srinivasan V, Mohamed M, Kato H. Melatonin in bacterial and viral infections with focus on sepsis: a review. Recent Pat Endocr Metab Immune Drug Discov. 2012 Jan;6(1):30-9. doi: 10.2174/187221412799015317. PMID: 22264213.

4. Sánchez-Barceló EJ, Mediavilla MD, Reiter RJ. Clinical uses of melatonin in pediatrics. Int J Pediatr. 2011;2011:892624. doi: 10.1155/2011/892624. Epub 2011 Jun 16. PMID: 21760817; PMCID: PMC3133850.

5. Lewy A. (2010). Clinical implications of the melatonin phase response curve. *The Journal of clinical endocrinology and metabolism*, *95*(7), 3158–3160. https://doi.org/10.1210/jc.2010-1031

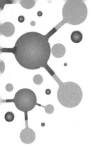

16

MELATONIN FOR DIABETES

We have discussed so many ways melatonin works to support energy through your mitochondria. When you look at various diseases like diabetes, which is a metabolic disorder dealing with energy, it's no surprise that our miracle molecule has shown to be effective in the management of diabetes both type 1 and 2. Besides supporting cellular energy, melatonin is important for the prevention of complications that are

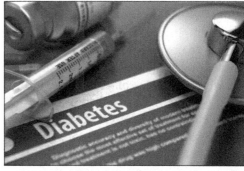

linked to the lack of sleep. Particularly poor sleep resulting from mental stress, hormonal imbalances, and immunological dysfunctions. It is surprising to note that type 2 diabetes is one of the major complications in people who suffer from insomnia. Insulin and melatonin are very intimately connected as we will dive into this science-rich chapter.

Melatonin lowers A1c

This study, 'Melatonin Use in Patients with Type 2 Diabetes and Insomnia' published in the Endocrine Web showed that melatonin supplementation cannot just help to improve the sleep pattern of patients with diabetes but also improve their glycemic control.

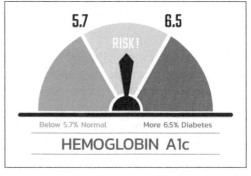

This study was conducted on 11 men and 25 women in a double-blind, randomized, crossover study design. The age of the participants was between 46 and 77 years. The study participants were treated with melatonin or a placebo for about three weeks during the 1st phase. This was followed by a one-week washout period, after which, the participants crossed over for 3 weeks of treatment with other preparations. This was the second phase of the research. All supplements were taken about 2 hours before bedtime for three weeks which might work best for lower melatonin dosing and is not necessary with supra physiological dosing schedules in my view.

During the extension period of 5 months, the study participants were administered melatonin in nightly doses. The sleep habits of these men and women were monitored objectively. The measures of certain markers for the assessment of glycemic control and inflammation were noted. The levels of the parameters measured at the baseline and also at the end of the study included fasting blood glucose, C-peptide, fructosamine, glycosylated hemoglobin (HbA1c), triglycerides, total cholesterol, high-density lipoprotein (HDL), and low-density lipoprotein (LDL) cholesterol, insulin, and some antioxidants.

Following about 5 months of melatonin use, it was noticed that the mean HbA1c was significantly lower in the test group as compared to the baseline. A significant improvement in the HbA1C levels was found in the patients suggesting that melatonin supplementation helped improve their diabetes control. There was a decline in the HbA1C level in patients who were treated with melatonin without any significant change in the HbA1C levels in the control group that was administered a placebo. The HbA1C level is considered one of the vital parameters of glycemic control in patients with diabetes. Having HbA1C levels within normal limits indicates a long-term improvement in the body's response to the treatment or other efforts like a change in the diet or lifestyle habits. HbA1C is believed to provide an average estimation of glycemic control over the past 3 months. The improvement in the HbA1C level in these patients has provided a strong foundation suggesting the efficacy of melatonin supplements for the management of diabetes.

The researchers concluded that the short-term use of melatonin might improve sleep maintenance in patients with type 2 diabetes and insomnia without interfering with the metabolism of glucose and lipids. But the long-term use of melatonin could produce a beneficial effect on the HbA1c levels, suggesting an improved glycemic control.[1]

What if diabetes is genetic? researchers have also discovered that increasing the levels of the sleep hormone melatonin through supplementation may reduce the ability of the insulin-producing cells in the pancreas to release insulin. Also, they have found that the effect could be stronger in patients who carry particular gene variants that are linked to a higher risk of type 2 diabetes.

These findings suggest the use of melatonin supplements could be helpful support in people having a genetic predisposition to developing diabetes. To begin with, it might seem to you that melatonin can make it worse for patients with diabetes to control their blood sugar levels as it reduces the ability of the tissues of the pancreas to release insulin. But this is not so. In fact, it can control how much insulin is released by the pancreas so that you can achieve optimum control over your blood sugar levels. And this is a highly unique effect of melatonin that is difficult or nearly impossible to achieve with any other treatment or drug. Trust me if Big Pharma could patent melatonin, it would be all over the news!

Patients who use melatonin supplements on a regular basis can achieve better control over their diabetes as this sleep hormone helps to regulate the secretion and release of insulin by your pancreas. It basically works by regulating the metabolic activities that are controlled by the body's circadian rhythm. The increased melatonin levels in the body ensure the various metabolic functions occurring in the body including the breakdown and absorption of sugars, production and release of insulin, and the production of *hunger hormones like ghrelin and leptin* are well controlled. This allows the body to regulate when and how much insulin is secreted in the body thereby improving glycemic control.

One consideration is if an individual was involved in intermittent fasting, they might find melatonin supplementation to help them fast through its insulin regulation, but also supporting hunger and cravings through ghrelin and leptin. Makes a good argument for melatonin during fasting programs like MitoFast.

These findings have been supported by one study that was recently published in the Hormone Molecular Biology and Clinical Investigation. This research, 'Hormone Molecular Biology and Clinical Investigation' explains the exact mechanism of action of melatonin that could help in the fight against type 1 and type 2 diabetes.[2]

According to the researchers who conducted this study, diabetes is commonly associated with the excessive production of free radicals during metabolic processes. The increased oxidative stress creates a state of imbalance between the body's natural antioxidants and free radicals. The excess free radicals can produce several harmful effects on the body's vital organs including the pancreas, resulting in cell death. It might reduce the ability of the pancreas to secrete insulin in the required amount in response to the increase in the levels of blood sugar. As a result, the elevated blood glucose level fails to fall, which should ideally have happened if insulin was released by the pancreas. This failure of the body to control the blood sugar levels as a part of its metabolic functioning can increase your risk of diabetes.

Moreover, melatonin might play a significant role in reducing oxidative stress by acting as an antioxidant. It is the body's own free radical scavenger that can attack and destroy the reactive oxygen species released during various metabolism processes because of which the damage to the cells of the pancreas is inhibited. This would restore the normal functions of the pancreas allowing this gland to start secreting insulin in adequate amounts to enable efficient glucose metabolism. This is how 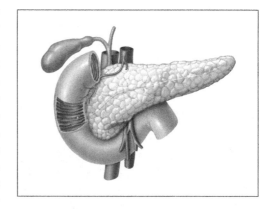 by using melatonin supplements, diabetes and its complications can be avoided.

Recall the mitochondria and the effect melatonin has on supporting that intracellular structure where energy is made? Well, this is the epicenter of where oxidation occurs and the cells in the pancreas are very metabolically active and when there is lots of energy being produced due to high energy demand you need lots of antioxidants to quench this process. This is where melatonin supports the pancreas and many other cells in your body. Melatonin may also stimulate the production of other antioxidants such as glutathione. These miracles of melatonin are one of the most effective natural anti-diabetic treatments people can choose in order to protect themselves against the risk of complications caused due to diabetes.[3] [4]

Why is melatonin considered the silent regulator of glucose homeostasis?

In human organisms, the circadian regulation for the metabolism of carbohydrates is essential for maintaining glucose homeostasis and ensuring optimum energy balance. An imbalance in glucose metabolism and insulin production has been linked to a variety of metabolic diseases including obesity, type 2 diabetes, metabolic syndrome, and cardiovascular diseases.

Melatonin, the pineal hormone, could serve as the key mediator molecule for integrating the cyclic environment and regulate the circadian distribution of the behavioral and physiological processes occurring in the body to promote the optimization of energy balance and blood glucose levels.

One study has reviewed the interplay between the modulatory physiological effects of melatonin on glucose homeostasis and the metabolic imbalance, from the endocrinological perspective.[5]

The remarkable effect of melatonin supplementation in the regulation of metabolic processes involved in the breakdown of glucose can be observed from the chronobiological perspective, considering this hormone to be a major synchronizer for maintaining the internal circadian order of the physiological processes occurring during energy generation.

This study, "Melatonin: A Silent Regulator of the Glucose Homeostasis" was conducted and published recently in 2017 with an aim to evaluate the role of melatonin as a natural molecule that can support carbohydrate metabolism in the body. Let us have a look at the findings of this study and what it has revealed about the functional synergism between melatonin and insulin.

Synergy between insulin & melatonin

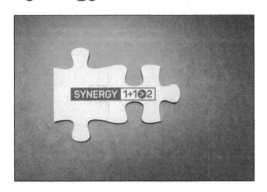

The scientific literature has stated that the first experimental injections of pineal extracts had led to hypoglycemia, indicating that the extracts might increase glucose tolerance, and support muscular and hepatic glycogenesis. In other words, if the extract mimics an active pineal and if the pineal is active such as at night while melatonin is high there is metabolic where you would expect better glucose regulation and tolerance.

The metabolic disruptions caused due to the absence of melatonin in patients with a pinealectomized state are characterized by the presence of a diabetogenic syndrome that can be depicted by reduced glucose tolerance as well as insulin resistance. Both of these states tend to be expressed peripherally in tissues such as the liver, fat cells, and skeletal muscles. The effects may also be evident centrally, at the level of the brain, or to be more precise the hypothalamus. This pathological picture could be reverted by using melatonin in the form of supplements through melatonin replacement therapy.

In addition to these dramatic findings, this study has also revealed that glucose intolerance, insulin resistance, and other metabolic disorders may be seen in certain pathological and physiological states associated with a reduction in melatonin levels in the body. These findings are observed in cases that are linked to the development of diseases as a result of aging, shift work, increase in environmental illumination during the nighttime, and the phenomenon of increased light pollution. Maybe we need to start wearing those blue blocking glasses?

The melatonin replacement therapy is expected to alleviate most of these abnormalities and restore health thereby promoting normal glucose metabolism in patients with diabetes.

By e mphasizing the functional synergism between insulin and melatonin, it is considered that pinealectomy-induced glucose intolerance and insulin resistance could be related to the mechanistic consequence of the decline in melatonin secretion. This is often perceived at the cellular level as a deficiency in the insulin-signaling pathways and the reduction in certain gene expressions and protein content. This study has shown that melatonin, by acting through the MT1 membrane receptors, can induce rapid tyrosine phosphorylation and stimulate the tyrosine kinase beta-subunits of insulin receptors. This can help in overcoming several intracellular transduction steps during the insulin-signaling pathways and help patients with diabetes achieve better control over their blood sugar levels.[6] In a nutshell you have melatonin receptors in your pancreas called MT-1 which connect melatonin to improved blood sugar control.

Melatonin's metabolic epigenetic regulation and pleiotropic effects

Melatonin produces a great influence on diabetes and the associated metabolic imbalances by regulating insulin secretion, and by scavenging the reactive oxygen species. It also protects the pancreatic β-cells of Langerhans that are known to be highly susceptible to oxidative damage.

It is universally accepted that industrial and social pressures, like working in shifts, can oppose the physiological circadian order that determines the occurrence of chronic illnesses, like diabetes.

In diabetes mellitus, the neurohumoral circadian rhythm is chronically impaired resulting in desynchronization of the cellular order in the body's healthy tissues as well as between the body and the external environment causing dysfunction between insulin and melatonin.

Diabetes mellitus has also been associated with a phase shift in the body's cardiac circadian clock. This is why; shift workers have an increased risk of diabetes that could be linked to the alterations in metabolic and cardiovascular intracellular circadian clock dysfunctions.

Loss of synchronization typically occurs due to sleep pattern and during the change in the exposure to light at different times of the day, including at night, due to a phenomenon called the "light-at-night pollution." In addition, changes in mealtimes can cause challenges with these natural synchronization issues. These forms of dys-synchronization are commonly observed in patients with diabetes mellitus, indicating the role of melatonin in triggering the development of this condition.

Moreover, the melatonin-insulin synergism is also evident in the form of the incubation of isolated visceral adipocytes, one of the peripheral functions of insulin being accentuated by the effect of melatonin.

This is proof that the adipose tissues are the peripheral targets of melatonin that help in the regulation of the body's overall metabolism including that of fats and carbohydrates. Similarly, it is demonstrated that melatonin activation by MT2 receptors in adipocytes can modulate the glucose uptake and absorption by these cells. Considering the physiology of adipose tissues, it is possible to demonstrate the synergistic effects of melatonin on the other actions of insulin in addition to its role in glucose uptake.

Insulin-induced synthesis of leptin and its release in the isolated adipocytes can also be potentiated by the effect of the MT1-mediated melatonin. This sleep hormone can regulate several other aspects of adipocyte biology, which can influence lipidemia, energy metabolism, and body weight, through its regulatory effect on lipolysis, adipocyte differentiation, lipogenesis, and fatty acids uptake.

These findings point to the possible role of melatonin in controlling insulin secretion, glucose and fat metabolism, glucose uptake by cells, and the reduction of oxidative damage. These studies have provided evidence linking the reduced melatonin levels due to reasons like working in shifts or an inability to get refreshing sleep to a higher risk of diabetes. This underlines the importance of replenishing the melatonin levels through supplementation to restore healthy metabolic functions and prevent the risk of diabetes.

Melatonin also exerts another unique effect on the metabolism of carbohydrates, considering the targets it stimulates for improving glucose uptake in the muscle cells by inducing the phosphorylation of the insulin receptor substrate-1 via MT2 signaling.

Also, melatonin therapy enables the MT2 receptors to be expressed in hepatocytes and elevates glucose release in the liver.

Another critical site for the actions of melatonin in reference to regulating energy metabolism includes the pancreatic islets wherein it influences the synthesis and release of insulin and glucagon.

Several immunocytochemical and molecular studies have demonstrated the presence of the melatonin receptors MT1/MT2 in the islets of Langerhans in the pancreatic tissue. The MT1 and MT2-mediated melatonin effect has been found to decrease the glucose-induced insulin secretion in the isolated pancreatic islets and insulinoma beta-cells.

Melatonin can influence the exocytosis of insulin by the β-cells as was demonstrated in experiments through the nonhydrolyzable GTP (guanosine-5′-trisphosphate) analog and a melatonin antagonist called the luzindole both of which have the potential to inhibit the melatonin effect on the secretion of insulin in the islets.

The intracellular signaling transduction pathways of the β-cell in the pancreas influenced by melatonin through the MT1 and MT2 membrane receptors also include cGMP, cAMP, and IP3 signaling mechanisms.

The activation of the receptors resulting in the inhibition of the forskolin- and glucose-induced insulin secretion, indicates that melatonin does work by inhibiting the cAMP and adenylate cyclase systems and helps to reduce the PKA content.

The pineal indolamine may induce the IGF-1 receptor phosphorylation that participates in maintaining the integrity of islet cells of the pancreas. Moreover, it has been suggested that melatonin may also stimulate glucagon secretion and synthesis. These findings further confirm the role of melatonin in diabetes management.

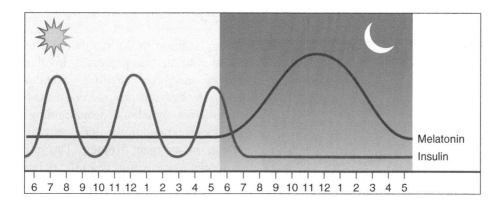

These actions of melatonin are essential for building the circadian profile of insulin release and secretion, and the synchronization of the pancreatic metabolic rhythm with the circadian rhythm. It should be noted that even insulin can regulate the melatonin synthesis by the pineal gland by potentiating the norepinephrine-induced melatonin secretion.

Interestingly, the link between melatonin and diabetes might be based on the observation that insulin production is inversely proportional to the melatonin concentration in the plasma. These 2 hormones, insulin, and melatonin, exhibit a well-regulated circadian rhythm, though there is a negative correlation between the dynamics of their syntheses.

The decrease in the abnormally regulated melatonin secretion has been related to a high risk of diabetes, which indicates that melatonin signals are critical for maintaining glucose homeostasis. In people with diabetes, endogenous glucose production and gluconeogenesis exhibit circadian rhythm that imposes an abnormality in the fasting blood glucose that does not exist in healthy individuals with normal levels of melatonin.

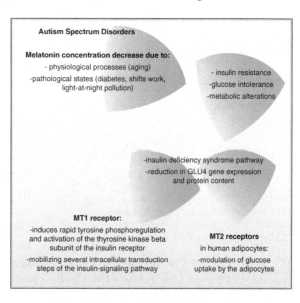

Melatonin can also inhibit the glucose-mediated release of insulin by the pancreatic cells emphasizing the activities it performs in supporting the functions of insulin. Besides EMF and chronic stress, the suppression of melatonin by nocturnal light exposure may work as a trigger for the development of type 2 diabetes in these cases as explained in the picture below:

Pathological consequences of melatonin depletion linked to diabetes

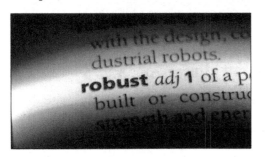

As an addition to the regulatory effect of melatonin on the processes involved in energy and carbohydrate metabolism, research has recently demonstrated that intrauterine metabolic programming may get disturbed due to the deficiency of melatonin in pregnant women. The children of mothers who suffer from the deficiency of melatonin may present with glucose intolerance and insulin resistance along with a delay in the glucose-induced secretion of insulin by the pancreatic islets. As a result, the risk of diabetes is higher in these children.

This provides a clear evidence that melatonin plays a vital role in metabolic epigenetic regulation. In other words, the environmental stresses causing a change in our genes can be avoided by having melatonin on board.

Robustness is the effect I would say best explains melatonin. Robustness is a major characteristic involved in the ability to adapt, survive, and reproduce.

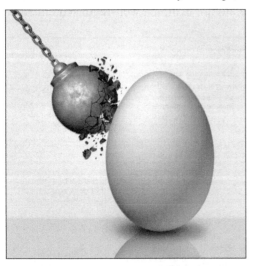

Metabolic dysfunctions are considered to induce a breakdown in the robustness of the biological systems, due to which the continuous maintenance of the body's physiological functions is disrupted. This can lead to internal disturbances in the body's metabolism resulting in the development of diabetes.

Moreover, melatonin can act as a powerful chronobiotic, in such cases, and regulate the metabolic processes such that the activity and the feeding phase of the daytime are synchronized with higher insulin sensitivity, and the rest of the fasting phase is synchronized with the insulin-resistant phase. In fact, melatonin can be the key mediator molecule in these mechanisms and induce nictemeral integration of the behavioral physiological processes. It can support the modulation of body weight regulation and energy balance, all of which are crucial for preventing diabetes.

A **chronobiotic is defined** as an agent that can cause phase adjustment of the body clock. Such a chronobiotic nature of energy metabolism and energy balance is often depicted by the 2 separated phases existing during a 24-hour period of the day and night cycle. The first phase is characterized by eating and the process of energy harvesting resulting in an increased energy intake, followed by its utilization, and storage. This period is associated with high glucose tolerance and a higher peripheral and central sensitivity to insulin. It is marked by an elevated secretion of insulin, with increased glucose uptake by insulin-sensitive tissues. It also leads to faster and more efficient glycogen synthesis, muscular and hepatic glycolysis, inhibition of hepatic gluconeogenesis, faster adipose tissue lipogenesis, and more efficient adiponectin production.

In contrast, the second phase, which is the rest and sleep phase of the day, is marked by a fasting period that requires the body to use the stored energy for maintaining and supporting cellular homeostasis. The energy is also used for exhibiting insulin resistance, accentuating hepatic glycogenolysis and gluconeogenesis, leptin secretion, and adipose tissue lipolysis.

Hormones other than melatonin that exert a modulatory effect on these cellular metabolisms, such as glucocorticoids, catecholamines, and growth hormone also present a circadian rhythmic fluctuation in their secretion and activities. Melatonin, by acting as an orchestrating factor in this circadian organization of metabolic processes, helps to prepare and modify the peripheral and central metabolic tissues so that they can respond to the action of these hormones efficiently.

It is these effects of melatonin that further help in regulating the metabolism of carbohydrates both in the daytime and night-time thereby protecting us against the risk of diabetes.

The anti-obesogenic effects of melatonin:
The Melatonin Darkness Diet

Melatonin has been shown to increase calorie usage! Investigators believe this increased calorie usage is due to more accumulation of brown fat. Unlike white fat (the most common type of body fat) that stores energy, brown fat contains many more mitochondria which make them more energy-producing. This powerful brown fat is very desirable and is a great source of energy when we need it. Especially for those following a ketogenic diet where they 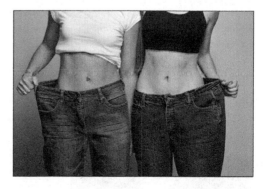 teach themselves to use fat as a fuel source versus the sugars in most carbohydrate-rich western diets.

We use whole body cryotherapy in our clinic and one of the biggest benefits of "Cryo" is this increased brown fat. This allows for an indirect benefit to the heart and brain as well as they can draw from this strong source of fuel.

Studies show animals who have had the pineal gland removed became overweight, and supplementation of melatonin reversed that weight gain. Furthermore, middle-aged fat animals given melatonin showed decreased weight and visceral fat late in life. These changes were not seen if melatonin was not given.

The anti-obesogenic effects of melatonin are, in part, the result of the regulatory role of this hormone on the balance of energy, mainly acting on the regulation of energy mobilization from the body's stores and energy expenditure through things like brown fat production.

It is demonstrated that in young and healthy individuals, melatonin supplementation therapy may reduce the long-term body weight gain and the extent of the visceral fat deposits. Keep in mind the visceral fat is the most stressful to the body and leads to more diseases.

Supplementation of melatonin can indeed lower your body weight. It is believed to work by inducing the reestablishment of circadian distribution of energy metabolism, and insulin signaling pathway reinstatement through melatonin receptors.

My weight loss challenge:

- Supplement with high-dose melatonin
- Try cryotherapy or even cold showers in addition to melatonin to increase brown fat.
- Use the ketogenic diet to teach your body to use fat as energy such as a 5:1:1 fasting/diet program (5 days of ketogenic, 24 hour fast, protein and carb loading day).
- Practice eating window of 6-10 hours each day so that fasting teaches your body to use fat as a fuel source.
- Consider the Mito Fast program.

Fasting for Diabetes

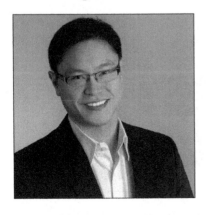

Dr. Jason Fung, the author of the book Diabetes Code, has shown fasting can make dramatic changes or cure diabetes. He has a program that has proven to reverse both type 1 and 2 diabetes. He considers diabetes type 2 as a cell full of glucose where it can't store anymore so the insulin receptors stop working.

Due to too many carbohydrates in the diet, your cells can become overloaded with sugar. By fasting the glucose out of our cells in the form of stored fat, we create a metabolic signal that allows insulin receptors to function properly.

His work has been revolutionary, and our clinic has embraced his finding by introducing more fasting protocols for our patients. Besides melatonin, I feel fasting, as well as a program that includes days of eating a ketogenic diet, makes good sense as a program to treat diabetes. A 5:1:1 program is where one would do a ketogenic diet 5 days a week followed by a 24 hour fast and then a carb-loading day. Dr. Fung currently uses 2-3 24hr fasting days per week as his core diabetes program.

It is clear these programs work more effectively with melatonin supplementation. These fasting and diet variation programs work well to keep the body working toward a balance that stresses the systems in a way that makes them stronger. It seems that maintaining the same diet each and every day is not the best strategy to live a long and healthy life. It comes back to hormesis, where stress in the right dosage gives a net gain in health. For more on Dr. Fung see his website here.

foreword by NINA TEICHOLZ

DR. JASON FUNG

author of The Obesity Code

THE

DIABETES

CODE

PREVENT AND

REVERSE

TYPE 2 DIABETES

NATURALLY

Ketogenic Diet & Diabetes

Metabolic flexibility is the key to a healthy body and healthy blood sugar. When I say metabolic flexibility what I mean is the ability to swing between creating cellular energy through both fast and proteins, and sugars and carbohydrates. These are 2 separate pathways, and the body typically becomes addicted to sugars and carbohydrates.

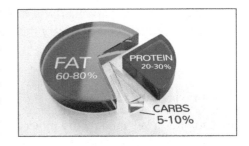

Imagine the difference between getting food out of your refrigerator versus having to go downstairs into your basement and pull food that is frozen and needs to be defrosted out of the freezer. There is much more energy in the freezer once you get it out and defrosted than there is in the refrigerator. This is the same thing that happens to us with regards to carbohydrates. Because we include them as the majority of the standard American diet it is common that the body becomes very efficient at using sugars and carbohydrates as fuel sources and simply stores the fat for later. Therefore, what I mean when I say metabolically flexible is that your body could either go to the freezer or to the refrigerator at will.

When folks first start venturing into a ketogenic diet, they will find themselves with their blood sugar crashing because they are unable to get the food out of the freezer. Once the body learns how to liberate that food out of the deep freeze then one can fast for extended periods of time or skip meals, and simply switch into ketosis where the body is using ketones from fat that is either through the diet or from stored sources in adipose cells.

In this study 'A low-carbohydrate, ketogenic diet to treat type 2 diabetes' a ketogenic improved glycemic control in patients with type 2 diabetes such that diabetes medications were discontinued or reduced in most participants.[7]

A ketogenic diet for type 1 diabetes may not be the best monotherapy. The fasting protocols that Dr. Jason Fung has developed appropriately combined with a ketogenic diet hold the most promise. A ketogenic diet alongside intermittent fasting or extended fasting, when combined with melatonin supplementation, is a winning combination.

Ben Azaidi founder of keto camp has recently released a book called Keto Flex. This book provides a lot of insight into some of the concepts regarding variations throughout the week in order to stress various systems and create metabolic flexibility. There are wide-reaching benefits to this approach including neurological health, gut and microbiome health, cardiovascular health, and of course metabolic resilience, which would play into diabetes quite well.

If you're going to be using hormesis, which is a stress that is provided in the right dosage stimulating the body to respond for a net gain in health, melatonin is your best friend in this instance. Melatonin is the primary support system the body relies on when there is stress. Remember the early research with the rodents where they were living stress-free, and the researchers couldn't see a difference with melatonin supplementation? It wasn't until they stressed the rodents in those tubes with the pinholes that they started to see melatonin's benefit, where it mitigated a variety of different diseases and extended lifespan in these rodents.

Including melatonin particularly in a high dose could be a powerful synergy alongside some of these more contemporary therapies for diabetes, such as fasting and a ketogenic diet.

Conclusion

Melatonin is a key modulatory molecule that can assure a healthy metabolism, optimization of energy balance, as well as body weight regulation.

Melatonin acts by potentiating both the peripheral and central insulin action by supporting the regulation of insulin-signaling pathways. Melatonin is also found to be responsible for maintaining adequate energy balance by regulating energy flow and energy expenditure by causing production of better brown fat.

Melatonin synchronizes the 2 major metabolic phases that exist 24-hour period of the day-night cycle including the activity/ feeding/wakefulness state against the rest/fasting/sleep phase. Basically, you're using energy during the day and storing it as you feed. During the night you are pulling energy in the form of glucose out to use to heal and repair the body.

The decline in the synthesis of melatonin can occur due to physiological processes such as aging, and pathologies associated with events like shiftwork and an illuminated environment during the night-time. This can induce insulin resistance, sleep disturbances, glucose intolerance, and metabolic circadian disorganization. This would depict a state of metabolic imbalance, and chrono-disruption aggravating the glycemic control and your general health.

The evidence that melatonin can induce insulin secretion and improve β-cell functions has provided a strong foundation supporting the use of melatonin supplements as an effective therapeutic approach for the reestablishment of glucose homeostasis. The scientific proofs support the evidence that melatonin replacement therapy, when carried out adequately, in terms of dosage, formulations, and the time of the administration, could contribute to maintaining efficient blood glucose levels in patients with diabetes and help restore the chronobiotic order needed for achieving a robust healthy state in the body.

Consider using fasting and ketogenic diet strategies for diabetes in addition to melatonin.

Reference

1. Garfinkel D, Zorin M, Wainstein J et al. Efficacy and safety of prolonged-release melatonin in insomnia patients with diabetes: a randomized, double-blind, crossover study. *Diabetes Metab Syndr Obes*. 2011; 4: 307-313. doi: 10.2147/DMSO.S23904.

2. Hormone Molecular Biology and Clinical Investigation (degruyter.com)

3. Melatonin: The diabetes treatment of the future? - De Gruyter Conversations

4. Espino, J., Pariente, J. A., & Rodríguez, A. B. (2011). Role of melatonin on diabetes-related metabolic disorders. *World journal of diabetes*, *2*(6), 82–91. https://doi.org/10.4239/wjd.v2.i6.82

5. Melatonin: A Silent Regulator of the Glucose Homeostasis | IntechOpen

6. American Medical Association (AMA). "Decreased melatonin secretion associated with higher risk of developing type 2 diabetes." ScienceDaily. ScienceDaily, 2 April 2013. <www.sciencedaily.com/releases/2013/04/130402162420.htm>.

7. Yancy, W.S., Foy, M., Chalecki, A.M. *et al.* A low-carbohydrate, ketogenic diet to treat type 2 diabetes. *Nutr Metab (Lond)* **2,** 34 (2005). https://doi.org/10.1186/1743-7075-2-34

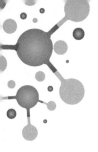

17

CANNABIS & SLEEP, MELATONIN'S POT CONNECTION

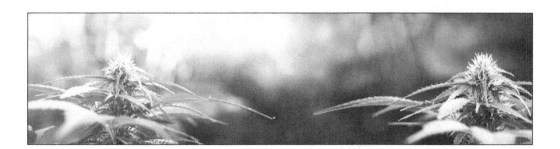

The exact relationship between melatonin and cannabis has only been recently discovered. The past few years have seen a growing interest in exploring the pot connection with melatonin and how it affects sleep.

The most important aspects that are worth further research include whether cannabis influences melatonin levels and if cannabis interacts with melatonin supplementation. Before we get into their convoluted relation, let's dive into some cannabis science first.

An introduction to Sleep & Cannabis

We have already discussed the importance of melatonin for regulating our sleep-wake pattern. The effect of cannabis on sleep is also well known, though it is undeniably complicated as the impact it produces depends on numerous factors such as the type of strain used, quantity, time of consumption, frequency of use, and so forth.

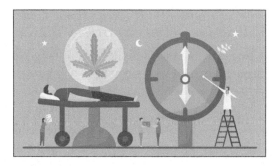

Since both melatonin and cannabis have the potential to influence sleep in different ways, the relationship between the two merits investigation in greater depth.

Melatonin, as we know, is a naturally occurring body-produced hormone, the main function of which is to regulate the circadian rhythm.

This graphic can help to clarify the various internal mechanisms of the body's circadian clock that are controlled naturally by melatonin and can be further influenced when a person consumes cannabis.

Cannabis & the sleep-wake cycle

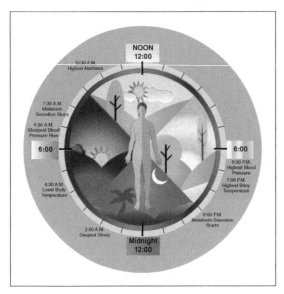

Rare mentions of melatonin with regard to cannabis are present in a 2017 study published in the Oregon Institute of Occupational Health Sciences.

In this, the research team has stated:

"Cannabis alters the sleep-wake cycle, increases the production of melatonin, and can inhibit the arousal system by activating cannabinoid type 1 (CB1) receptors in the basal forebrain and other wake-promoting centers."[1]

The study has further states that "Investigations have shown that the major psychoactive compound in cannabis, Δ9-tetrahydrocannabi-nol (THC), can decrease sleep onset latency in naïve users or at low doses for experienced users (eg, 70 mg/day); but, higher doses for experienced users increased sleep latency and wake after sleep onset.[2],[3],[4] *Indeed, frequent cannabis users (≥5 uses/week for 3 months and lifetime use ≥2 years) are reported to have shorter total sleep duration, less slow-wave sleep, worse sleep efficiency, and longer sleep onset compared to controls.*[5] *The contrasting benefits of THC exposure may represent the biphasic influence of THC on CB1 receptors whereby acute use causes more activation of CB1 receptors and tendency toward sleep, but long-term use results in desensitization of the CB1 receptor and decreased downstream signaling."*

Using THC in a dose higher than 70 mg per day, more than 5 days a week, might result in an increase in your sleep latency period. In high doses, THC can produce a stimulatory

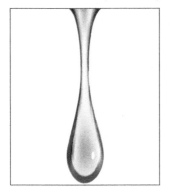

effect on the arousal system of the brain which will make it difficult to fall asleep after you hit the bed.

Also, frequent cannabis users who use it regularly for more than 2 years might also develop more serious chronic sleep issues. This happens because THC in cannabis can shorten the total sleep duration, slow-wave sleep, and worsen sleep efficiency[6]. It can also prolong your sleep onset latency period as was observed in the participants of the study who were given THC against those who were given only a placebo.

The contrasting benefits of cannabis usage based on the duration and dosage represent the biphasic influence of THC on the CB1 receptors whereby its acute or short-term use causes the activation of these receptors and an improved tendency toward sleep, whereas its long-term or chronic use in higher doses results in the desensitization of the receptors resulting in reduced downstream signaling.

The contrasting benefits of THC exposure may represent the biphasic influence of THC on CB1 receptors whereby acute use causes more activation of CB1 receptors and tendency toward sleep. Still, long-term use results in desensitization of the CB1 receptor and decreased downstream signaling[7].

CB-1 receptors have opposing effects where they can either excite or inhibit the brain. CB1 receptors excite the brain through inhibiting GABA (an inhibitory neurotransmitter) and inhibit the brain via inhibiting glutamate (an excitatory neurotransmitter). It can also affect the body's sleep-wake system through these CB1 receptors present in the brain.

The increased secretion of melatonin[8] might help to improve the quality and duration of your sleep. It may also promote these effects further by creating an inhibitory effect on the parts of the brain that are more active when you are alert, which is usually in the daytime. This suggests that the use of cannabis in the evening hours might complement the benefits of melatonin supplements. Cannabis can suppress the level of alertness by inhibiting the activities of the arousal system, thus allowing you to enjoy a more restful sleep.

The investigations have further shown that tetrahydrocannabinol (THC), which is a major psychoactive compound in cannabis, can also reduce your sleep-onset latency period when cannabis is used by naïve users or at a very low dose by experienced users. It indicates that the sleep-promoting effect of cannabis may get somewhat neutralized by the effects of THC due to its excitatory effects through glutamate. When cannabis is consumed in a very high dose of 70 mg before bedtime, it will prevent an efficient sleep-promoting effect. On the contrary, very low doses are needed for regular users to achieve this effect. THC seems to have a positive effect on your sleep latency period, time to fall asleep. However, length and quality are other stories. THC users have a shortened reported sleep duration across the board[9].

To get a better idea of how long it would be safe to use cannabis, let us check what another study has to say about this. One study, "Sleep disturbance in heavy marijuana users," published in Sleep in 2008[10], showed that the recently abstinent but heavy marijuana users had a difference in their polysomnographic (PSG) values compared to that of a drug-free control group. It should be noted here that cannabis is the genus of which marijuana is the species.

During this study, a group of participants was carefully selected based on their history of marijuana usage. The heavy marijuana users who had discontinued the drug intake were selected for the study inclusion and later matched to a control group with no history of drug abuse or usage in any form. The questionnaire data was collected before the cessation of the use of marijuana. The polysomnographic study was conducted in a core sleep laboratory for two consecutive nights after the discontinuation of marijuana use.

The results of this study helped explain how the duration of use of marijuana could affect sleep. The marijuana users included in this study showed wide differences in their PSG measures, including a lower total sleep time and reduced slow-wave sleep. These parameters showed a sharp decline compared to that in the participants of the control group on both nights. The participants with a history of drug use also showed reduced sleep efficiency, a longer sleep onset period, and shorter REM latency compared to those in the control group on the second night of the study. Most of the sleep continuity parameters were worse for the marijuana group than the control group on the second night, indicating that the overall quality of sleep became worse in the marijuana group. This study suggested that the benefits of cannabis are likely to continue to decline with repeated or long-term usage[11].

Besides poor sleep, inadvertent use of cannabis is also linked to a higher risk of several other conditions such as depression and poor motivation.

This study has also quoted older research from 1986. This study, "Effects of Tetrahydrocannabinol on Melatonin Secretion in Man," was published in the journal, Hormone and Metabolic Research. It was aimed at observing the melatonin levels in 9 male volunteers, aged between 29 to 33 years, after consuming a cannabis joint containing THC or a regular cigarette without any THC[12].

This study found that the participants who used the cannabis joint had a significant rise in their melatonin blood levels. There are two additional aspects that the researchers have cited about the impact of cannabis or THC on melatonin levels in this study. These aspects include the frequency of use and the quantity of cannabis consumed, which makes sense as regular users will down-regulate their endocannabinoid receptors sites, whereas more and more THC is needed to achieve the same effects[13].

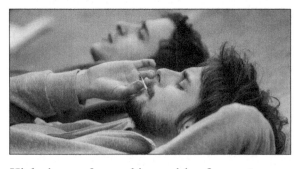

According to the analysis, this study showed that THC might lessen the time needed to fall asleep, especially in occasional users. It may also produce a similar effect for frequent users when used in a lower dose. Again, this is due to the receptor sites being wide-open in occasional users.

High doses of cannabis used by frequent users may cause increased sleep latency or longer time to fall asleep. It would also shorten the duration of sleep, increase disruptions in sleep, and lessen deep sleep or slow-wave delta sleep.

Why THC in high doses causes Sleep disturbances.

In this study[14], 'Cannabidiol Counteracts the Psychotropic Side-Effects of Δ-9-Tetrahydrocannabinol in the ventral hippocampus through Bidirectional Control of ERK1–2 Phosphorylation,' they discuss the negative impact THC can have on the brain and the chemistry. The ventral hippocampus (VH, temporal part) is involved in the control of emotional and anxious behaviors.[15] This ventral hippocampus is considered a part of your limbic brain. The limbic system supports a variety of functions, including emotion, behavior, long-term memory, and olfaction[16].

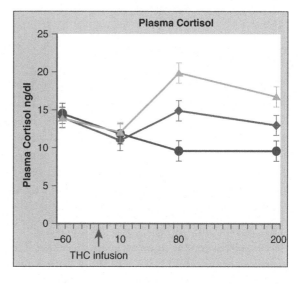

Emotional life is which is largely housed in the limbic system, critically aids the formation of memories[17]. The ventral hippocampus (VHC) has been related to anxiety behaviors and has a high expression of cannabinoid-1 (CB1) receptors[18].

Consistent with the literature, Δ-9-THC increased plasma cortisol levels. Δ-9-THC increases ACTH and cortisol levels via CB-1 receptor activation within the paraventricular nuclei, and either directly or indirectly (via other neurotransmitters) modulates corticotrophin-releasing hormone (CRH) secretion[19]. Δ-9-THC produces an early and brief increase followed by a predominantly inhibitory effect on prolactin release[20], which is mediated by CB-1R activation of tuberoinfundibular (TIDA) DA neurons. The lack of a significant inhibitory Δ-9-THC effect on plasma prolactin in this study may be explained by the brief period of observation[21]. The poor sleep with higher THC dosing or with chronic users may be the cortisol, or it may be the fatiguing of the inhibition through desensitization of the CB1 receptor and decreased downstream signaling within both the ventral hippocampus and the inhibition of glutamate[22]. Since THC also inhibits GABA, there could be a shift where this predominates, leaving you with little GABA to buffer against excitation in the brain. GABA is the brain's primary inhibitory neurotransmitter, whereas it is the master brake system. Poor GABA signaling will lead to anxiety

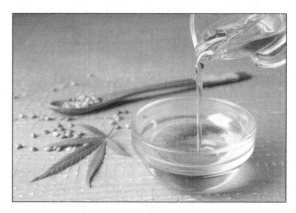

and overexcitation, thus interrupting quality sleep. There is another form of THC called Delta 8 THC. Most cannabis that is available has Delta 9 THC. Delta 8 THC might be the answer for those that want to use cannabis with the desired effects from THC late at night. We will get into that shortly.

THC & CBD for Sleep.

THC has a tendency, at higher doses, to cause over-excitation, and as we have seen in the literature, the higher doses of THC can inhibit quality sleep. CBD seems to be somewhat of a natural antidote to balance THC. A study published in the Journal of Clinical Psychopharmacology in 2014 has helped us understand the impact of cannabis on melatonin secretion with better clarity. This study, "Effect of Delta-9-tetrahydrocannabinol and cannabidiol on nocturnal sleep and early-morning behavior in young adults," was aimed at assessing the effects of cannabis extracts on nighttime sleep, early-morning performance, sleepiness, and memory[23].

The participants of this study included eight healthy volunteers (four males and four females between the ages of 21 to 34 years). The four treatment protocols adopted in this study were placebo, THC combined with cannabidiol (CBD) both in the doses of 5 mg each, Delta-9-tetrahydrocannabinol (THC) in a dose of 15 mg, and THC with CBD both in the doses of 15 mg each. These formulations were administered with the help of an oro-mucosal spray during the 30-minute period after 10 pm. The electroencephalogram of the participant was recorded during the sleep period between 11 pm, and 7 am. The performance of participants along with their sleep latency and the subjective assessment of mood and sleepiness was measured after 8:30 am (about 10 hours after the administration of the formulation).

There were no effects observed in the 15 mg THC group for nocturnal sleep. The concomitant administration of drugs (5 mg of THC with 5 mg of CBD or 15 mg of THC with 15 mg of CBD), caused a decrease in stage 3 of sleep (deep sleep). The higher dose combination was found to improve wakefulness. The next day, those who took a 15 mg dose of THC showed impaired memory with their sleep latency reduced and an increase in sleepiness and change in moods. The participants who were treated with a lower dose combination had their reaction time improved. They had a faster reaction time on a digital recall task. With the higher dose combination, participants reported improved sleepiness and a change in moods. Those who were given 15 milligrams of THC appeared to be sedated, while those treated with 15 mg of CBD appeared to have 'alerting' properties as CBD increased their awake activities during sleep, which counteracted the sedative activities of 15 mg of THC. This study showed how variable doses of CBD and THC could produce a unique impact on different parameters of sleep as well as wakefulness and cognitive functions during the daytime[24].

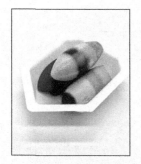

It's advisable to include CBD with any of your THC dosings. Whether taking cannabis for sleep or other benefits, studies seem to support the combination of the two. Keep in mind that the natural plant has many different cannabinoids besides just CBD. Nature has packaged the natural plant in a way that seems to be superior to dosing with the individual isolates of THC or CBD. This is why a full-spectrum extract is processed with a CO2 extraction so that the Terpenes are preserved and will provide the highest quality product and effect for you. Besides the entire family of cannabinoids, there are multiple Terpenes that are present in cannabis, such as linalool. As only one example of many Terpenes found in cannabis flowers, linalool is the primary active ingredient in lavender. There have been numerous studies to show that lavender supports sleep. In this study, oral lavender oil preparation (80 mg/day) showed a significant beneficial influence on the quality and duration of sleep in 221 patients suffering from anxiety disorders[25]. Another great sleep terpene is myrcene. Many high CBD strains naturally contain this sleep-promoting and sedating terpene. Controlled studies on humans are lacking for myrcene's sedative effects; however this effect is well established in the animal literature. People have been using hops as a human sleep aid for centuries because hops have very high myrcene levels[26].

So, what you want to look for is a full-spectrum hemp extract that has been processed to preserve the natural terpenes. Why hemp? Hemp is a strain of cannabis that has been specially bred to have a low level of Delta 9 THC that is within the legal limits. This is ideal because then you have the full gift that nature intended to provide together versus individual components that have been made chemically in the lab.

THC, Deep Sleep & Glymphatic's

Research shows that higher THC levels will inhibit deep sleep. We know from the research that the primary activator to the Glymphatic's is deep sleep. Therefore, there will be a negative effect on the Glymphatic's with high THC dosing[27]. It is dosing later in the day

> "It could be very beneficial for sleep to combine melatonin with linalool, CBD, and just a hint of THC. The high-dose melatonin product called sandman made by MitoZen.com is just this plus magnolia extract and glutathione."

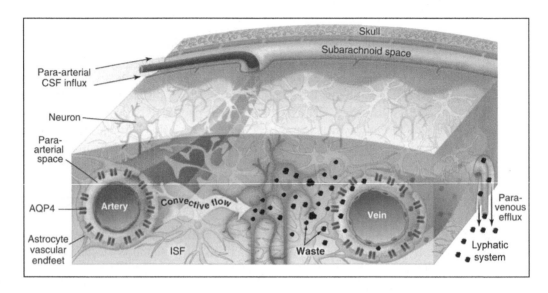

such as after dinner that will have more of an impact on your sleep cycles. Let's revisit the Glymphatic system. Just like the lymphatic system in the body, this system is there to keep your brain more like a river versus a swamp. Swamps are going to attract more microbial growth as well as there won't be as much nutrient delivery and toxic removal. Studies show the Glymphatic's, when not properly activated on a regular basis, leads to many neurological conditions such as Parkinson's disease, Alzheimer's disease, poor recovery from traumatic brain injuries, early cognitive decline, and any neurologic disease that results in the accumulation of proteins such as tau protein, alpha-synuclein, and beta-amyloid. The good news is that it is possible to clear many of these proteins and reverse these conditions with the right natural approach. The key to this is activating autophagy which is cellular eating and recycling. We've discussed this in prior chapters but let's review it again. Autophagy comes from the Greek word to self-eat. It is a mechanism whereby the body switches into a cleaning and recycling phase. This is where it identifies old dead and dying cells or cellular components and clears them up, and uses them as building blocks to create fresh, new high-functioning cells or cellular components. Among the most important cellular components is your mitochondria. One-third of your body weight is mitochondria. These are small structures in all of your cells that produce energy from glucose and oxygen. Without these functions, you would not survive even a second. The recycling of mitochondria is called mitophagy. In this research, the role of melatonin in the regulation of autophagy and mitophagy is reviewed[28]. The author discusses signaling through oxidation and how melatonin is the premier antioxidant that plays a vital role in both signaling and protecting your body from dysfunctional mitochondria[29].

In the study, melatonin attenuated traumatic brain injury-induced inflammation: a possible role for mitophagy. Melatonin treatment activated mitophagy through the mTOR pathway, then attenuated TBI-induced inflammation. Furthermore, treatment with melatonin significantly ameliorated neuronal death and behavioral deficits after TBI, while 3-methyladenine reversed this effect by inhibiting mitophagy[30].

> **Dr John's Comment:**
> **Using Melatonin & Fasting to improve your brain.**

I thought we would review this a little to try and get some perspective on how to properly take care of your brain so that you avoid serious problems in the future. Besides minimizing high THC strains later in the day, it would be important to also consider minimizing any protein accumulation through properly activating the Glymphatic's and Autophagy at the same time. It's about cleaning it up (Autophagy) and then mobilizing it out of the brain (Glymphatic's)[31]. Both of these systems are important to consider simultaneously. This is why the body is wise to place deep sleep in the same zone as the fasting state. Fasting is the primary activator of mTOR, which is the primary signaling gene for autophagy [32]. These are why eating habits like intermittent fasting, such as narrowing your eating window to between 6 to 10 hours each day are so important. Longer fasts also make good sense, such as a full 3-to-5-day water fast. I am also an advocate of a weekly 24- hour fast where one goes from lunch to lunch. As I mentioned in earlier chapters, I often will recommend patients use intermittent fasting, a weekly 24-hour fast, and the monthly 3-to-5 day fast for three months straight. This is a typical strategy that I start many of my patients on that are dealing with a chronic condition. This can also be used for people looking to achieve higher levels of health. One of the reasons that I designed the Mito Fast was to give structure for either a 24-hour fast or a

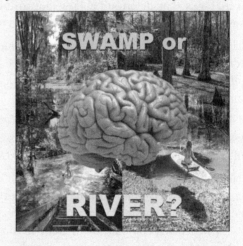

3-to-5 day fast as well as certain nutrients that activate signaling factors that can accentuate the benefits prior to during and after a fast. Taking melatonin while fasting allows for proper Glymphatic activation. It is important to clear out these recycled and broken-down protein components from the brain. Besides these protein components, there are also microbes and toxins that the brain's immune system needs to clear out.

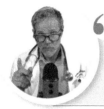

> *Dr John's Comment: On a side note, many times these proteins like tau are actually there to protect your brain as they wrap around microbes and toxins like flypaper to wall them off from causing damage to your nerves.*

While we're on the subject of Autophagy and in light of this chapter on cannabis, an interesting fact is that one of the ways cannabis has been shown to work against cancer is its ability to regulate the autophagy of cancer cells, such as discussed in this study. "Various studies reported a cannabinoid-induced autophagy mechanism in cancer and non-cancer cells."[33]

What happens if you mix weed & melatonin?

Most of the studies performed to assess the combined effects of melatonin and cannabis were focused on determining how they influenced sleep. Studies have linked cannabis use to several health benefits, including increased melatonin production and improved sleep onset!

The first effects of the combined use of melatonin and cannabis were experienced in the form of sensations described as closed-eye hallucinations (also called the closed-eye visualizations)[34], along with an ability to experience a feeling of being 'high' and visualizing intense dreams.

These closed-eye hallucinations have been reported to resemble a dream-like state wherein the users tend to vividly visualize certain thoughts that go through their heads often, especially while they are still awake[35] [36].

The second effect of the combined use of cannabis and melatonin was undoubtedly fascinating. It was found to affect a majority of cannabis users. The effect is commonly described as the complete absence of dreams. This effect has also been experienced by users who often complained of frequent dreams that interfered with their sleep. But, after continued use of melatonin and cannabis, they noticed an adaption to this and a return to normal sleep patterns.

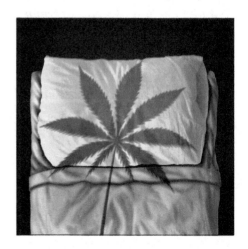

The absence of dreams may happen because of the ability of cannabis to prolong the deep-sleep stage of sleep. It reduces the time a person usually spends in the REM (rapid-eye-movement) phase of sleep, which is the period where intense dreaming usually occurs[37].

This study has suggested that the use of cannabis, by prolonging the deep-sleep stage of sleep, can shorten the REM phase, which causes users to stop seeing any dreams. Moreover, the lack of dreaming may be seen as beneficial for people, for instance, those with PTSD who suffer from recurring haunting nightmares. I personally feel these people need to be coached through these experiences so that they can move through them versus running away from them. In our clinic, we will do ketamine-assisted psychotherapy which is a way for people to fully uncover what's in their subconscious. REM is the sleep stage when the subconscious is sorting out all the events of the day and how they relate to your current mental database. Both THC and alcohol are very detrimental to this REM sleep, and therefore, many people with chronic addiction do not mentally or emotionally develop properly.

> **Dr John's Comment:**
> **Dr John's Advice to Improve your Brain,**
> **Protection again high THC usage.**
>
> *We all have those friends or maybe family members that don't seem to have matured mentally or emotionally over the years while we have made significant changes ourselves. Maybe it's you that haven't grown mentally or emotionally? If so, you're in luck because you can use strategies that increase something called BDNF. BDNF stands for brain-derived neurotrophic factor and is one of the primary signaling factors for repair and regeneration in your nervous system. You can use strategies to increase BDNF to catch up on four years of stress to your brain by using some of the suggestions here that will increase BDNF. The heat from saunas, intense physical exercise, various mushrooms like lion's mane and hericium erinaceus, reducing stress and inflammation (melatonin), and ambient sun exposure also correlated with BDNF[38]. Socialize because isolation appears to lower your BDNF levels[39]. Plants that are rich in polyphenols and other antioxidants are beneficial for your BDNF levels, like in Lucitol[40]. Eating plenty of high-quality protein can help your brain stay healthy as you age[41]. Go Keto, because Beta-hydroxybutyrate, a ketone your liver produces when you eat a very-low-carb diet or ketogenic diet, appears to increase brain BDNF levels[42]. Dark chocolate, blueberries, and extra-virgin olive oil are high-polyphenol foods that are proven to increase BDNF and support brain health [43][44][45][46]. Eat more fish as the omega 3s in fatty fish increase BDNF levels[47][48]. Take the peptide semax. Also, high dose melatonin, fasting, meditation, and activities that are new and novel such as learning a new sport like stand-up paddleboarding promote neuroplasticity. However, it would be best to go lighter on THC if you choose not to pay particular attention to this section. Add a few of these suggestions into your weekly activities to buffer the stress that the high THC is creating.*

What about Delta 8 THC?

A new form of THC is emerging called Delta 8 or Δ*8* THC. Unlike the more common Δ*9* THC, Δ*8* is legal in most states. Δ*8* THC has a less intense effect making it more desirable for many users that find the more common Δ*9* to be a bit too much for them.

A 1973 study examined the effects of delta-8 THC on sleep in cats[49], showing promising results. The study found that delta-8 THC induced sedation in cats, causing fewer and longer paradoxical sleep or REM episodes. This means that delta-8 caused longer REM (rapid eye movement) episodes, which are important to the sleep cycle because they stimulate parts of the brain essential for learning and memory. The researchers conclude that delta-8 might have clinically useful sedative-hypnotic properties. The study also found that delta-8 THC did not elicit inappropriate behavior because it lacks the "psychotomimetic effects" (paranoia) commonly produced by delta-9 THC[50].

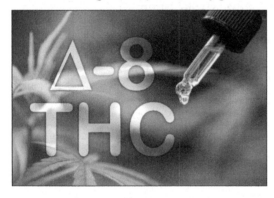

NeuroDiol begins manufacturing DeltaDiol[51] this year in an attempt to provide folks with an option that they can purchase right on the Internet. No need to go to a government-controlled pharmacy where many people find limited options due to tight regulations. It seems many of the negative aspects of THC we discussed earlier would be much less prevalent using Δ*8* versus Δ*9*. Although more research needs to be done, it seems obvious that the gentle nature of the Δ*8 THC* is healthier.

Bullets for Keeping your brain healthy:

- Heat from saunas
- Physical exercise
- Mushrooms like Liones Maine and Hericium erinaceus
- Reducing stress and inflammation (melatonin)
- Sun exposure
- Socialize and avoid isolation
- Plants that are rich in polyphenols and other antioxidants
- Eating plenty of high-quality protein
- Ketogenic Diet
- Eat more fish
- Take the peptide semax.
- High dose melatonin

- Fasting,
- Meditation & Breathing Exercises
- New and novel activities to promote neuroplasticity
- Go lighter on THC

Conclusion:

It seems pretty clear from the research that it may be best to take a small amount of THC in a full-spectrum hemp extract tincture in the morning if you were over 40 years old. The evidence is very clear that it will likely prevent degenerative neurological diseases as well as assist in creating some balance in the central nervous system. As far as sleep, a very low amount of THC with a very high CBD content 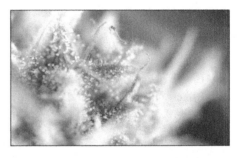 is the answer. There may be occasions that one will need help to fall asleep. However, you will sacrifice your deep sleep if you overdo it with the THC. In my practice, I will often dose people with a high dose of melatonin as well as a little bit of full-spectrum hemp that has very low THC and high CBD. If they continue to have difficulty with their sleep, I will ramp up the CBD content, sometimes up as high as 100+ milligrams. For those regular cannabis users, you might consider laying off the high THC strains, especially after dinner time. I think there's a strong argument that over time, this is going to create some significant health problems. The importance of deep sleep cannot be underestimated. Deep sleep is associated with all of the repair and regeneration of your body as well as the Glymphatic system as we've discussed in other chapters. The Glymphatic system is the brain's detox and gutter system, just like the lymphatic system is to the rest of the body. Primarily activated with deep sleep, neglect of the system will cause a buildup in toxins and proteins in the brain that could lead to brain fog, mental confusion, memory issues, and as it progresses, degenerative neurological may occur due to the buildup of various proteins in the brain that would normally be cleaned out with the Glymphatics. The Glymphatic and THC are at odds with each other. When you pick up a high THC strain after dinner, you're making a choice that results in the nerves in your brain swimming in their own poop, basically. Besides considering the Glymphatics, we also discussed the importance of activating Autophagy as a cleanup and recycling mechanism that should be considered an important mechanism during deep sleep. These Autophagy signaling factors can be improved with fasting as well as certain plant extracts such as those contained within Phase 2 of the Mito Fast. The purpose of this fasting protocol is to stack both fastings while also taking certain plant extracts such as resveratrol, fisetin, and pterostilbene. Besides fasting, there's a strong argument to take super physiological doses of melatonin if you are a regular cannabis user to curb this inhibition to deep sleep. I always recommend that people track their sleep so that they know exactly what their sleep scores are based on the choices they make. Once you have a decent baseline of your REM, deep sleep, and heart rate variability or HRV, you can see how these various substances affect your specific sleep variables. Lastly, I would also suggest, when consuming strains of cannabis for sleep, that one paid particular attention to strains that are high in Linalool or Myrcene. Very few cannabis **strains** contain a **high** amount of **linalool. However,** Zkittlez, Kosher Kush, and Do-Si-Dos all contain **linalool** as their third most abundant terpene. Strains with **high myrcene** content include Blue Dream, AK-47, and OG Kush. I'm going to include a bullet list of brain-supporting strategies for my "Stoner›› readers out there.

Reference

1. Bowles, Nicole & Herzig, Maya & Shea, Steven. (2017). Recent legalization of cannabis use: Effects on sleep, health, and workplace safety. Nature and Science of Sleep. Volume 9. 249-251. 10.2147/NSS.S152231.

2. Nicholson AN, Turner C, Stone BM, Robson PJ. Effect of Delta-9-tetrahydrocannabinol and cannabidiol on nocturnal sleep and early-morning behavior in young adults. J Clin Psychopharmacol. 2004 Jun;24(3):305-13. doi: 10.1097/01.jcp.0000125688.05091.8f. PMID: 15118485.

3. Tassinari, C.A. & Ambrosetto, Giovanni & Peraita-Adrados, Maria & Gastaut, H.. (1976). The neuropsychiatric syndrome of delta-9-tetrahydrocannabinol and cannabis intoxication in naive subjects: A clinical and polygraphic study during wakefulness and sleep. The Pharmacology of Marihuana. 357-382.

4. Feinberg, Irwin & Jones, Reese & Walker, James & Cavness, Cleve & Floyd, T.. (1976). Effects of marijuana extract and tetrahydrocannabinol on electroencephalographic sleep patterns. Clinical pharmacology and therapeutics. 19. 782-94. 10.1002/cpt1976196782.

5. Bolla, K. I., Lesage, S. R., Gamaldo, C. E., Neubauer, D. N., Funderburk, F. R., Cadet, J. L., David, P. M., Verdejo-Garcia, A., & Benbrook, A. R. (2008). Sleep disturbance in heavy marijuana users. *Sleep*, *31*(6), 901–908. https://doi.org/10.1093/sleep/31.6.901

6. Bolla, K. I., Lesage, S. R., Gamaldo, C. E., Neubauer, D. N., Funderburk, F. R., Cadet, J. L., David, P. M., Verdejo-Garcia, A., & Benbrook, A. R. (2008). Sleep disturbance in heavy marijuana users. *Sleep*, *31*(6), 901–908. https://doi.org/10.1093/sleep/31.6.901

7. Bowles, N. P., Herzig, M. X., & Shea, S. A. (2017). Recent legalization of cannabis use: effects on sleep, health, and workplace safety. *Nature and science of sleep*, *9*, 249–251. https://doi.org/10.2147/NSS.S152231

8. Lissoni, Paolo & Resentini, M & Mauri, R & Esposti, D & Esposti, G & Rossi, D & Legname, Giuseppe & Fraschini, Franco. (1986). Effects of Tetrahydrocannabinol on Melatonin Secretion in Man. Hormone and metabolic research = Hormon- und Stoffwechselforschung = Hormones et métabolisme. 18. 77-8. 10.1055/s-2007-1012235.

9. Kesner Andrew J., Lovinger David M., Cannabinoids, Endocannabinoids and Sleep, Frontiers in Molecular Neuroscience; vol 13, 2020, pp125; https://www.frontiersin.org/article/10.3389/fnmol.2020.00125 DOI=10.3389/fnmol.2020.00125

10. Bolla KI, Lesage SR, Gamaldo CE, Neubauer DN, Funderburk FR, Cadet JL, David PM, Verdejo-Garcia A, Benbrook AR. Sleep disturbance in heavy marijuana users. Sleep. 2008 Jun;31(6):901-8. doi: 10.1093/sleep/31.6.901. PMID: 18548836; PMCID: PMC2442418.

11. Bolla KI, Lesage SR, Gamaldo CE, Neubauer DN, Funderburk FR, Cadet JL, David PM, Verdejo-Garcia A, Benbrook AR. Sleep disturbance in heavy marijuana users. Sleep. 2008 Jun;31(6):901-8. doi: 10.1093/sleep/31.6.901. PMID: 18548836; PMCID: PMC2442418.

12. Lissoni, Paolo & Resentini, M & Mauri, R & Esposti, D & Esposti, G & Rossi, D & Legname, Giuseppe & Fraschini, Franco. (1986). Effects of Tetrahydrocannabinol on Melatonin Secretion in Man. Hormone and metabolic research = Hormon- und Stoffwechselforschung = Hormones et métabolisme. 18. 77-8. 10.1055/s-2007-1012235.

13. Lissoni P, Resentini M, Mauri R, Esposti D, Esposti G, Rossi D, Legname G, Fraschini F. Effects of tetrahydrocannabinol on melatonin secretion in man. Horm Metab Res. 1986 Jan;18(1):77-8. doi: 10.1055/s-2007-1012235. PMID: 3005151.

14. Roger Hudson, Justine Renard, Christopher Norris, Walter J. Rushlow and Steven R. Laviolette, Effects of Δ-9-Tetrahydrocannabinol in the Ventral Hippocampus through Bidirectional Control of ERK1–2 Phosphorylation,Journal of Neuroscience 30 October 2019, 39 (44) 8762-8777; DOI: https://doi.org/10.1523/JNEUROSCI.0708-19.2019

15. Gulyaeva, N.V. Ventral hippocampus, Stress and Psychopathology: Translational implications. *Neurochem. J.* **9,** 85–94 (2015). https://doi.org/10.1134/S1819712415020075

16. Sense of smell - Wikipedia

17. Limbic system - Wikipedia

18. A.C. Campos, F.R. Ferreira, F.S. Guimarães, J.I. Lemos,Facilitation of endocannabinoid effects in the ventral hippocampus modulates anxiety-like behaviors depending on previous stress experience, Neuroscience, Volume 167, Issue 2,2010,Pages 238-246, ISSN 0306-4522, https://doi.org/10.1016/j.neuroscience.2010.01.062. (https://www.sciencedirect.com/science/article/pii/S0306452210001545)

19. D'Souza, D., Perry, E., MacDougall, L. *et al.* The Psychotomimetic Effects of Intravenous Delta-9-Tetrahydrocannabinol in Healthy Individuals: Implications for Psychosis. *Neuropsychopharmacol* **29,** 1558–1572 (2004). https://doi.org/10.1038/sj.npp.1300496

20. D'Souza, D., Perry, E., MacDougall, L. *et al.* The Psychotomimetic Effects of Intravenous Delta-9-Tetrahydrocannabinol in Healthy Individuals: Implications for Psychosis. *Neuropsychopharmacol* **29,** 1558–1572 (2004). https://doi.org/10.1038/sj.npp.1300496

21. D'Souza, D., Perry, E., MacDougall, L. *et al.* The Psychotomimetic Effects of Intravenous Delta-9-Tetrahydrocannabinol in Healthy Individuals: Implications for Psychosis. *Neuropsychopharmacol* **29,** 1558–1572 (2004). https://doi.org/10.1038/sj.npp.1300496

22. Haspula D, Clark MA. Cannabinoid Receptors: An Update on Cell Signaling, Pathophysiological Roles and Therapeutic Opportunities in Neurological, Cardiovascular, and Inflammatory Diseases. *International Journal of Molecular Sciences*. 2020; 21(20):7693. https://doi.org/10.3390/ijms21207693

23. Nicholson AN, Turner C, Stone BM, Robson PJ. Effect of Delta-9-tetrahydrocannabinol and cannabidiol on nocturnal sleep and early-morning behavior in young adults. J Clin Psychopharmacol. 2004 Jun;24(3):305-13. doi: 10.1097/01.jcp.0000125688.05091.8f. PMID: 15118485.

24. Nicholson AN, Turner C, Stone BM, Robson PJ. Effect of Delta-9-tetrahydrocannabinol and cannabidiol on nocturnal sleep and early-morning behavior in young adults. J Clin Psychopharmacol. 2004 Jun;24(3):305-13. doi: 10.1097/01.jcp.0000125688.05091.8f. PMID: 15118485.

25. Koulivand, P. H., Khaleghi Ghadiri, M., & Gorji, A. (2013). Lavender and the nervous system. *Evidence-based complementary and alternative medicine : eCAM, 2013*, 681304. https://doi.org/10.1155/2013/681304

26. Myrcene: What Is It and What Are Its Effects? | Terpenes (cannigma.com)

27. Mendelsohn AR, Larrick JW. Sleep facilitates clearance of metabolites from the brain: glymphatic function in aging and neurodegenerative diseases. Rejuvenation Res. 2013 Dec;16(6):518-23. doi: 10.1089/rej.2013.1530. PMID: 24199995.

28. Ana Coto-Montes, Jose Antonio Boga, Sergio Rosales-Corral, Lorena Fuentes-Broto, Dun-Xian Tan, Russel J. Reiter,Role of melatonin in the regulation of autophagy and mito-phagy: A review,Molecular and Cellular Endocrinology, Volume 361, Issues 1–2,2012,Pages 12-23,ISSN 0303-207, https://doi.org/10.1016/j.mce.2012.04.009.(https://www.sciencedi-rect.com/science/article/pii/S0303720712002626)

29. Ana Coto-Montes, Jose Antonio Boga, Sergio Rosales-Corral, Lorena Fuentes-Broto, Dun-Xian Tan, Russel J. Reiter,Role of melatonin in the regulation of autophagy and mito-phagy: A review,Molecular and Cellular Endocrinology, Volume 361, Issues 1–2,2012,Pages 12-23,ISSN 0303-207, https://doi.org/10.1016/j.mce.2012.04.009.(https://www.sciencedi-rect.com/science/article/pii/S0303720712002626)

30. Lin, C., Chao, H., Li, Z., Xu, X., Liu, Y., Hou, L., Liu, N. and Ji, J. (2016), Melatonin atten-uates traumatic brain injury-induced inflammation: a possible role for mitophagy. J. Pineal Res., 61: 177-186. https://doi.org/10.1111/jpi.12337

31. Rasmussen, M. K., Mestre, H., & Nedergaard, M. (2018). The glymphatic pathway in neu-rological disorders. *The Lancet. Neurology, 17*(11), 1016–1024. https://doi.org/10.1016/S1474-4422(18)30318-1

32. Sengupta S, Peterson TR, Laplante M, Oh S, Sabatini DM. mTORC1 controls fasting-in-duced ketogenesis and its modulation by ageing. Nature. 2010 Dec 23;468(7327):1100-4. doi: 10.1038/nature09584. PMID: 21179166.

33. Yun CW, Lee SH. The Roles of Autophagy in Cancer. Int J Mol Sci. 2018 Nov 5;19(11):3466. doi: 10.3390/ijms19113466. PMID: 30400561; PMCID: PMC6274804.

34. Closed-eye hallucination - Wikipedia

35. Melatonin and Weed: What Happens When You Mix Them (greencamp.com)

36. Lissoni P, Resentini M, Mauri R, Esposti D, Esposti G, Rossi D, Legname G, Fraschini F. Effects of tetrahydrocannabinol on melatonin secretion in man. Horm Metab Res. 1986 Jan;18(1):77-8. doi: 10.1055/s-2007-1012235. PMID: 3005151.

37. A23.1.full.pdf (bmj.com)

38. Molendijk, M. L., Haffmans, J. P., Bus, B. A., Spinhoven, P., Penninx, B. W., Prickaerts, J., Oude Voshaar, R. C., & Elzinga, B. M. (2012). Serum BDNF concentrations show strong seasonal variation and correlations with the amount of ambient sunlight. *PloS one*, *7*(11), e48046. https://doi.org/10.1371/journal.pone.0048046

39. Zaletel I, Filipović D, Puškaš N. Hippocampal BDNF in physiological conditions and social isolation. Rev Neurosci. 2017 Jul 26;28(6):675-692. doi: 10.1515/revneuro-2016-0072. PMID: 28593903.

40. Sangiovanni, E., Brivio, P., Dell'Agli, M., & Calabrese, F. (2017). Botanicals as Modulators of Neuroplasticity: Focus on BDNF. *Neural plasticity*, *2017*, 5965371. https://doi.org/10.1155/2017/5965371

41. Glenn, J. M., Madero, E. N., & Bott, N. T. (2019). Dietary Protein and Amino Acid Intake: Links to the Maintenance of Cognitive Health. *Nutrients*, *11*(6), 1315. https://doi.org/10.3390/nu11061315

42. Hu E, Du H, Zhu X, Wang L, Shang S, Wu X, Lu H, Lu X. Beta-hydroxybutyrate Promotes the Expression of BDNF in Hippocampal Neurons under Adequate Glucose Supply. Neuroscience. 2018 Aug 21;386:315-325. doi: 10.1016/j.neuroscience.2018.06.036. Epub 2018 Jun 30. PMID: 29966721.

43. Dias, G. P., Cavegn, N., Nix, A., do Nascimento Bevilaqua, M. C., Stangl, D., Zainuddin, M. S., Nardi, A. E., Gardino, P. F., & Thuret, S. (2012). The role of dietary polyphenols on adult hippocampal neurogenesis: molecular mechanisms and behavioural effects on depression and anxiety. *Oxidative medicine and cellular longevity*, *2012*, 541971. https://doi.org/10.1155/2012/541971

44. Sangiovanni, E., Brivio, P., Dell'Agli, M., & Calabrese, F. (2017). Botanicals as Modulators of Neuroplasticity: Focus on BDNF. *Neural plasticity*, *2017*, 5965371. https://doi.org/10.1155/2017/5965371

45. Socci, V., Tempesta, D., Desideri, G., De Gennaro, L., & Ferrara, M. (2017). Enhancing Human Cognition with Cocoa Flavonoids. *Frontiers in nutrition*, *4*, 19. https://doi.org/10.3389/fnut.2017.00019

46. Williams CM, El Mohsen MA, Vauzour D, Rendeiro C, Butler LT, Ellis JA, Whiteman M, Spencer JP. Blueberry-induced changes in spatial working memory correlate with changes in hippocampal CREB phosphorylation and brain-derived neurotrophic factor (BDNF) levels. Free Radic Biol Med. 2008 Aug 1;45(3):295-305. doi: 10.1016/j.freeradbiomed.2008.04.008. Epub 2008 May 5. PMID: 18457678.

47. Gómez-Pinilla F. (2008). Brain foods: the effects of nutrients on brain function. *Nature reviews. Neuroscience*, *9*(7), 568–578. https://doi.org/10.1038/nrn2421

48. Pawełczyk, T., Grancow-Grabka, M., Trafalska, E. *et al.* An increase in plasma brain derived neurotrophic factor levels is related to n-3 polyunsaturated fatty acid efficacy in first episode schizophrenia: secondary outcome analysis of the OFFER randomized clinical trial. *Psychopharmacology* **236,** 2811–2822 (2019). https://doi.org/10.1007/s00213-019-05258-4

49. Marshall B. Wallach, Samuel Gershon, The effects of Δ8-THC on the EEG, reticular multiple unit activity and sleep of cats, European Journal of Pharmacology,Volume 24, Issue 2,1973,Pages   172-178,ISSN   0014-2999,https://doi.org/10.1016/0014-2999(73)90068-X(https://www.sciencedirect.com/science/article/pii/001429997390068X)

50. Marshall B. Wallach, Samuel Gershon, The effects of Δ8-THC on the EEG, reticular multiple unit activity and sleep of cats, European Journal of Pharmacology,Volume 24, Issue 2,1973,Pages   172-178,ISSN   0014-2999,https://doi.org/10.1016/0014-2999(73)90068-X(https://www.sciencedirect.com/science/article/pii/001429997390068X)

51. DeltaDiol™ Super Concentrate - Mitozen Scientific

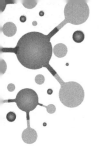

18

MELATONIN FOR THE MANAGEMENT OF LIVER DISORDERS

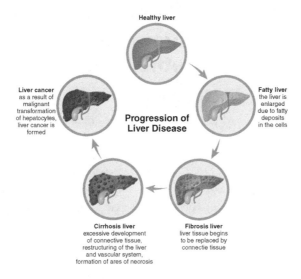

Your liver is the organ that filters your blood and is one of the primary ways we detoxify ourselves. It's not a big surprise that melatonin would have a powerful action on this organ as this is an area of high metabolism and cellular energy production. This energy creates the need to buffer the by-products of creating energy, which is known as oxidation. Melatonin is the primary antioxidant that protects us along with glutathione and they are of the utmost importance for a healthy liver.

The liver also plays a crucial role in digestion, metabolism, and energy production. It also helps to regulate the processes involved in energy release and utilization, which is why it is considered an essential organ for improving energy levels and maintaining good health and fitness.

Here is a brief discussion about melatonin's functions that help to regulate the metabolic processes performed by the liver. We will also discuss whether melatonin can be helpful in the management of liver diseases.

Melatonin and circadian rhythms in liver diseases: Functional roles and potential therapies

One study, "Melatonin and circadian rhythms in liver diseases: Functional roles and potential therapies", published in the Journal of Pineal Research in 2019 has provided evidence linking melatonin to healthy liver functions. This study was conducted to understand the liver's independent circadian rhythm and expression and how it is regulated by melatonin[1].

Several studies have already revealed the strong association between circadian rhythms and various hepatic diseases. The risk of developing these diseases could be linked to the disruption in the rhythm or the clock gene expressions, which make a person prone to develop liver steatosis, cancer, and inflammation[2]

The effect of the disruptions in the circadian rhythms leading to liver diseases are summarized in the table below:

Effects	Associated disease	Model
Elevation of gut permeability	ALD	Nighttime workers with moderate alcohol drinking[20]
Elevated liver damage and steatosis	ALD	Liver-specific *BMAL1* knockout mice with alcohol feeding[25,26]
Increased glucose tolerance	NAFLD	Rats with light exposure at night[32]
Increased body weight and adipose tissue	NAFLD	Rats with delayed feeding[33]
Increased hepatic lipid accumulation	NAFLD	Mice with HFD at daytime[34]
Impaired lipid metabolism	NAFLD	Liver-specific *BMAL1* knockout mice[37]
Elevated liver damage	Cholestasis	BDL rats with complete light[64]
High HCC development	HCC	Jet-lagged mice[78]
High incidence of complications	IRI	Patients with liver transplantation at night[99]

It is known that melatonin, being a natural and robust antioxidant, could protect the liver against the effect of alcohol intake and excessive fat accumulation. These unhealthy dietary and lifestyle habits contribute to the production of reactive oxygen species in the body, thereby worsening oxidative stress responsible for causing inflammatory and cancerous changes in the liver tissues.

This study specifically demonstrated that melatonin administration would minimize the oxidative stress-induced damage in the liver while also improving the symptoms of hepatic diseases.

There is accumulating evidence suggesting that restoring your circadian rhythm and its expressions through melatonin supplementation might offer a promising therapeutic strategy for patients diagnosed with liver diseases. Melatonin has a functional role and has significant therapeutic potential to restore proper circadian rhythm and buffer oxidative stress, which improves liver conditions[3].

There is an association between melatonin secretion and circadian rhythms and the development of liver diseases that could be avoided through melatonin supplementation. Does this mean that you can go out and drink like it's New Year's every day? Probably not the best idea but at the end of this chapter, I will make some suggestions on how to properly support yourself for those nights out on the town.

Take a look at the graph below and see all of the ways that Melatonin administration can provide benefits.

Effects	Dose	Associated disease	Model
Increase of circulating white blood cells	10 mg/kg/day	ALD	Mouse with ethanol injection[29]
Decreased liver damage	10 or 15 mg/kg/day	ALD	Pregnant rat with ethanol gavage[30]
Decreased oxidative and ER stress	500 µg/kg/day	NAFLD	Ob/ob mice[40]
Improved steatosis and insulin resistance	100 mg/kg/day	NAFLD	HFD mice[41]
Decreased de novo lipogenesis	10-50 mg/kg	NAFLD	HFD mice[42]
Increase of brown adipose tissue mass and activity	3 mg/day	NAFLD	Patients with melatonin deficiency[44]
Restored mitochondria functions	10 or 20 mg/kg/day	NAFLD	HFD mice[49,50]
Improved gut microbiota diversity	108 mg/kg/day	NAFLD	HFD mice[52]
Improved liver conditions	2 mg/g/day	PSC	$Mdr2^{-/-}$ mice[65]
Improved liver conditions	5 mg/kg/day	Bile duct injury	Rats with TAA administration[66]
Decreased liver damage and steatosis	2.5-20 mg/kg/day	Toxin-induced liver damage	Rats with CCl_4 administration[67,68]
Improved clock gene expression	5 or 10 mg/kg/day	Toxin-induced liver damage	Mice with CCl_4 administration[71]

Melatonin administration changes the expression level of something called "clock genes." Though the detailed mechanism is still not completely understood, these expression changes in the "clock genes" improve your circadian rhythms and are believed to contribute to the therapeutic benefits of melatonin for the liver.

Melatonin treatment can help restore mitochondrial function in the liver cells called the hepatocytes and even inhibit the deposition of lipids. See more detail on this in Chapter 8 on Cardiology. These hepatic cells can also transmit pro-inflammatory cytokines. If you've been following this book, you now know how melatonin is produced in all of your mitochondria as a reaction to buffer cytokines or inflammation resulting from stress at the cellular level. Melatonin administration would target this form of unfavorable cell-to-cell communication occurring between hepatic cells. Without this buffering system, a much faster progression of liver diseases occurs.

Melatonin may also limit the release of free radicals in the damaged liver tissues, which would protect the healthy part of the liver against the adverse effects linked to oxidative stress. The favorable changes expected to occur in the liver cells following melatonin administration also include improved communication between liver cells. This communication happens through small extracellular vesicles. These vesicles are secreted from different liver cells. Several forms of extracellular vesicles such as exosomes, apoptotic bodies, microvesicles, and microparticles are categorized based on their specific particle sizes and biogenesis. Extracellular vesicles also contain certain cellular mediators, such as DNAs, proteins, and RNAs, that can transfer these mediators into the recipient cells. This mechanism, which enables cell-to-cell communication mediated by extracellular vesicles plays a critical role in the pathophysiology of hepatic diseases.

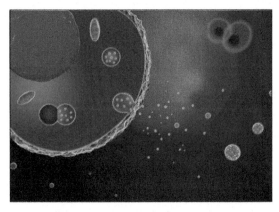

Just imagine the wide range of communication that needs to occur in a liver doing hundreds of jobs and coordinating all of the events to maintain healthy blood levels. It's not always good to have more communication going on, as that could also indicate future problems. For instance, some hepatic cells can produce a higher number of vesicles during lipid-induced liver damage. These extracellular vesicles may contain TRAIL (tumor necrosis factor-related apoptosis-inducing ligand) that could regulate the growth of cancer tissues within the liver cells through cell-to-cell communications[4].

By targeting the activities of these vesicles, Melatonin could help restore healthy cell-to-cell communication and so help to inhibit or minimize the spread of cancer. This form of activity triggered by melatonin is beneficial for patients diagnosed with hepatic cancers and those who suffer from liver diseases triggered by alcohol and fatty foods.

Keep in mind; it's not fat that's the enemy; it's the type of fat. They are good fats, and they're bad fats. Some of the worst fats that are destructive to the liver are vegetable oils that have been heated up and made rancid. If you eat out at restaurants often, it's impossible to avoid these. They're also in many baked goods and chips that are commercially available. Avoiding these bad fats is one of the most important things we can do to live longer and be more vital. These fats find their way into our cell membranes which causes problems with communication and up-regulates cytokines. With this idea in mind, it's easy to understand the relationship between melatonin, liver disease, and fats that cause inflammation. Good fats are monounsaturated and polyunsaturated fats like linoleic,

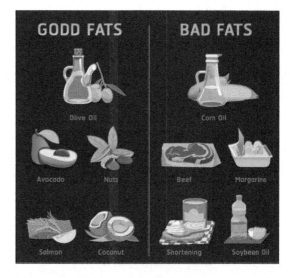

alpha-linoleic, or omega fatty acids such as EPA & DHA. Not all saturated fats are bad for you, especially if you're not consuming many carbohydrates. Carbohydrates cause a lot of oxidation and inflammation, which then interact with fats, making things worse. Many studies show that people on a low-carb diet do not have all of the negative consequences seen with high carbohydrate diets along with a high-fat diet.

Research on melatonin therapies has provided evidence showing the benefits of this hormone in improving liver functions. In human trials, daily melatonin supplementation in a dose of 3 mg for at least three months has been shown to cause an increase in the brown adipose tissue mass.

> ## Dr John's Comment:
>
> *Since we know that the negative consequences of inflammation and oxidative stress to the liver, this could be reversed to some extent by regular use of melatonin supplements. Using melatonin reduces inflammation in the hepatocytes allowing them to start functioning efficiently. Remember when we talked about cytokines and inflammation only allowing the mitochondria to produce 10% of the energy due to converting to aerobic glycolysis versus using the Krebs cycle? That means inflammation can starve your liver of 90% of its energy. Restoring energy to this organ will improve lipid metabolism, carbohydrate metabolism, enzyme secretion, hormones, and so on.*

> **Dr John's Comment:**
>
> *"There is brown fat and white fat in your body. When you were young, you had a lot of brown fat, but when you become old, much of the fat becomes white. The basic difference between the two is that brown fat is very rich in mitochondria and what's called metabolically active fat. This means it's a better source of energy for you when you are in a fasting state and you require pulling energy out of your fat storage. Keep in mind that when you are sleeping, you are in a fasted state, and this is when you are getting your energy. "*

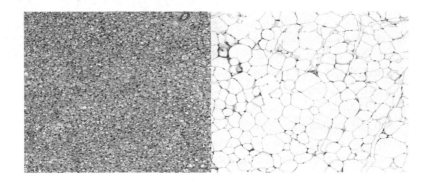

Left is mitochondrial rich brown fat and right is white fat.

A higher accumulation of white fat is noted in patients with a marked melatonin deficiency.

In addition, melatonin is also shown to regulate circadian rhythms. The secretion of melatonin is rhythmic and periodic in healthy individuals. This is why; there is a growing consensus that melatonin, when used as a supplement, must mimic a similar rhythmic dosage. When administered in this form, such that the dosages of melatonin are in sync with the optimal production of natural melatonin in the body, patients are expected to derive higher benefits.

The favorable effects of melatonin supplementation used rhythmically based on the body's sleep-wake would also provide hepatic benefits by promoting the functions of the liver and protecting you against liver diseases including liver cancer, alcoholic hepatitis, fatty liver disease, and cirrhosis.

Another study provided an in-depth explanation about the effects of melatonin on the liver concerning liver injuries caused by toxins. This study, "Effects of Melatonin on Liver Injuries and Diseases," published in the International Journal of Molecular Sciences in 2017, was conducted to assess whether melatonin could help protect the liver against the toxic effects of heavy metals and drugs[5]. We live in an incredibly toxic world today. There are thousands of manufactured chemicals floating around our environment, and it's up to your liver to filter these and protect us from them. Chemical pollutants, heavy metals, prescription drugs in our drinking water can all induce liver damage. Liver diseases involve various liver pathologies, such as hepatic steatosis, hepatitis, fatty liver, fibrosis, cirrhosis, and even hepatocarcinoma. Despite all the research performed over the past several decades, there are very few therapy choices for managing liver injuries due to toxins and heavy metal poisoning. Big Pharma is working hard to discover new treatments that could be effective and safe to reverse and block liver injuries. If only melatonin could be patented, it would be a major blockbuster prescription for liver disease, among many others. But unfortunately for Big Pharma, and fortunately for us, God owns the patent for melatonin.

A recent study showed that melatonin could be used for the prevention and treatment of liver injuries. These findings are based on summaries about the potential role of melatonin in reversing liver damage while paying particular attention to its mechanism of action[6].

The Protective Effect of Melatonin on Chemical-Induced Liver Injuries

Environmental toxins and chemical pollutants can create adverse effects on our liver. The beneficial role of melatonin on liver damage induced due to these chemical pollutants like organic compounds, mycotoxins, and metals is clear.

Positive results were seen in experimental models of CCl4 (carbon tetrachloride)-induced liver injuries and melatonin where CCl4 can induce acute and chronic liver damage. In acute liver injuries induced due to the exposure to CCl4, the levels of lipid peroxide (LPO), lipid hydroperoxides (LOOH), malondialdehyde (MDA), and triglyceride (TG) were found to be increased. In contrast, the levels of all the good stuff such as glutathione (GSH) concentrations were found to be reduced. Several other parameters linked to the functions of the liver were found to be adversely affected in patients who had developed serious toxicity due to the exposure to CCl4[7].

This study shows that melatonin supplementation could lessen the signs of liver injury. A reduction in the concentrations of hepatic liver enzymes can also be reversed to some extent by undergoing treatment with melatonin supplements. The activities of SOD, GSSG-R, CAT, and the rise in LPO levels and hepatic XO activities were found to be attenuated following melatonin administration in a dose of 10, 50, or 100 mg per kg body weight in a dose-dependent manner[8].

These findings mean that using melatonin regularly would offer an effective way to protect yourself against the adverse effects of chemical poisoning. It will reduce damage to the liver due to harmful chemicals and toxins and enable you to avoid the risk of acute and chronic hepatic diseases. Regular use of melatonin may also help to improve your liver functions by reducing inflammation and oxidative stress caused by these chemicals. This will also help to enhance the production of digestive enzymes in your liver and improve your digestion. Moreover, toxic chemicals like CCl4 are also known to cause mitochondrial alterations by inducing oxidation of the intramitochondrial glutathione. These toxins can also cause the inhibition of some enzymes that support digestion and metabolism, like succinate dehydrogenase (complex II), and modify the levels of plasma nitric oxide, which may alter the blood supply to your liver and other vital organs.

Melatonin supplements given in a dose of 10 mg per kg body weight will reverse these changes. It will improve the mitochondrial GSH-Px (GSH peroxidase) activities and prevent the excessive rise in nitric oxide levels. This will also help to ensure optimum availability of proteins in your body and reduce your risk of diseases that arise due to protein malnourishment[9][10].

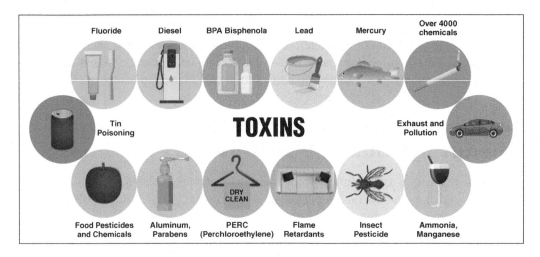

Nutrient absorption, as we get older, becomes a real problem. Besides our gut getting weaker, so we're not absorbing as much, we're also not able to assimilate these if your liver is not working correctly. This is one of the reasons that many alcoholics have poor muscle mass. Regular use of melatonin might hold the key to ensuring that toxins entering your body are buffered and removed so that they don't create widespread inflammation in your body and liver disease.

For those bodybuilders or anti-aging enthusiasts who enjoy growth hormone, melatonin can increase the expression of growth hormone or IGF-I[11]. Melatonin could also improve the health of the cell membranes in your liver. Melatonin regulates the transfer of molecules across different cells and tissues in the liver, thereby promoting its normal functions.

Besides protecting the liver against the toxicity induced by CCl4, melatonin is also effective for preventing liver damage linked to exposure to benzene and toluene, both of which are common chemical pollutants[12]. These chemicals are among the many in camp Lejeune when I was young and thus, exposed to them in the drinking water. I will dive into this more in the chapter where we talk about melatonin for children.

These chemicals are known to produce a detrimental effect on humans as well as animals. Benzene can cause impairment in liver functions by inducing disruptions in the lipid peroxidation of microsomes and mitochondria. Cadmium (Cd) is another common toxic substance found in the environment. It is known to cause hepatotoxicity in humans and animals. Exposure to cadmium can induce severe histopathological changes, including the loss of normal structural integrity of the liver parenchymatous tissues, cellular degeneration, cytoplasmic vacuolization, and cellular necrosis. It can also result in the congestion of the blood vessels, destruction of the cristae mitochondria, formation of fat globules, and glycogen depletion. These toxic effects of cadmium on the liver could be counteracted with the help of melatonin treatment. Cadmium exposure can also produce cytotoxicity that can disrupt the mitochondrial membrane potential and increase reactive oxygen species (ROS). It may also reduce the mitochondrial mass and the mitochondrial DNA content. Accumulation of cadmium in the liver tissues can also worsen oxidative stress and inflammation[13]. I would expect to see a lot of white fat with someone that has heavy metal toxicity, especially with cadmium.

Melatonin supplementation, in these cases, can reduce liver injury and minimize oxidative damage and inflammation by stimulating the mechanisms that decrease serum levels of ALT and AST and by inhibiting the production of pro-inflammatory cytokines. It is also believed to work by preventing the action of NLRP3 and alleviating oxidative stress while attenuating hepatocyte death[14].

After recovering from Lyme disease, I found out mold illness was a big part of my getting sick and that my house had mold. A lot of toxins can be released from these mold species that find their way to the liver. The broad category for this illness is biotoxin illness. Mycotoxins are the secondary metabolites that are produced in the body by some toxigenic fungi. The species commonly known to produce these toxins include aflatoxins, trichothecenes, fumonisins, ochratoxin A, zearalenone, and patulin. Among these mycotoxins, ochratoxin A and aflatoxins have a higher potential to induce liver injuries. It is known that aflatoxins can produce chronic mutagenic, carcinogenic, teratogenic effects, and acute inflammatory effects. Melatonin has also been found to protect the liver against these types of mycotoxins, and it can help restore healthy activities of the liver and allow this organ to support digestive functions and metabolism more efficiently[15].

The effects of melatonin in the management of non-alcoholic fatty liver disease (NAFLD)

The benefits of melatonin supplementation for improving your liver health are not limited to its ability to protect this vital organ against the damage caused by heavy metals and toxins. It can also help reduce the symptoms of non-alcoholic fatty liver disease and prevent the progress of this condition. I always say it's either toxins or infec-

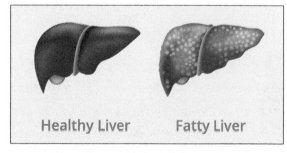

Healthy Liver   Fatty Liver

tions that are the root of all diseases. I think even though they are finding cases where no cause for fatty liver is identified, it's most likely related to one of those even though it's not apparent. Genetics also causes people to have poor detox pathways resulting in weak liver function, which could also be at the cause but much more rarely, in my opinion. A study showed benefits to patients diagnosed with this condition when treated with melatonin. The study, "The Effects of Melatonin in Patients with Nonalcoholic Fatty Liver Disease: A Randomized Controlled Trial," was published in the Advanced Biomedical Research in 2017[16].

This study was designed to assess the effects of melatonin on the development and progression of non-alcoholic fatty liver disease compared to placebo. NAFLD (Non-alcoholic fatty liver disease) is a chronic liver condition defined by excessive accumulation of fats in the liver in the forms of triglycerides. In most cases, more than 5% of hepatocytes show variations or abnormalities on histological examination. NAFLD has been recently recognized as one of the major liver diseases affecting people worldwide[17].

Worldwide, the incidence of NAFLD in the general population ranges between 9% to 37%. It is estimated that the incidence of NAFLD in the adult population is from 30% to 40% and that nearly 40% of people with NAFLD tend to have NASH (non-alcoholic steatohepatitis). Recent studies in some countries have reported that the prevalence of NAFLD in the general population is nearly 20- 30%[18].

The molecular mechanisms underlying the progression of NAFLD are not entirely understood. But, insulin resistance, cytokine imbalances, and oxidative stress are the known key pathophysiological mechanisms that can trigger and worsen NAFLD development. Of course, when one looks deeper to ask the question, what's causing the cytokines? I would offer infections such as with Epstein Barr Virus, and the accumulation of biotoxins from mold may be at the root of these cases. These factors have explained the transformation of NAFLD when the liver is also affected by other conditions like simple steatosis and NASH. It also explains the interaction of free radicals with certain cellular constituents that may result in the hepatocyte's peroxidative deterioration resulting in the impairment of liver function. Treatment methods that may efficiently reduce both the apoptosis and oxidative stress in hepatocytes to reverse or inhibit the further progress of NAFLD, such as the case with melatonin, make sense.

This study specifically tried to assess the benefits of melatonin in terms of how this molecule could help to protect the liver tissues against the abnormal changes caused by NAFLD. The research revealed that the lipid peroxidation inhibitory and the hypocholesterolemic effects of melatonin (also shown in some previous studies) could effectively relieve NAFLD symptoms[19].

Dr John's Comment:

"Consider the carbohydrates as gasoline on fire causing the fats to go rancid right in your bloodstream. Many of the refined carbohydrates, in particular, create a tremendous amount of inflammation in the body. These bad fats also find themselves in your cell membranes for up to two years, interfering with your cells' ability to communicate and receive proper signaling from your hormones. I am a big proponent of a high-fat diet such as the ketogenic diet. Although I don't practice this diet every day of the week, it is the primary diet I eat. I believe in having carbohydrate loading days, but I do not consume any of the more dangerous fats."

It may also help reduce the levels of cholesterol and triglycerides in your blood and prevent the most common precursor of NAFLD, which is diet-induced hypercholesterolemia. Please keep in mind the standard American diet includes lots of carbohydrates. So when you combine carbohydrates with fats, it will get you in trouble.

The antioxidant and anti-inflammatory properties of melatonin could be a great support for your liver to fight against NAFLD. The antioxidant action of melatonin will ensure the free radicals that can accelerate liver damage and erode into the healthy hepatocytes at a rapid speed are destroyed much sooner before they can produce any adverse effect. So, this will leave your liver with improved efficiency to recover and repair the damaged tissues. This faster healing of the damaged cells will help your liver function more normally within a shorter period.

The anti-inflammatory action of melatonin would enhance the results further by simply modifying the response of the liver to the pro-inflammatory substances released by the immune cells. It will alter the immune response such that the substances that can worsen liver damage, like cytokines, are no longer produced by the immune cells in higher quantities. This form of anti-inflammatory effect created by melatonin supplements can play a crucial role in allowing you to recover faster. It would help inhibit further damage to the liver and support the processes involved in repairing the damaged tissues or hepatocytes. So, your road to recovery would be smoother with melatonin.

Within a short duration of starting the use of melatonin supplements, you'll find a remarkable improvement in your liver functions evident in the form of better digestion. A study aimed at determining the effect of melatonin on some biochemical parameters in patients diagnosed with NAFLD has revealed similar findings. A total of 100 patients who were histopathologically diagnosed with NAFLD were grouped into two categories. Among these, the first group of patients was treated with oral melatonin, while the other group was treated with a placebo. The doses were given three times daily for three months, that's all-day dosing[20] [21].

The collected data included the weight of the patient, waist measurements, DBP (diastolic blood pressure), SBP (systolic blood pressure), ALT (alanine aminotransferase), AST (aspartate aminotransferase), and hsCRP (high sensitive C-reactive protein). Additionally, the fatty liver grade and the side effects were also measured at the baseline and after the treatment period using a standardized clinical chemistry technique.

Dr John's Comment:

"Dr. Frank Shallenberger taught me to dose patients both day and night when the extra support is needed. He emphasized this with cancer patients and with degenerative neurological patients, and I would assume that he would be a proponent for this with anybody that has a severe liver condition."

Before the treatment, the average of the waist, weight, SBP, ALT, DBP, AST, and hsCRP of the participants of both the case group and the placebo or control group were in a similar range. After treatment with either melatonin or placebo, significant differences were noted in these parameters of patients in both groups indicating the effectiveness of melatonin in the management of liver diseases. After the treatment, the fatty liver grade was found to be statistically improved. This showed the remarkable therapeutic effect produced by melatonin in patients of the case group. This study has provided valuable findings that could pave the way for devising better treatment strategies for patients with moderate to severe complications linked to liver diseases[22].

Melatonin supplementation as a promising adjunct for the management of liver disease

New research has suggested that melatonin supplementation could work as a promising adjunct for the treatment of patients with liver diseases. One study[23], "Dietary Melatonin Supplementation Could Be a Promising Preventing/Therapeutic Approach for a Variety of Liver Diseases," published in the Nutrients in 2018 has revealed that including melatonin supplements in the treatment plan for cirrhosis, alcoholic and non-alcoholic fatty liver, and even liver carcinoma could improve the outcomes considerably.

Chronic liver diseases like cirrhosis and hepatic carcinoma are a global problem, with oxidative stress, inflammation, and mitochondrial dysfunctions being the primary mechanisms responsible for their progression. According to this review published in Nutrients, researchers have demonstrated that melatonin supplements may offer promising therapy in the prevention and treatment of these diseases by acting as a natural antioxidant, anti-inflammatory, and anti-carcinogenic agent.

Melatonin is basically an indoleamine whose main role is to regulate the functions of the neuro-immuno-endocrine systems of our body. This hormone is often used for supporting sleep and for its antioxidant properties in the management of cancer. But, this study has demonstrated its wide-reaching benefits that could help in promoting recovery of patients with serious life-threatening complications of liver diseases, including hepatic failure.

The common issues linked to liver health could be attributed to the age-related decline in the body's normal physiological functioning and the wear and tear of healthy tissues. After childhood, particularly in the elderly, the secretion of melatonin decreases considerably, possibly due to inflammation and degenerative changes in the pineal gland, as well as the decline in cellular functions in all organs of the body. These abnormal changes could be related to chronic liver diseases, which is why increasing your use of melatonin supplementation might be important for you during this phase.

The common alterations in hepatic diseases are the result of fibrosis, steatosis, carcinogenesis, and inflammation. Liver fibrosis is reversible to some extent, and so, regression of hepatic diseases at this stage could be a critical strategy for preventing the progression of diseases.

Melatonin supplementation in a dose of 10 mg per day has been proven to increase the plasma melatonin levels significantly while reducing the levels of liver enzymes in patients with degenerate and fibrotic changes in the liver, demonstrating the benefits of this hormone in the management of liver diseases.

Researchers have revealed that melatonin supplementation could improve hepatic mitochondrial functions, reduce oxidative stress, and enhance mitochondrial functions. Melatonin in the hepatic cells can also play a protective role on the mitochondrial dysfunctions and help to inactivate fibrogenesis, preventing further fibrosis considerably or reversing the pre-existing fibrotic or pro-fibrotic changes to some extent[24].

Other nutritional supplements that could be beneficial for your liver health include fish oil and probiotics. Probiotics have been shown to decrease liver fat and improve the activities of liver enzymes. Probiotics are also likely to be the most effective in inhibiting bacterial translocation and controlling the effect of intestinal microbiota on hepatic functions. Fish oil supplements can exert an anti-inflammatory action and restore insulin sensitivity, which is considered important as we need to understand liver diseases are linked to obesity and diabetes. This suggests that including the use of melatonin supplements in your treatment plan along with the use of supplements containing fish oil and probiotics could help you recover faster and reduce your risk of life-threatening complications.

It is also essential to encourage a restricted diet that is low in or completely devoid of carbohydrates. Adequate exercise to promote faster weight loss can further enhance the benefits of melatonin supplements in these patients. Patients with established liver diseases usually have a higher nutritional demand than what could typically be obtained from their diet alone. So, they should also consider using nutritional supplements containing vitamins, minerals, and antioxidants to mitigate the pathogenesis of the disease[25].

The application of phytomelatonin for the treatment of liver diseases

As far as the therapeutic strategies for managing liver diseases are concerned, the role of the person's diet is another well-established factor. Melatonin, identified as one of the hormones secreted in the body of humans, was also discovered in plants and named phytomelatonin.

These substances can produce a positive effect on the liver during aging and even in pathological conditions. In particular, it's essential for us to understand that the amount of melatonin produced by the pineal gland decreases during our lifetime. Also, its reduction in the blood may be related to the increased risk of developing pathological conditions in which the mitochondrial dysfunctions at the cellular level and oxidative stress play a key role. Moreover, it has been suggested that phytomelatonin containing foods might provide a source of dietary melatonin. So, their ingestion through supplements or balanced diets may be sufficient to confer the health benefits of this hormone.

I came across one research[26], "Dietary Melatonin Supplementation Could Be a Promising Preventing/Therapeutic Approach for a Variety of Liver Diseases," published

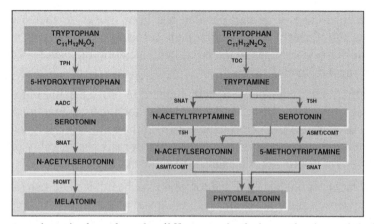

in the Nutrients in 2018 that was aimed at assessing the role of plant-based melatonin in the management of liver diseases.

In this study, the classification of hepatic diseases and the overview of some of the most important aspects of melatonin and phytomelatonin, based on the differences in their synthesis, and their presence in foods, were evaluated. This study also focused on assessing the role of melatonin and phytomelatonin in health and diseases.

The findings of this study have suggested that supplementing with both melatonin and phytomelatonin could be considered critical for preventing diseases affecting the liver. The potential beneficial effects of melatonin and phytomelatonin in the management of liver diseases with respect to their molecular mechanisms of actions can be viewed in this picture below:

This study further revealed that Melatonin, in the form of N-acetyl-5-methoxytryptamine, can be a highly conserved form of indoleamine molecule that is found in all microorganisms and even in plants and animals. And the best part is that it is considered a safe molecule since it forms part of the body's natural physiological processes and is produced naturally in the body. In fact, several human and animal studies have reported that the short-term use of melatonin does not lead to any adverse effects, even when used in extreme doses. Here is yet another source supporting supraphysiological dosing. They also concluded that the long-term melatonin treatment might not cause any severe adverse effects[27].

The benefits of melatonin for controlling elevated liver enzymes

One of the primary functions of the liver is to produce specific enzymes that help in the digestion of food and support metabolism. These enzymes are produced in the liver in the required amounts to maintain metabolic activities. An increase or decrease in the secretion of these enzymes could affect the health of the liver. It may also lead to disruptions in the digestive and metabolic processes occurring in the body.

Some medications are known to produce severe side effects which can affect liver function due to the secretion of enzymes. Statins are the most commonly implicated group of drugs in this regard. Several studies have revealed that the regular use of statins could affect the liver heath and cause disturbances in the production of these enzymes. Luckily, melatonin supplementation is helpful in controlling these side effects of statins and restoring healthy levels of liver enzymes.

One research study[28], 'The Effects of Melatonin on Elevated Liver Enzymes during Statin Treatment,' published in the BioMed Research International in 2017, has provided insights into the benefits of melatonin supplementation for protecting the liver against the adverse effects caused by statins.

Statins are the groups of medications commonly prescribed to patients who suffer from increased cholesterol levels. These drugs are used widely for modifying fat metabolism to control lipid abnormalities and protect the patient against the risk of cardiovascular diseases such as hypertension, stroke, and heart attacks.

These medications reduce cholesterol levels and prevent or slow down the development of atherosclerosis. This can help to reduce the risk of heart attacks and stroke that usually occur due to the compromised blood supply to the cardiac muscles or brain, respectively, as a result of the narrowing of the arteries caused by atherosclerosis.

While these drugs are effective to some extent for preventing atherosclerosis and reducing cholesterol levels, they do cause serious long-term side effects, most of which are linked to liver health. This study was aimed at assessing the role of melatonin supplements in reversing or preventing these side effects and to check whether this hormone could regulate the production of liver enzymes in patients who are using statins for the treatment of high cholesterol.

The research into how to minimize the side effects of statins is important, seeing as studies have revealed that statins cause an increase in the levels of liver enzymes, particularly alanine aminotransferase and aspartate. An assessment of the usefulness of melatonin for counteracting these adverse hepatic events has revealed favorable results.

This research program included 60 patients between the ages of 47 and 65 years. Among these, 41 were women, and 19 were men, all of whom were diagnosed with hyperlipidemia and were taking statins like atorvastatin or rosuvastatin in a dose of 20 to 40 mg a day. The patients were allocated randomly in two groups. The first group was treated with the same statin they were taking earlier with a daily standardized dose of 20 mg along with melatonin supplements. The second group of patients took statins along with placebo in the same dose and same time of the day.

The follow-up lab testing of the liver enzymes was performed to assess the levels of AST, ALP, GGT, and ALT following the treatment for 2, 4, and 6 months. The results of this study have shown that Melatonin can exert a strong hepatoprotective effect in patients using statins and prevent disruptions in the liver functions caused due to the abnormal rise in the secretion of these enzymes. This marks the need to use melatonin supplements in conjunction with statins to minimize the risk of side effects and protect the liver functions while maintaining healthy metabolic and digestive functions.[29][30]

How Emotions and Organs are Connected in Traditional Chinese Medicine

In traditional Chinese medicine (TCM), emotions and physical health are intimately connected. This integrated mind-body approach to health and healing operates in a dynamic loop where emotions impact the health of the body and vice versa. For example, according to TCM theory, excessive irritability and anger can affect the liver and result in multiple ailments, including menstrual pain, headache, redness of the face and eyes, dizziness, and dry mouth. Alternatively, an imbalance in the liver can result in stormy moods.

Diagnosis in traditional Chinese medicine is highly individualized. Once an impaired organ system and/or emotional imbalance is identified, the unique symptoms of the patient determine the practitioner's treatment approach.

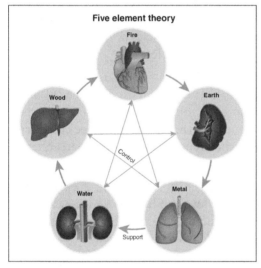

Traditional Chinese medicine has been practiced for over 2,000 years, and its use in the United States as part of complementary healthcare has grown dramatically over the last few decades. In fact, from 2002 to 2007, there was a 50% increase in acupuncture use, from around 8 million to over 14 million people accessing this treatment[31].

TCM is based on the principle that mental and physical well-being are intricately entwined. In turn, practitioners believe that optimal health is governed by balancing a person's qi (vital life force) with the complementary forces of yin (passive) and yang (active) and the five elements of fire, water, earth, wood, and metal[32].

In TCM, it is believed that emotional imbalances can act as both symptoms and causes for physical issues. Additionally, mental health conditions are linked to specific physical ailments of key organs. According to traditional Chinese medicine, emotions are narrowed down to five basic feelings that are each associated with a corresponding element and organ in the body:

- • Anger with the liver
- • Fear with the kidney
- • Joy with the heart
- • Sadness and grief with the lung
- • Worry with the spleen

For example, under the TCM theory, breast distension, menstrual pain, and irritability during menses are treated with certain herbs and acupuncture points that target the liver. Headaches, dizziness, excessive anger, and redness of the face point to an alternative type of liver pattern and are treated in a different way[33].

Digestion and the processing of nutrients are primary functions of this vital organ[34].In TCM, the liver is associated with anger, depression, and the below physical symptoms:

- • Emotions: Anger, resentment, frustration, irritability, bitterness, and "flying off the handle."
- • Liver function: Involved in the smooth flow of energy and blood throughout the body; regulates bile secretion and stores blood; is connected with the tendons, nails, and eyes
- • Symptoms of liver imbalance: Breast distension, menstrual pain, headache, irritability, inappropriate anger, dizziness, dry, red eyes, and other eye conditions, and tendonitis
- • Liver conditions: Liver qi stagnation, liver fire

Melatonin and weight loss

Weight loss has been frequently associated with the use of melatonin supplementation. This benefit could be attributed to the activation and recruitment of brown adipose tissue by melatonin that converts energy stored in fats into heat. This property of melatonin could be effective in the management of fatty liver diseases. It may also support the faster recovery of obese patients with hepatic diseases, as excessive fat deposition in different body tissues triggers inflammation and can be a strong headwind to healthy weight loss. Melatonin, by reducing body fat, would decrease inflammation and allow healthy weight loss in a shorter duration.

Signs of a Stressed Liver

The following symptoms listed might suggest your liver function might be overstressed: Acid reflux, bloating and gas, constipation, skin and/or eyes that are yellowish (a symptom of jaundice), inability to lose weight, high blood pressure, moodiness, anxiety, or depression, Dark urine or circles under the eyes, Rosacea, chronic fatigue, excessive sweating, bruise easily and poor appetite.

Besides melatonin, you can support your liver through a few lifestyle changes. Follow these four natural liver-friendly suggestions.

1. Remove Toxic Foods from Your Diet

Limit processed foods, hydrogenated oils, refined sugar; most convenience foods are toxic to your liver. Hydrogenated oils, also known as "trans fats," have higher levels of saturated fat. The chemical structure of the oil itself has been altered to increase its shelf-life. Consumption of trans fats dramatically increases stress on your liver. Nitrites, commonly found in convenience foods, fast foods, lunch meats, and many wines, are not liver-friendly. These harmful chemicals are used to preserve foods.

Besides dietary toxins, you might avoid toxin exposure from your cosmetics, laundry detergent, and fabric softeners, personal care products, drinking municipal water, working with industrial solvents and paints without gloves.

2. Nutrients that Support your Liver

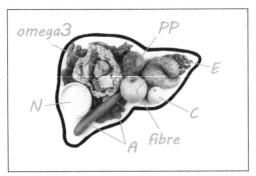

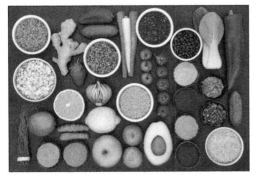

Milk Thistle is considered the "primero" of detoxifying and liver-protecting herbs. Milk thistle helps to eliminate the buildup of chemicals, heavy metals, prescription medications, environmental pollutants, and alcohol in the liver. Milk thistle helps to reduce the negative effects on the liver after chemotherapy and radiation. The active ingredient silymarin helps to strengthen the cell walls in the liver while supporting healthy regeneration[35].

Bitter Herbs can improve both phase 1 and 2 detoxification. Bitter herbs are the cornerstone of herbal medicine due to their powerful liver support. A range of physiological responses occurs following stimulation of the bitter receptors of the tongue. The bitter taste stimulates the specific bitter taste buds at the back of the tongue to stimulate the parasympathetic nervous system to trigger a number of reflexes. These reflexes are important to the digestive process and general health. The following are great bitter herbs: Chicory, Coriander, Dandelion, Endive, Horehound, Mint, Sorrel, Milk thistle, Beet, Wild lettuce, Wormwood, Angelica, Chamomile, Goldenseal, Rue, Yarrow, and Horseradish. Burdock and Dandelion teas are great options to help detox your liver. They both have a natural diuretic effect, allowing your liver to eliminate toxins more quickly.

Glutathione is the main nutrient that supports the phase 2 liver detox pathways where we neutralize chemicals and drugs. Glutathione's sulfur helix wraps around toxins and chaperones them out of the body. Like melatonin, glutathione is poorly absorbed, and suppository and liposomal administration is far superior. NAC is another nutraceutical that can be taken, and its benefits are due to its conversion into glutathione. Glutathione and melatonin can make an excellent combination together and are synergistic. Turmeric supports healthy liver tissue and liver metabolism.

3. Drink Raw Vegetable Juice

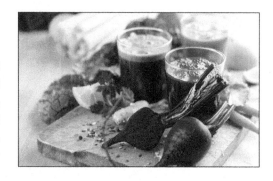

Juicing your veggies has the added benefit of making the vegetables easier to digest and more readily available for absorption, taking some stress off your liver. Vegetables are ideal for liver cleanses and include beet, dandelion, cabbage, parsley, celery, cauliflower, and Brussels sprouts.

4. Eat liver or take Desiccated Liver.

Liver from grass-fed cattle or organic chicken is rich in vitamins A and B, folic acid, choline, iron, copper, zinc, chromium, and CoQ10. Although I find the taste of liver difficult to stomach, it is one of the most nutrient-dense foods you can eat.

5. Morning Liver Detox Protocol

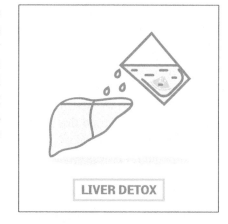

LIVER DETOX

Fat-soluble toxins will become trapped in the enterohepatic biliary circulation (EHC). Toxins will become dissolved in your bile acids and they will cycle over and over from the liver to the small intestine and back to the liver. To bind these and clear them, you can drink the following morning drink. In addition to this, it can be helpful to take a binder before bed as your bile has a strong release during the first few hours of sleep.

1. Juice 1 organic lemon into 6-8 oz of spring water.

2. Add 1 tsp of Glycine

3. Drink with a binder such as BIND from Revelation Health, or if you have a chronic illness, you might consider getting a prescription for cholestyramine from your doctor for a 30-day liver cleanse.

6. Gallbladder Flush

You will need the following in order to do this cleanse: 1 bottle of phos drops from Standard Process, 3 grapefruits or 6 lemons, one 8 oz. bottle of olive oil. Take 30 drops of Phos Drops diluted in 8 ounces of spring water three times a day for 3-6 days before doing the Gallbladder Flush.

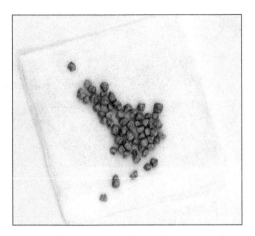

On the evening of the gallbladder flush, make sure to have finished all of your phos drops for this day before starting the flush). Begin by juicing your choice of lemon or grapefruit. You will need at least 6 oz. of cold squeezed juice (4 oz. to mix with olive oil and 2 oz. to drink after). It can help to have a glass with 2 oz. of juice to drink immediately after the oil/juice mixture. Place the 4 oz. of juice with the 4 oz. of olive oil. Stir and drink quickly. Then drink 2 oz. of lemon or grapefruit juice. Go directly to bed and lie on your back with your head and upper body propped up for at least 20 minutes before going to sleep. After 20 minutes, you can assume your normal sleeping position. In the morning, you will notice a number of hard green stones in your bowel movement. These could be stones from your gallbladder, along with stones created by the olive oil soaking up your bile and the toxins held within it.

Conclusion

Over the years, I've had to support my liver. When I was very sick with Lyme disease and mold illness, my liver and gallbladder seemed to take a significant amount of stress due to the infection and toxicity of the biotoxins that were released from all of these microbes. Early on, I began to experiment with glutathione suppositories and noticed this was one of the first things I tried that gave me significant improvement. I would take the suppositories before bed and wake up with less inflammation, more energy, and less brain fog. As a result, GlutaMax was created. These were the early days in the development and formulations of a number of the suppositories that are now produced now by MitoZen.com such as Sandman which is MitoZen's glutathione and melatonin suppository.

Supplementing with melatonin (& glutathione) can be of benefit to support the liver and also to aid the liver in recovering from a variety of different diseases that affect the liver. Due to the first-pass metabolism of melatonin in the liver, melatonin taken orally as in traditional melatonin supplements can render the majority of that melatonin useless. Melatonin is mainly metabolized in the liver, broken down in phase 1 liver detox by the cytochrome P450 enzyme. Melatonin is then conjugated to sulfate, released as 6-sulfatoxymelatonin, and excreted out of the body. Due to the liver being a hot zone in your body where toxins need to be either eliminated or neutralized, it's no surprise that there is also a higher incidence of oxidation and energy needs. These stress zones are where melatonin can give us support. Due to all of the toxins in our environment, it is impossible to avoid them, which leads me to conclude that most people could use some support with melatonin supplementation. I've given some excellent strategies for liver cleanses and gallbladder flushes, as well as nutraceutical considerations. Glutathione, NAC, and milk thistle are among my favorites.

Don't ignore the fact that emotions are tied to the liver, specifically hostility, anger, and rage. They are only two emotional states. The first being love and the other being fear. Hostility, anger, and rage are always hiding underneath the fear. Doing work to uncover subconscious thoughts and beliefs that might be running some of these emotional programs could also be a benefit to support your liver.

Reference

1. Sato, K, Meng, F, Francis, H, et al. Melatonin and circadian rhythms in liver diseases: Functional roles and potential therapies. *J Pineal Res.* 2020; 68:e12639. https://doi.org/10.1111/jpi.12639

2. Sato, K, Meng, F, Francis, H, et al. Melatonin and circadian rhythms in liver diseases: Functional roles and potential therapies. *J Pineal Res.* 2020; 68:e12639. https://doi.org/10.1111/jpi.12639

3. Rafael Bruck, Hussein Aeed, Yona Avni, Haim Shirin, Zipora Matas, Mark Shahmurov, Ilana Avinoach, Galina Zozulya, Nir Weizman, Ayala Hochman, Melatonin inhibits nuclear factor kappa B activation and oxidative stress and protects against thioacetamide induced liver damage in rats,Journal of Hepatology,Volume 40, Issue 1,2004,Pages 86-93,ISSN 0168-8278, https://doi.org/10.1016/S0168-8278(03)00504-X.(https://www.sciencedirect.com/science/article/pii/S016882780300504X)

4. Yulyana Yulyana, Berwini B. Endaya, Wai H. Ng, Chang M. Guo, Kam M. Hui, Paula Y.P. Lam, and Ivy A.W. Ho.Stem Cells and Development.Jul 2013.1870-1882.http://doi.org/10.1089/scd.2012.0529

5. Zhang JJ, Meng X, Li Y, Zhou Y, Xu DP, Li S, Li HB. Effects of Melatonin on Liver Injuries and Diseases. Int J Mol Sci. 2017 Mar 23;18(4):673. doi: 10.3390/ijms18040673. PMID: 28333073; PMCID: PMC5412268.

6. Zhang JJ, Meng X, Li Y, Zhou Y, Xu DP, Li S, Li HB. Effects of Melatonin on Liver Injuries and Diseases. Int J Mol Sci. 2017 Mar 23;18(4):673. doi: 10.3390/ijms18040673. PMID: 28333073; PMCID: PMC5412268.

7. Bonomini F, Borsani E, Favero G, Rodella LF, Rezzani R. Dietary Melatonin Supplementation Could Be a Promising Preventing/Therapeutic Approach for a Variety of Liver Diseases. *Nutrients.* 2018; 10(9):1135. https://doi.org/10.3390/nu10091135

8. Mortezaee, K, Khanlarkhani, N. Melatonin application in targeting oxidative-induced liver injuries: A review. *J Cell Physiol.* 2018; 233: 4015– 4032. https://doi.org/10.1002/jcp.26209

9. Microsoft Word - Document2 (immunehealthscience.com)

10. Chen Y-C, Sheen J-M, Tiao M-M, Tain Y-L, Huang L-T. Roles of Melatonin in Fetal Programming in Compromised Pregnancies. *International Journal of Molecular Sciences.* 2013; 14(3):5380-5401. https://doi.org/10.3390/ijms14035380

11. Kireev, R.A., Vara, E. & Tresguerres, J.A.F. Growth hormone and melatonin prevent age-related alteration in apoptosis processes in the dentate gyrus of male rats. *Biogerontology* **14,** 431–442 (2013). https://doi.org/10.1007/s10522-013-9443-6

12. Zhang JJ, Meng X, Li Y, Zhou Y, Xu DP, Li S, Li HB. Effects of Melatonin on Liver Injuries and Diseases. Int J Mol Sci. 2017 Mar 23;18(4):673. doi: 10.3390/ijms18040673. PMID: 28333073; PMCID: PMC5412268.

13. Cao, Z, Fang, Y, Lu, Y, et al. Melatonin alleviates cadmium-induced liver injury by inhibiting the TXNIP-NLRP3 inflammasome. *J Pineal Res.* 2017; 62:e12389. https://doi.org/10.1111/jpi.12389.

14. Cao, Z, Fang, Y, Lu, Y, et al. Melatonin alleviates cadmium-induced liver injury by inhibiting the TXNIP-NLRP3 inflammasome. *J Pineal Res.* 2017; 62:e12389. https://doi.org/10.1111/jpi.12389.

15. Iranshahi, Milad & Etemad, Leila & Shakeri, Abolfazl & Badibostan, Hasan & Karimi, Gholamreza. (2020). Protective activity of melatonin against mycotoxins-induced toxicity: a review. Toxicological & Environmental Chemistry. 101. 1-16. 10.1080/02772248.2020.1731751.

16. Pakravan H, Ahmadian M, Fani A, Aghaee D, Brumanad S, Pakzad B. The Effects of Melatonin in Patients with Nonalcoholic Fatty Liver Disease: A Randomized Controlled Trial. Adv Biomed Res. 2017 Apr 17;6:40. doi: 10.4103/2277-9175.204593. PMID: 28503495; PMCID: PMC5414412.

17. Watanabe, S., Yaginuma, R., Ikejima, K. *et al.* Liver diseases and metabolic syndrome. *J Gastroenterol* **43,** 509 (2008). https://doi.org/10.1007/s00535-008-2193-6

18. Shira Zelber-Sagi, Roni Lotan, Amir Shlomai, Muriel Webb, Gil Harrari, Assaf Buch, Dorit Nitzan Kaluski, Zamir Halpern, Ran Oren, Predictors for incidence and remission of NAFLD in the general population during a seven-year prospective follow-up, Journal of Hepatology, Volume 56, Issue 5, 2012, Pages 1145-1151, ISSN 0168-8278, https://doi.org/10.1016/j.jhep.2011.12.011. (https://www.sciencedirect.com/science/article/pii/S0168827812000499)

19. Pan, M., Song, Y.-L., Xu, J.-M. and Gan, H.-Z. (2006), Melatonin ameliorates nonalcoholic fatty liver induced by high-fat diet in rats. Journal of Pineal Research, 41: 79-84. https://doi.org/10.1111/j.1600-079X.2006.00346.x

20. Pakravan, H., Ahmadian, M., Fani, A., Aghaee, D., Brumanad, S., & Pakzad, B. (2017). The Effects of Melatonin in Patients with Nonalcoholic Fatty Liver Disease: A Randomized Controlled Trial. *Advanced biomedical research*, 6, 40. https://doi.org/10.4103/2277-9175.204593

21. Liver enzymes in patients diagnosed with non-alcoholic fatty liver disease (NAFLD) in Veracruz: a comparative analysis with the literature (openaccessjournals.com)

22. Pakravan, H., Ahmadian, M., Fani, A., Aghaee, D., Brumanad, S., & Pakzad, B. (2017). The Effects of Melatonin in Patients with Nonalcoholic Fatty Liver Disease: A Randomized Controlled Trial. *Advanced biomedical research*, 6, 40. https://doi.org/10.4103/2277-9175.204593

23. Bonomini, F., Borsani, E., Favero, G., Rodella, L. F., & Rezzani, R. (2018). Dietary Melatonin Supplementation Could Be a Promising Preventing/Therapeutic Approach for a Variety of Liver Diseases. *Nutrients*, *10*(9), 1135. https://doi.org/10.3390/nu10091135

24. Bonomini, F., Borsani, E., Favero, G., Rodella, L. F., & Rezzani, R. (2018). Dietary Melatonin Supplementation Could Be a Promising Preventing/Therapeutic Approach for a Variety of Liver Diseases. *Nutrients*, *10*(9), 1135. https://doi.org/10.3390/nu10091135

25. New review shows melatonin supplementation may be a promising adjunct for liver disease (designsforhealth.com)

26. Bonomini, F., Borsani, E., Favero, G., Rodella, L. F., & Rezzani, R. (2018). Dietary Melatonin Supplementation Could Be a Promising Preventing/Therapeutic Approach for a Variety of Liver Diseases. *Nutrients*, *10*(9), 1135. https://doi.org/10.3390/nu10091135

27. Bonomini, F., Borsani, E., Favero, G., Rodella, L. F., & Rezzani, R. (2018). Dietary Melatonin Supplementation Could Be a Promising Preventing/Therapeutic Approach for a Variety of Liver Diseases. *Nutrients*, *10*(9), 1135. https://doi.org/10.3390/nu10091135

28. Chojnacki C, Błońska A, Chojnacki J. The Effects of Melatonin on Elevated Liver Enzymes during Statin Treatment. Biomed Res Int. 2017;2017:3204504. doi: 10.1155/2017/3204504. Epub 2017 May 29. PMID: 28630863; PMCID: PMC5467275.

29. Chojnacki, C., Błońska, A., & Chojnacki, J. (2017). The Effects of Melatonin on Elevated Liver Enzymes during Statin Treatment. *BioMed research international*, *2017*, 3204504. https://doi.org/10.1155/2017/3204504

30. Leonardo Baiocchi, Tianhao Zhou, Suthat Liangpunsakul, Lenci Ilaria, Martina Milana, Fanyin Meng, Lindsey Kennedy, Praveen Kusumanchi, Zhihong Yang, Ludovica Ceci, Shannon Glaser, Heather Francis, and Gianfranco Alpini, Possible application of melatonin treatment in human diseases of the biliary tract, American Journal of Physiology-Gastrointestinal and Liver Physiology 2019 317:5, G651-G660

31. How Emotions and Organs Are Connected in Chinese Medicine (verywellmind.com)

32. Traditional Chinese Medicine & Acupuncture (practicalpainmanagement.com)

33. Traditional Chinese Medicine & Acupuncture (practicalpainmanagement.com)

34. Traditional Chinese Medicine & Acupuncture (practicalpainmanagement.com)

35. Ladas EJ, Kroll DJ, Oberlies NH, Cheng B, Ndao DH, Rheingold SR, Kelly KM. A randomized, controlled, double-blind, pilot study of milk thistle for the treatment of hepatotoxicity in childhood acute lymphoblastic leukemia (ALL). Cancer. 2010 Jan 15;116(2):506-13. doi: 10.1002/cncr.24723. PMID: 20014183; PMCID: PMC3542639.

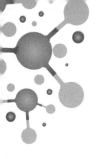

19

MELATONIN & CANCER

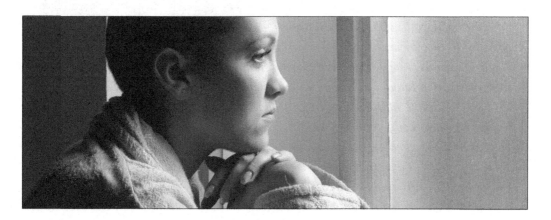

Cancer can be a devastating disease. On Thanksgiving day 2019, I lost one of my best friends. His name was Tim Brown and he had a unique story where the love of his life suddenly died of a heart attack one evening when they returned from dinner. He and Sidra

were in the midst of the most powerful love affair and this loss was such a major emotional blow to Tim that it caused him severe depression and anxiety. Tim noticed a growth in his cervical lymph nodes just before this happened but once the depression settled in, Tim had no motivation to seek care for himself. His immune system was negatively affected by the emotional trauma of losing the love of his life and the cancer had no problem aggressively metastasizing throughout Tim's entire body. It started in his colon and had already metastasized to his lymph nodes in his neck just before his love so suddenly and unexpectedly died. Tim presented to my clinic prior to the lab results of

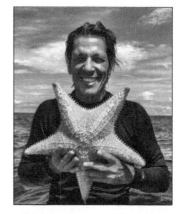

the biopsy and we began using the best therapies I knew of to support cancer such as IV Ozone, IV Vitamin C, Hyperthermia, mitochondria support such as NAD+, fasting, ketosis and, of course, supra physiologic melatonin doses both day and night. Sadly, it was too late for Tim by the time we started working together and I knew that in my heart of hearts. I even told him he might consider some preparation for death by using psychedelics such as psilocybin, similar to the end-of-life approaches used in Canada[1]. As difficult as that

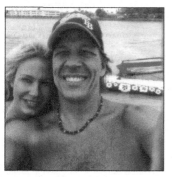

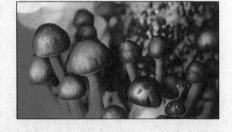

> **Dr John's Comment:** *It's important to consider this for terminal cases as it's the time for them to dive into their own spiritual awakening and deeper connection with their personal truth, within whatever religion or belief system they subscribe to. For some, death is seen as a new beginning and for some it is seen as the end. I personally subscribe to the Buddhist view of multiple lives, and reincarnation. Looking back, I wish Tim had the ability to utilize psychedelic medicines such as psilocybin. The research on end-of-life care, especially coming out of Canada, is very impressive. During these psychedelic sessions, people have a mystical experience with a divine consciousness. It's experiencing the end of life before the end of life. The light at the end of the tunnel is spoken about so many times by folks that died and came back. A feeling of complete love and oneness are often associated with this experience. I have experienced this myself in a clinical and professional setting and it was life changing. Studies reveal these patients become less fearful of death after this type of journey. There are similar studies being done with MDMA. In our office, we use ketamine assisted psychotherapy which could also be utilized, however this particular psychedelic medicine would not be my medicine of choice for an end of life journey compared to MDMA or psilocybin. See NeuroJourneys.com for information on this subject [2].*

conversation was, he was surprisingly open to discussing this but I could also tell there was still a lot of fight in him to beat the disease.

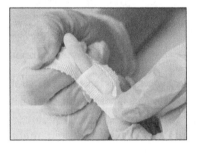

I started Tim on 200 mg melatonin suppositories immediately each night. I even dosed Tim with 200 mg melatonin suppositories during the day. In this chapter, we're going to take a deep dive into why I would consider this. We're going to discuss why the mitochondria is at the core of all cancers and how Dr. Otto Warburg in the 1940's revealed much of which is still being ignored by our medical community. His discoveries about oxygen and how the mitochondria makes energy in a cancer cell versus a normal cell changed the way we understood cancer and the "Warburg Effect" is the commonly used phrase in research. You might go back to Chapter 3 where we took a deep dive into melatonin in the mitochondria. We will discuss how melatonin works directly within the "Warburg Effect" in this chapter[3].

I would never suggest using melatonin as a mono therapy against cancer or any other disease. I think most alternative practitioners would agree with me that a multi therapeutic approach will yield the best results. I will try to include many of these other therapeutics in this chapter to give the reader a clear idea as to what best practices might look like in an alternative setting for the treatment of cancer. One of the top physicians and pioneers in this field, in my opinion, is Dr. Frank Shallenberger out of Reno, Nevada. He is both a close friend and colleague as well as one of the inspirations for writing this book.

The Cancer Cascade

Back in the very early 2000s, I used to hold cooking classes at Whole Foods and I would lecture on the cancer cascade. I would break cancer down and demonstrate how it's a process that takes time to develop and is not something that spontaneously occurs in the body. Cancer needs the right conditions to manifest itself. It's the end result of a chronic stressful state to the cells causing the cells to switch their method of making energy from one normal process fusing oxygen and glucose that creates either 36 or 38 ATP's, to another. These ATP's are the currency of energy for each cell. It is produced in the mitochondria through a process called the Krebs cycle or the TCA cycle. When a cell is under stress such that it overwhelms its ability to buffer that stress, it will switch to a much more primitive way of making energy called aerobic glycolysis or fermentation. This process will yield about 10% of the energy that would otherwise be created through the Krebs cycle.

Otto Warburg observed this effect, suggesting that defects in mitochondrial function may be at the core of cancer development. Mitochondria

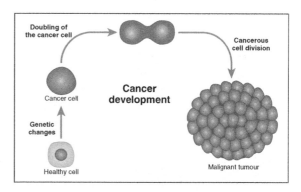

Simplistic view of cancer. Genetic changes seems to be out of out control. What happens leading up to this? What drives this?

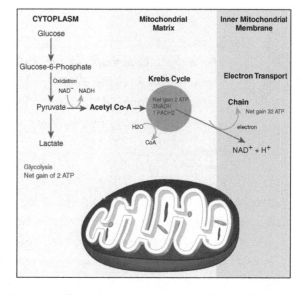

create energy, provide building blocks for new cells and tissues, and control stressful oxidation through melatonin. As we have explored in our chapter on mitochondria (Chapter 3), melatonin is produced in all of your mitochondria as a buffer against oxidative stress due to cytokines, which prevents this switch to aerobic glycolysis. In cancer, the mitochondrial tricarboxylic acid (TCA) cycle enzymes switch and begin to produce cancer promoting substances or oncogenic metabolites. This leads to a negative selection for pathogenic mitochondrial genome mutations. Basically, your body starts to produce more dysfunctional mitochondria. Mitochondria play a central and multi-functional role in malignant tumor progression, and targeting mitochondria with therapies such as with using high dose melatonin provides an excellent therapeutic opportunity that should not be ignored[4].

What are the primary causes of this cascade that leads to so much stress in the mitochondria that it influences the entire cell to switch to a cancer cell? Modern medicine views cancer as a genetic problem and this may be partially true. There are problems with a myopic view of cancer since epigenetics are the most important factors, and not the genetics themselves, which mean the ability to adapt and resist stress. Don't be fooled, stress is the cause of all disease including cancer as it up regulates inflammatory cytokines. Spending too much time in the danger zone is what creates disease or dis-ease, a lack of ease in the body. Melatonin expands both the comfort zone and the hormetic zone at a cellular level. Looking at the view of dis-ease from an oxidation standpoint, stress increases the need for energy and at the same time can squelch the normal production of energy. As stated before, this is through the "Warburg Effect" that the cell must begin making energy through aerobic glycolysis yielding a fraction (10%) of the energy it once enjoyed. At this point, there is also runaway oxidation and the cells are overwhelmed with the inability to quench the excess oxidation from the cytokines and the limited energy supply resulting from the shift from TCA to aerobic glycolysis. There are a number of antioxidants that are important and can support this but no other is more important than melatonin.

Dr John's Comment: In the 1980s the Reagan administration made some radical changes to research funding . As a result, 85% of the studies are now conducted by bio pharmaceutical companies that are researching their own drugs. Statistics on this are showing that these studies are 24% more likely to report favorable effects of their compound and 89% less likely to report side effects of the compound being studied. When 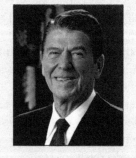 reading through the various studies on melatonin and cancer, you'll find a number of studies where chemotherapeutics were used in tandem with melatonin. Keep this in mind when looking at that data because melatonin may be the trojan horse for these chemotherapy agents. Too bad they are not also looking at the comparison of melatonin alone versus the combination with the chemo agent they sell. I would guess the results may be better without the chemo in a number of them!

Melatonin Stops the Cancer Cascade

Stress causes cancer and melatonin buffers the cells against stress. Melatonin is produced in the mitochondria in order to deal with stress. Recall we discussed the original research on melatonin where they were looking at rodent models that were living in a stress-free status. They gave the mice melatonin and did not see a big difference between the group that received melatonin versus the group that did not. It wasn't until later when they used small tubes to confine the rodents to a small space to create stress. It was then that they observed all of the amazing benefits of melatonin which were not seen nor necessary when no stress exists. Melatonin is there primarily for us to deal with stress. An absence of stress is simply not the case for most of us. Besides pushing ourselves mentally, emotionally and physically with technologies to become ultra productive, we have exposure to tens of thousands of man-made toxins and poor quality food containing low vitamin and nutrient values. Air pollution is a significant stressor that I don't feel gets enough attention. We are bombarded by harmful microwaves or EMF from our Wi-Fi, cell phone, cell phone towers and all of the electronics that have Wi-Fi and Bluetooth built into them. These EMF's are melatonin killers as explained in Chapter 14. Then, there are microbes and biotoxins, some of which were man-made such as Lyme disease which was created on Plum Island by the Nazi scientists who were brought into the USA after World War II[5]. There is also COVID-19 that was shown to be synthetically produced for "gain of function" experiments in a lab in Wuhan China. One unique stressor I think warrants comment here is mold illness. Water-damaged buildings and the toxic effect that mold can create in the body can lead to many diseases including cancer. Scientists have conducted studies where they looked at mold when exposed to EMF. What they found was that there was a heightened state that the mold would go into that would lead it to become more toxic and harmful to humans. It's almost like the mold was angry when exposed to the Bluetooth and Wi-Fi signals such that it becomes aggressive and attacks its hosts.

Lack of quality sleep leads to poor recovery from stress. Due to the regenerative cycle the body goes into during sleep, sleep provides a powerful stress buffer. Melatonin will be present during this quality sleep which is a core reason we even look at sleep to begin with. When sleep is absent, then many other stressors can be magnified greatly. Light pollution stress is one of those, especially at night after inhibiting our melatonin and circadian rhythm. Blue light pollution is a powerful stressor to our sleep.

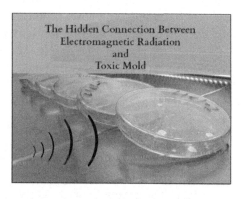

The Hidden Connection Between Electromagnetic Radiation and Toxic Mold

Indeed, there are stressors in today's world that go beyond our ability to adapt with the faculties that we were born with, thus there is a need to turn to things like melatonin to support us in today's radically challenging and stressful environment. This becomes most important for people that have cancer and are looking to support themselves through the process of healing and extending their life.

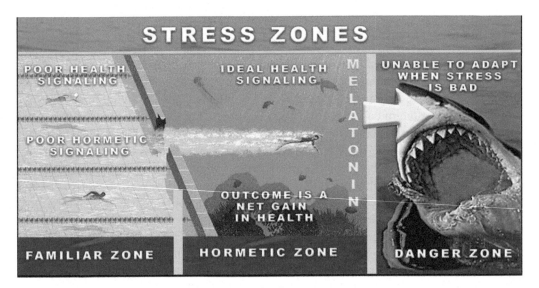

These are the 3 zones. The most beneficial zone is called the hormetic zone where all the growth & healing occurs. Melatonin allows you to go deeper into the danger zone, allowing your body to receive more stress before the body is unable to adapt and it results in harm. Too much time in the danger zone may develop into cancer.

Mitochondrial Stress, Inflammation & Cancer

One thing that all of these stressors have in common is their ability to up-regulate cytokines in the body. Cytokines or inflammatory molecules are the result of stress. An inflammatory cytokine is a type of cytokine (a signaling molecule) that is secreted from immune cells and certain other cell types that promotes inflammation. Inflammatory cytokines are predominantly produced by T helper cells (Th) and macrophages that are involved in the upregulation of inflammatory reactions[6]. The cytokines are primarily the following: interleukin-1 (IL-1), IL-12, IL-18, tumor necrosis factor alpha (TNF-α), interferon gamma (IFNγ), and granulocyte-macrophage colony stimulating factor (GM-CSF). Excessive and chronic production of inflammatory cytokines contribute to inflammatory diseases that have been linked to different diseases such as cancer.

Because all of the main stressors ultimately lead to increased inflammatory signaling in the body, we must consider both the volume of the stressor as well as the ability of the body to buffer that stressor. There is a zone just around what's called a familiar zone where you get into something called the hormetic zone. If you get outside of the hermetic zone then that means your stressors have exceeded your body's ability to quench that level of inflammation and oxidation.

The real cause of cancer is the failure to have an adequate epigenetic adaptation to stress/inflammation/cytokines resulting in an energy source shift of the mitochondria (TCA to aerobic glycolysis). There are a few anti-cancer mechanisms that melatonin uses such as anti angiogenic effects to cancer cells, apoptosis (cellular death) of cancer cells, and induction of cancer cell differentiation, autophagy (cellular eating) of cancer cells, and a significant reduction of tumor cell proliferation. Next, we will dive into the details of these anti-cancer mechanisms.

Anti Angiogenesis

Anti-angiogenesis is one of the major mechanisms which melatonin exerts its anti cancer effects. Upregulation of angiogenesis is a main feature of tumor progression and spread. Anti-angiogenesis is a massive positive step in any anti cancer therapy program. Melatonin employs a few mechanisms to starve cancer cells of needed nutrients and oxygen. Cancer is really slowed due to hypoxia induced factor-1α (HIF-1α) and the genes under its control, such as vascular endothelial growth factor (VEGF). These are the primary targets of melatonin for inhibition of angiogenesis. Melatonin hinders HIF-1α thereby preventing VEGF expression and also prevents the formation of HIF-1α, phospho-STAT3 and CBP/p300 complex which is involved in the expression of angiogenesis genes[7].

VEGFR2's activation and expression is yet another anti-angiostatic property of melatonin. Melatonin also inhibits endothelial cell migration, endothelial cell invasion, and endothelial cell tube formation[8].

Melatonin Activates Cancer Cell Apoptosis.

Melatonin induced PUMA up-regulation. The technical way it works is through ER Stress. This endoplasmic reticulum stress-mediates a protein called C/EBP and the p53-independent pathway. Activating this pathway has greatly impressed scientists interested in novel approaches to cancer therapy. These strategies demonstrate that up-regulation of PUMA contributes to the sensitizing effect of melatonin on apoptosis (cellular death) of cancer cells[9].

Shift in Mitochondrial Energy Production

Melatonin, its precursor, and its metabolites target mitochondrial function and alter oxidative phosphorylation in human melanoma cells. Several studies have shown the presence of melatonin in the mitochondrial compartments of cells. The implication of this is that the effects of melatonin on cancerous cells may be due to their regulation/energy metabolism, which either depends on mitochondria or that cytosolic glycolysis for ATP synthesis which is mostly used by cancer cells.

Differentiation of Cancer cells

A recent study demonstrated that treating head and neck cancer with a combination of melatonin and rapamycin significantly activated mitophagy by regulating mitochondrial function[10]. Another study indicated that melatonin specifically induces cancer cell differentiation[11].

Autophagy in cancer and Melatonin

We have spoken about autophagy before in other chapters and as I've explained previously, it's a process of cellular eating. This becomes a very important strategy of the body when cells like cancer cells begin to form because it is important for those to be cleaned up and autophagy is one of those mechanisms. Numerous studies have demonstrated that melatonin supplementation leads to the progressive accumulation of autophagosome vacuoles, which causes disruptions in the cellular membranes and organelles of cancer cells which cause rapid destruction of these cells[12].

Inhibition of Cellular proliferation

The authors found that melatonin could significantly reduce tumor cell proliferation while inducing a decrease in the clonogenic and self-renewal abilities of tumor cells. Melatonin was capable of inhibiting the growth of SK-MEL-1 cancer cells. This is one of the several physiological effects ascribed to melatonin. The growth-inhibiting property of melatonin on melanoma cells is related to changes in the normal cell cycle and increased levels of tyrosinase, the primary enzyme responsible for regulating melanogenesis activity[13]. Now that we have this foundation, let's start to look at some of the research that has been done specifically on melatonin on various cancers.

Research on Melatonin & Cancers
Melatonin & Brain Tumors

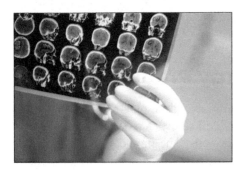

The safety and efficacy of melatonin in the management of brain tumors has been demonstrated.

Melatonin has shown immense promise in the management of cancers and tumors of various organs and systems. It is also found to be effective for treating specific tumors affecting the brain, including Glioblastoma.

Glioblastoma (GBM) is an intransigent and aggressive form of a brain tumor that is extremely challenging to treat. Researchers are trying to find a better treatment that will help patients with GBM recover faster. Melatonin has shown encouraging results in this regard.

The study, 'Melatonin's Antineoplastic Potential Against Glioblastoma' published in "The Cells" in March 2020[14], has reported the anti-tumor effects of melatonin is effective against GBM when used alone or in combination with anticancer drugs.

Notably, this study shows that melatonin could help to reduce the proliferation of GBM-inducing cells (GICs), which are similar to stem cells isolated from the patients with GBM.

It is no surprise that no significant adverse effects were observed with the use of melatonin in animals and human studies, even when used in extremely high doses to treat GBM.

This study has also shown that melatonin can be used as a promising multitasking supplement for supporting the efficacy of GBM therapy. Something they also found which should really be considered an important part in all cancer applications is that melatonin can reduce the side effects of chemotherapy and radiotherapy, which can be brutal and really breaks down the body such that it has trouble recovering post therapy. Like all diseases, sleep is usually impacted and melatonin also improves patients' sleep. Poor sleep can have an impact on cancer, as well as help with the brutal chemo and radiation. Melatonin also showed an overall boost to brain functions from the damage of the tumor and even the mental, emotional stress due to the diagnosis of the tumor.

Researchers who conducted this study have suggested that these advantages of melatonin are highly important and should not be underestimated while treating patients with chemotherapy-related illness. These benefits may substantially improve the patient's quality of life. I wonder why melatonin isn't the standard of care in cancer treatments with the upside and lack of side effects reflected in the research such as in this study?

The primary benefit of melatonin, in this case, is literally, the destruction of GSCs, which are the cell subpopulation responsible for the development, relapse, progression, and therapeutic resistance of GBM tumor. The authors found that melatonin could significantly reduce tumor cell proliferation while inducing a decrease in the clonogenic and self-renewal abilities of tumor cells.

Moreover, cell death was observed in GBM-affected cells that were treated with melatonin along with ultrastructural features of autophagy (which we discussed in an earlier chapter). By supporting autophagy, melatonin could help in the rapid elimination of cancer cells from the body by cells that can attack and engulf them. Melatonin supplementation also led to the progressive accumulation of autophagosome vacuoles, which caused disruptions in the cellular membranes and organelles of cancer cells causing rapid destruction of these cells. These changes brought about by melatonin helped to destroy abnormal cells in GBM thus supporting patient recovery. I would consider fasting and a ketogenic diet in cases like these and some of my colleges are doing just this in their cancer clinics. Upregulating signaling for autophagy using fasting is a big thrust of research. Keep in mind, all the big-Pharma research is focused on patentable specific molecules, which in my opinion, will not be the answer to this problem as a more comprehensive approach involving natural substances and relatively free therapies such as fasting don't attract the attention of these biopharmaceutical companies. Therefore, it is not likely we will see a protocol that makes the most sense based on the structure of our current healthcare model. Just like the situation with Alzeihmers and the work Dale Bredeson did with his research, there needs to be more complex plans that include multiple strategies to effect the biology[15].

Another study[16], 'Melatonin in Cancer Management: Progress and Promise' published in 'Cancer Research' in 2006 has revealed that melatonin can improve life expectancy in patients who have developed brain metastases. This means melatonin could help to protect the brain tissues that have been affected due to the metastasis or spread of cancer cells from other organs of the body.

This study was specifically focused on assessing the effect of melatonin in the management of advanced solid tumors in the brain. In this trial, 50 patients diagnosed with brain metastases whose condition had progressed under initial therapy were treated with supportive care alone or a combination of melatonin and supportive care. It showed that the survival rate improved in patients who were treated with melatonin against those who received only supportive care. There was also a significant difference in the mean survival time of patients treated with melatonin against those who didn't.

This study also discussed the results of another trial in patients diagnosed with untreatable metastatic solid tumors in the brain who were treated with a daily dose of 20 mg oral melatonin along with low doses of antitumor cytokines, IL-12 and IL-2. The anticancer immune response of cytokines and lymphocyte proliferation were found to be significantly higher following melatonin treatment. These studies have shown the potential of melatonin in the treatment of advanced solid tumors with brain metastases. Again, I would argue the addition of fasting and a ketogenic diet may be considered in these cases and may have further benefit[17].

Another study[18], 'Five Year-Survival with High-Dose Melatonin and Other Antitumor Pineal Hormones in Advanced Cancer Patients Eligible for the Only Palliative Therapy,' published in the 'Research Journal of Oncology' in 2018 has shown that using high doses of melatonin could slow down cancer progression linked to the deficiency of some mechanisms responsible for the natural immune response.

This theory is based on the concept that cancer-related immunosuppression depends only on the alternation of immune cells and the loss of the neuroendocrine regulation and anti-tumor response by the immune cells, which are primarily inhibited by the hormones secreted by the pineal gland, primarily melatonin.

Dr. John's Comment Box

Wow! "Melatonin's the primary activator of anti-tumor responsiveness of the immune system." They stated that in this study! That should have been on CNN, NBC and Fox, you would think. Maybe someone doesn't want you to know about it? I want you to know about it and that's why I'm writing this book!"

Finally, cancer progression has also been shown to be associated with a progressive decline in the endocrine dysregulation of the pineal gland. So, what the researchers worked out during this study was they simply provided what they called "endocrine oncostatic pineal replacement therapy" to counteract cancer growth and improve the survival of patients. This theory proved to be successful as the results of the endocrine oncostatic pineal replacement showed promise with the known pineal hormones like melatonin. This improved the survival and slowed cancer growth even in patients for whom no other treatment option was available. I say, "Why just limit this to those cases when it's so effective[19]?"

Breast Cancer

The use of melatonin in treating breast cancer has been extensively studied. According to Cohen et al., the "Role of pineal gland in etiology and treatment of breast cancer," 1978, a reduction in the function of the pineal gland correlates to a higher risk of breast cancer. This is due to an increased exposure time for circulating estrogens[20].

The hypothesis of Cohen et al. is based on the following observations: (i) countries that have a low incidence of pineal calcification have the lowest incidence of breast cancer

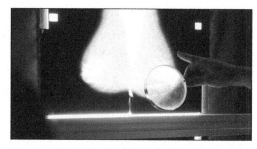

(less fluoride in municipal water), (ii) patients that take chlorpromazine, which increases the levels of melatonin in the body, have lower risks of breast cancer, (iii) according to in-vitro data, melatonin may directly impact breast cancer cells, (iv) melatonin may also directly impact the production of estrogen due to its presence on human ovarian cells[21].

A systematic review of randomized controlled trials of melatonin in solid cancer tumor patients was conducted by Mills et al., in 2005. The results were promising, showing that there are positive effects of using melatonin as the sole treatment or as an adjunct in cancer treatment[22].

The unblinded, controlled trials involved 643 patients in the same hospital. The effects of melatonin resulted in a reduction in the risk of death at one year. While 1-year survival isn't great as there's a mean recurrence time of seven years, melatonin appears effective in the treatment of breast cancer. The effect of melatonin was consistent with dose and type of cancer.

They, like all other studies, also concluded that there were no adverse effects reported from the use of melatonin. Due to its tremendous safety profile, melatonin can be used extensively in clinical trials and studies[23]. Melatonin can be used as the sole treatment option or in combination with other available cancer therapies and treatments.

In a randomized trial of 40 ER-negative, post-menopausal, breast cancer patients, melatonin and tamoxifen combined showed better outcomes for partial response and 1-year survival than using just tamoxifen. A study conducted by Lissoni et al., "A randomized study of tamoxifen alone versus tamoxifen plus melatonin in estrogen receptor-negative heavily pretreated metastatic breast-cancer patients," demonstrated the amplification effect melatonin has on tamoxifen in the treatment of cancer[24].

Tamoxifen can reduce the risk of breast cancer in post-menopausal and premenopausal women. It is one of the best treatments for breast cancer available. According to the randomized trial, melatonin can enhance the effects of tamoxifen, coupled with its own anti-cancer effects, to increase the 1-year survival of cancer patients.

A daily dose of 20 mg melatonin was administered orally in combination with tamoxifen to one group, and another group received just tamoxifen alone, also 20 mg daily. While no complete response was observed, the partial response in the group that received both tamoxifen and melatonin was higher than the group that received just tamoxifen. The 1-year survival percentage was also higher.

The group on both tamoxifen and melatonin did not record any drug-related toxicity and was also relieved of anxiety and depression. This is due to its neurological support as the heart and the nervous system are the most metabolically sensitive to energy via mitochondria so it's no surprise we see many other comorbidities in cancer also improve when melatonin is given as a supplement[25].

Ovarian cancer

A leading cause of death among women with genital tract disorders[26]. Even with all the advancements of chemotherapy and surgeries, little has been done to change the prognosis in this subset of cancers. Due to that fact, melatonin should be considered due to its anti-ovarian cancer mechanisms. Studies have reported the anticancer effect of melatonin on ovarian cancer, and the underlying mechanisms include inducing apoptosis and cell cycle arrest and immune regulation[27].

Cervical cancer

Cervical cancer is the second leading cause of female tumors worldwide[28]. Several studies have reported the anticancer effect of melatonin on cervical cancer. Melatonin could reduce cervical cancer cell viability in-vitro, and suppress cervical adenocarcinoma metabolism in-vivo[29].

Endometrial cancer

Endometrial cancer, like breast cancer, is an estrogen-dependent neoplasia, and its incidence is rapidly increasing worldwide[30,31] There have been a few studies showing the anti-cancer effect of melatonin on endometrial cancer[32,33].

Skin Cancer

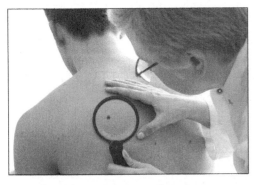

A study conducted in 2010 by Cabrera et al., "Melatonin decreases cell proliferation and induces melanogenesis in human melanoma SK-MEL-1 cells," found that melatonin was capable of inhibiting the growth of SK-MEL-1 cells. This is one of the several physiological effects ascribed to melatonin[34].

Melanoma is a form of skin cancer that occurs when the melanocytes, cells that control the pigment in the skin, become cancerous. This condition is the most severe form of skin cancer and also one of the deadliest cancers in the world.

The growth-inhibiting property of melatonin on melanoma cells is related to changes in the normal cell cycle and raised tyrosinase, the primary enzyme responsible for regulating melanogenesis activity.

Melatonin, its precursor, and its metabolites target mitochondrial function and alter oxidative phosphorylation in human melanoma cells. Several studies have shown the presence of melatonin in the mitochondrial compartments of cells. The implication of this is that the effects of melatonin on cancerous cells may be due to their regulation/energy metabolism, which either depends on mitochondria or that cytosolic glycolysis for ATP synthesis that is mostly used by cancer cells.

The results of this study suggest the use of melatonin, its precursor, and metabolites in melanoma treatment, either as a stand alone or combined with currently available targeted therapies.

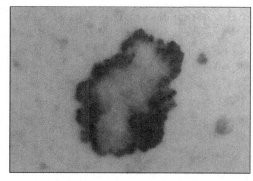

Dr. John's Comment: Basically, they say that melatonin might be effective just by itself for one of the deadliest cancers known, melanoma. They also point out what I've been writing about extensively regarding how the energy within the mitochondria is shifted to the inefficient form called aerobic glycolysis in cancer versus the normal effective TCA cycle.

Liver Cancer

Liver cancer is the second most common cause of cancer death globally, and hepatocellular carcinoma (HCC) is the main liver cancer (70%-80%), which is one of the most frequent cancers with the highest incidence worldwide [35,36]. Sadly, surgery remains the most "medically"effective treatment for patients with HCC, but it is only reasonable for a limited number of cases. Some will cry out for an effective chemotherapeutic drug even though chemo has not shown to be the therapeutic breakthrough our broken medical system wished for[37]. The effects of melatonin on liver cancer have been reported in several studies. Melatonin inhibits the process of hepatocarcinogenesis (liver cancer) through a few pathways. There is a pro-apoptotic (via modulation of COX-2/PI3K/AKT pathway, Bcl-2/Bax ratio, activation of ER stress) which is a cell-destroying mechanism. Then, there are also anti-angiogenesis and anti-invasive effects melatonin uses which makes it a considerable asset in managing cancers in the liver and other tissues of the body.

Renal cancer

Renal cancer is very aggressive. It is the third most common urologic cancer and accounts for 3% of adult cancers. It does have a male predominance (sex ratio 3/1)[38]. The research on melatonin's anticancer effect on renal cancer is summarized. The mechanism underlying was elucidated as inducing upregulation of p53-upregulated modulator of apoptosis[39].

Collectively, inducing apoptosis and inhibiting metastasis are the main effects of melatonin on renal cancer cells. Moreover, concomitant melatonin administration with other therapies might be an effective clinical choice for patients with renal cancer, given that melatonin showed enhancement effects on other anticancer agents.

Lung cancer

Lung cancer is one of the deadliest cancers one can encounter. Lung cancer is the second most frequent cancer in males[40] . Non-small-cell lung cancer (NSCLC) is a primary form of lung cancer[41] and the published literature suggests that the disruption of melatonin rhythm could increase the NSCLC incidence[42]. In several pharmaceutical funded studies, melatonin has been reported to be a potential therapeutic strategy for lung cancer. Melatonin enhances the effects of radiotherapy and some anticancer drugs and I bet if it was used by itself the results might even be better. Melatonin likely works well without these harmful therapies and in more alternative circles, melatonin is combined with less harmful approaches such as hyperthermia, high-dose vitamin C, ketogenic diet and insulin potentiation therapy. Keep in mind that the only reason companies will fund this type of research is if they have the ability to capture an income source on the other side. I can only imagine how attractive melatonin would be as a combination therapy with a molecule I had a patent on. It's only likely to make my molecule look that much better. I say this as I am a bit biased to more natural approaches. However, one study did show melatonin's effect was more significant when it was used as an adjuvant therapy than being used alone for lung cancer using two different chemotherapy agents: doxorubicin & gefitinib. Berberine is a natural extract which has been shown to up-regulate autophagy of cancer cells when radiation is used against cancer[43]. The enhancement of autophagy with melatonin adds to the therapeutic effects of berberine for its beneficial role in the treatment of lung cancer[44].

Gastric cancer

Gastric cancer ranks second among malignant tumors worldwide[45]. Several studies point out the mechanisms in which melatonin creates inhibition of gastric cancer. We mentioned this when we first discussed the anti-angiogenic effect of melatonin that gives it a great mechanism in fighting cancer. Melatonin inhibits HIF-1α accumulation and endogenous VEGF generation through inhibition of RZR/RORγ in hypoxic SGC-7901 cells where it will inhibit the proliferation of gastric cancer cells[46]. Melatonin inhibited angiogenesis in an SGC-7901 gastric cancer cell line [148]. Melatonin was able to inhibit cell viability, clone formation, cell invasion, and induce apoptosis of gastric cancer cell lines through the suppression of NF-κB. Melatonin has inhibitory effects on cellular proliferation and pro-apoptotic effects on a gastric adenocarcinoma cancer cell line called SGC7901 [47]. Gastric cancer cells SGC7901 cultured with melatonin showed more differentiated morphologic phenotype as compared with untreated cells. Melatonin also up-regulated enzymes that promote dedifferentiation in gastric tissue[48].

Indeed melatonin has been shown to be a powerful inhibitor of the growth of gastric cancer cells. The main mechanisms include inhibiting angiogenesis so the cancer cells starve, promoting cellular cancer apoptosis, and immunoregulation to enroll your immune system in the fight against cancer.

Pancreatic cancer

This is the cancer that took out Steve Jobs, the creator of Apple. It is a highly lethal disease with a relatively low 5-year survival rate[49, 50]. It responds poorly to radiotherapy and chemotherapy because the tumor cells are particularly resistant to apoptosis[51].

In a study, melatonin exhibited a highly inhibitory effect on cellular proliferation of pancreatic carcinoma cells. This was seen partly due to a strong up-regulation in the anti-angiogenic effect of melatonin. When melatonin for pancreatic cancer was studied there was a significant decrease in VEGF[52]. Melatonin reduced viability of pancreatic tumor cells through inducing changes of mitochondrial activity[53]. Melatonin alone exhibited growth inhibition on a pancreatic cancer cell line SW-1990. The mechanism melatonin uses is through the downregulation of Bcl-2 and upregulation of Bax[54]. Melatonin also enhanced cytotoxicity and apoptosis induced by 3 different chemotherapeutic agents (5-fluorouracil, cisplatin and doxorubicin) in pancreatic cancer cells[55].

Melatonin improved antitumor activity of capecitabine in pancreatic cancer. This next fact is shocking. What they did is take a toxic drug known to cause pancreatic cancer called N-nitrosobis (2-oxopropyl) amine and used it to measure the effectiveness of melatonin compared to a drug used to treat pancreatic cancer called capecitabine. Of course, when given alone the cancer risk dropped all the way to 33% where it was only 66% with the drug capecitabine. However, in the group treated with a combination of capecitabine and melatonin, only 10% of animals showed pancreatic adenocarcinoma formation[56].

In general, melatonin has shown inhibition on the growth of some pancreatic cancer cells.

Colorectal cancer

Melatonin has shown anticancer against various colorectal cancers. A study showed that melatonin increased ROS levels and decreased cellular viability of human colorectal carcinoma cells[57]. Melatonin's anti-cancer effects are associated with its antioxidative and anti-inflammatory activities. Melatonin counteracts the oxidative by inhibiting the nitric oxide production in cultured colon cancer cells[58] . In another study, cell proliferation was suppressed significantly and apoptosis was induced by melatonin on colorectal cancer [59]. Another study showed that melatonin inhibits tumor cell growth and progression of colon carcinoma[60]. Another study determined there is a strong interaction between cell death and cellular senescence in human colorectal cancer cells which is induced by melatonin [61]. There is a significant decrease in mRNA expression of melatonin receptor MT1 in colorectal cancer compared with the healthy adjacent mucosa tissue[62]. Melatonin has also shown synergistic effects with other anticancer agents on colorectal tumors. The combination of ursolic acid and melatonin led to an enhanced antiproliferative and pro-apoptotic activity in colon cancer cell lines[63]. Melatonin is a great therapeutic strategy for colorectal cancer, since it could reduce the progression of colorectal cancer. The underlying mechanisms include: regulation of CaMKII, ET-1, Nrf2 signaling pathways, and induction of ACF.

Melatonin Radiation & Chemo

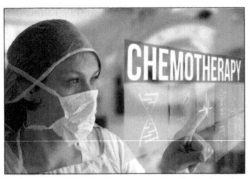

This study[64], "Melatonin as Adjuvant Cancer Care With and Without Chemotherapy: A Systematic Review and Meta-analysis of Randomized Trials," was conducted by Seely et al., in which the authors of the study systematically reviewed the effects of melatonin on 1-year survival, complete and partial response, stable disease, and toxicity. The study included 21 randomized clinical trials that all dealt with solid tumors. The results of these trials showed improved effects for complete response, partial response, and stable disease. In clinical trials where melatonin was combined with chemotherapy, there was increased 1-year survival and better complete response, partial response, and stable disease. They then concluded that melatonin may be beneficial to cancer patients already on other forms of cancer therapies by increasing the chances of survival and lowering the negative effects associated with chemotherapy.

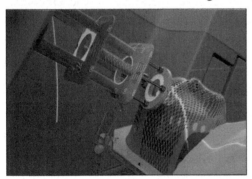

Incidentally, this same study also found melatonin to be useful in reducing the incidence of several other conditions, including alopecia, anemia, asthenia, and thrombocytopenia. Of course, if you've been following this, this doesn't come as any surprise to you due to melatonin's wide reach to rejuvenate the body and protect it from stress.

Another meta-analysis by Wang et al[65]., "The efficacy and safety of melatonin in concurrent chemotherapy or radiotherapy for solid tumors: A meta-analysis of randomized controlled trials," was conducted in 2012 to observe the effects of melatonin treatment on tumor remission,   1-year survival, and the side effects of radiochemotherapy.

This meta-analysis involved eight eligible randomized controlled trials and 761 patients with solid tumor cancer. In the trials, a daily dose of 20 mg melatonin was used orally, combined with chemotherapy or radiotherapy.

The meta-analysis results showed that melatonin improved the complete and partial remission rate and 1-year survival rate. The effects of melatonin were consistent across different types of cancers. Melatonin also significantly reduces radiation and chemotherapy-related side effects, like neurotoxicity, thrombocytopenia, and fatigue. There were no reports of any adverse effects.

The low toxicity of melatonin treatment is one of the most significant benefits of melatonin, as it ensures that further and larger tests can be conducted to determine the extent of melatonin's effects on cancer.

Melatonin & Lung Cancer

Lissoni et al. conducted published "Randomized Study with the Pineal Hormone Melatonin versus Supportive Care Alone in Advanced Non-Small Cell Lung Cancer Resistant to a First-Line Chemotherapy Containing Cisplatin" in 1992 to compare the effects of just melatonin and supportive care in lung cancer[66]. The dose of melatonin used daily was 10 mg taken orally. The study involved 63 lung cancer patients, with 31 taking melatonin and 32 receiving just supportive care. The results of the study showed that patients taking just melatonin had a higher 1-year survival percentage and also better disease stabilization. As consistent with melatonin treatment and therapy, there weren't adverse effects and drug-related toxicities. Patients treated with melatonin even showed better performance status than patients on supportive care.

Melatonin & Colon Cancer

Colon cancer was studied where melatonin was used in combination with another drug in cancer treatment, Interleukin-2. This was proven by Barni et al. in a 1995 study, "A Randomized Study of Low-Dose Subcutaneous Interleukin-2 Plus Melatonin versus Supportive Care Alone in Metastatic Colorectal Cancer Patients Progressing under 5-Fluorouracil and Folates[67]."

5-fluorouracil is one of the drugs of choice in treating various cancers, with colorectal cancer being the most impacted by the drug. Active metabolites of 5-fluorouracil disrupt DNA and RNA synthesis through a mechanism involving the folate metabolic pathway.

Interleukin-2 can generate an anti-cancer immune response and may be an effective agent in treating advanced colon cancer. Interleukin-2 is typically used in cancer treatments at high doses, but the amplification property of melatonin on Interleukin-2 may lead to the use of low—dose subcutaneous Interleukin-2 in metastatic colorectal cancer patients progressing under 5-fluorouracil.

In this study by Barni et al., fifty cancer patients were evaluated for survival time percentage and response. The trial was randomized, with some patients receiving just supportive care, while other patients received low-dose subcutaneous Interleukin-2 and melatonin. A relatively high dose of melatonin was used for the study, 40mg per day, taken orally. High to them, however if you've been reading this book, you might not think this is so high. The results of the study showed a significantly higher 1-year percentage in patients that received melatonin and Interleukin-2.

Here is another study showing the effectiveness of melatonin combined with agents for the treatment of colorectal cancer. The study, "Biomodulation of cancer chemotherapy for metastatic colorectal cancer: a randomized study of weekly low-dose irinotecan alone versus irinotecan plus the oncostatic pineal hormone melatonin in metastatic colorectal cancer patients progressing on 5-fluorouracil-containing combinations" was conducted by Cerea et al.[68]

A combination of melatonin and irinotecan led to better results of partial remission plus stable disease than patients that received just irinotecan. The dose of melatonin used in the 30-patient study was 20 mg. Here again there were no adverse effects or drug-related toxicities from the use of melatonin in combination with low-dose irinotecan.

Prostate Cancer & Melatonin

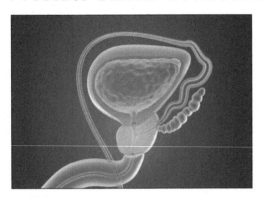

Prostate cancer is the second most common cancer and a leading cause of cancer mortality in men[69]. In addition, melatonin could cause phenotypic changes, mainly neuroendocrine differentiation, thereby sensitizing human prostate cancer cells to apoptosis induced by cytokines, such as TNF-α or TRAIL[70]. Melatonin treatment could inhibit proliferation of prostate cancer cells by resynchronizing dysregulated circadian rhythm circuitry[71]. Melatonin could inhibit cell growth of both androgen-dependent and androgen-independent prostate cancer[72]. Melatonin works against prostate cancer through its anti-angiogenic effects. Melatonin significantly suppressed the expression of angiogenesis-related proteins HIF-1α, HIF-2α and VEGF[73]. Melatonin also has anti-proliferative effects on prostate cancer cell lines and the mechanisms involved is the inactivation of NF-κB, via melatonin MT1 receptors.[74,75]. Another study documented that melatonin suppressed HIF-1α, thus melatonin acts as a potent anti-cancer supplement for prostate cancer therapy[76]. Sirt1 is a NAD+-dependent compound and is overexpressed in prostate cancer cells[77]. Melatonin significantly suppressed Sirt1 activity in multiple human prostate cancer cell lines, accompanied by a significant reduction in the proliferative potential of prostate cancer cells[78]. This next study was done by using only increasing daytime blue light. The blue light increased nocturnal melatonin and will enhance the inhibition on prostate cancer growth on male nude rats, as shown by decreased tumor growth rates, tumor cAMP levels, aerobic glycolysis (you should be very familiar with this mechanism which is also called the Warburg effect) [79]. Besides, oral administration of melatonin significantly inhibited prostate cancer tumorigenesis as characterized by reduction in prostate and genitourinary weight, serum IGF-1/IGFBP3 ratio, and mRNA and protein levels of PCNA and Ki-67, which were accompanied with a significant reduction in Sirt1[80]. Many studies will support the use of melatonin in the prevention and treatment of prostate cancer. Melatonin exerts an antiproliferative activity on androgen-independent prostate cancer cells. Melatonin is commonly used as a primary substance to postpone the relapse of hormone-refractory prostate cancers[81].

In this paper titled "Inflammation, infection, and prostate cancer" the author describes how both inflammation and infection are at the root cause of many prostate cancer's. I would argue that infection and toxicity are the main root causes of inflammation in the body in general[82]. Direct antibiotic injections to the prostate have been shown to be of benefit with some cases of both prostate cancer as well as prostate hypertrophy. In our clinic, we use a direct ozone injection into the prostate gland along with the use of melatonin suppositories. When you consider the location of the suppository in relation to the prostate, this route of administration makes good sense.

Conclusion

Cancer can be a devastating disease. There is a specific cascade of events that leads to cancer that often happens many years before the cancer is diagnosed. Looking at the various stressors that we outlined in this chapter can help both the doctor and the patient to identify helpful strategies to reduce these various stressors in order to design an ideal environment for cancer patients to slow or reverse cancer. Melatonin should be considered as a support for all cancer patients. There are very few substances, if any, that can hold a candle to melatonin's repertoire of ammunition against cancers of all types. Melatonin has anti-angiogenic properties, which starve cancer cells, as well as anti-proliferative effect on cancer cells, cancer cell apoptosis effect, and anti cancer cell differentiation. It also shifts the mitochondria energy status supporting an anti cancer effect. Could you just imagine if a patent was able to be issued for melatonin against cancer? Do you think this would be on commercials on TV? I offer it would be a household name for all its benefits on cancer! There are no negative effects with melatonin and the upside is simply too great to ignore. Higher doses of melatonin should be considered for individuals living with cancer. Delivery methods such as using a suppository or taking it in a liposomal route would be more effective than a standard oral form due to the poor oral absorption. Dosing both day and night may be helpful. Daytime dosing is possible for most individuals. Since only about 20% of the population will have a difficult time with melatonin during the day due to the fact that light suppresses the sleepiness effects of melatonin. This leaves 80% of the population to enjoy daytime dosing with little side effects such as grogginess or fatigue. Unfortunately, few physicians are properly trained abou melatonin making it difficult for many patients to find an educated doctor to guide them with a melatonin dosing schedule. My best suggestion would be to give this book to your doctor or healthcare practitioner so they can become educated. If you're a physician yourself, maybe do your part and pass this book on to other healthcare practitioners especially those treating cancer.

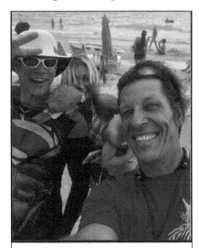

One of the few pics I have with Tim. I have no clue who the girl in the back is! LOL

Reference

1. In Canada, End-of-Life Therapy May Be the Path to Legal Psilocybin (filtermag.org)

2. (11) The Neuro Journey | Facebook

3. Liberti MV, Locasale JW. The Warburg Effect: How Does it Benefit Cancer Cells? Trends Biochem Sci. 2016 Mar;41(3):211-218. doi: 10.1016/j.tibs.2015.12.001. Epub 2016 Jan 5. Erratum in: Trends Biochem Sci. 2016 Mar;41(3):287. Erratum in: Trends Biochem Sci. 2016 Mar;41(3):287. PMID: 26778478; PMCID: PMC4783224.

4. Leon J, Acuña-Castroviejo D, Sainz RM, Mayo JC, Tan DX, Reiter RJ. Melatonin and mito-chondrial function. Life Sci. 2004 Jul 2;75(7):765-90. doi: 10.1016/j.lfs.2004.03.003. PMID: 15183071.

5. Interview: U.S. bioweapon lab suspected of source of lyme disease: expert (bignewsnetwork. com)

6. Chong MM, Metcalf D, Jamieson E, Alexander WS, Kay TW. Suppressor of cytokine sig-naling-1 in T cells and macrophages is critical for preventing lethal inflammation. Blood. 2005 Sep 1;106(5):1668-75. doi: 10.1182/blood-2004-08-3049. Epub 2005 May 17. PMID: 15899915.

7. Talib, W. H., Alsayed, A. R., Abuawad, A., Daoud, S., & Mahmod, A. I. (2021). Melatonin in Cancer Treatment: Current Knowledge and Future Opportunities. *Molecules (Basel, Switzerland)*, *26*(9), 2506. https://doi.org/10.3390/molecules26092506

8. Goradel NH, Asghari MH, Moloudizargari M, Negahdari B, Haghi-Aminjan H, Abdollahi M. Melatonin as an angiogenesis inhibitor to combat cancer: Mechanistic evidence. Toxicol Appl Pharmacol. 2017 Nov 15;335:56-63. doi: 10.1016/j.taap.2017.09.022. Epub 2017 Sep 30. PMID: 28974455.

9. Li J, Lee B, Lee AS. Endoplasmic reticulum stress-induced apoptosis: multiple pathways and activation of p53-up-regulated modulator of apoptosis (PUMA) and NOXA by p53. J Biol Chem. 2006 Mar 17;281(11):7260-70. doi: 10.1074/jbc.M509868200. Epub 2006 Jan 6. PMID: 16407291.

10. Shen YQ, Guerra-Librero A, Fernandez-Gil BI, Florido J, García-López S, Martinez-Ruiz L, Mendivil-Perez M, Soto-Mercado V, Acuña-Castroviejo D, Ortega-Arellano H, Carriel V, Diaz-Casado ME, Reiter RJ, Rusanova I, Nieto A, López LC, Escames G. Combination of melatonin and rapamycin for head and neck cancer therapy: Suppression of AKT/mTOR pathway activation, and activation of mitophagy and apoptosis via mitochondrial function regulation. J Pineal Res. 2018 Apr;64(3). doi: 10.1111/jpi.12461. Epub 2018 Jan 9. PMID: 29247557.

11. Lee, W-J, Chen, L-C, Lin, J-H, et al. Melatonin promotes neuroblastoma cell differentiation by activating hyaluronan synthase 3-induced mitophagy. *Cancer Med*. 2019; 8: 4821– 4835. https://doi.org/10.1002/cam4.2389

12. Talib, W. H., Alsayed, A. R., Abuawad, A., Daoud, S., & Mahmod, A. I. (2021). Melatonin in Cancer Treatment: Current Knowledge and Future Opportunities. *Molecules (Basel, Switzerland)*, *26*(9), 2506. https://doi.org/10.3390/molecules26092506

13. Perdomo J, Quintana C, González I, Hernández I, Rubio S, Loro JF, Reiter RJ, Estévez F, Quintana J. Melatonin Induces Melanogenesis in Human SK-MEL-1 Melanoma Cells Involving Glycogen Synthase Kinase-3 and Reactive Oxygen Species. *International Journal of Molecular Sciences*. 2020; 21(14):4970. https://doi.org/10.3390/ijms21144970

14. Moretti E, Favero G, Rodella LF, Rezzani R. Melatonin's Antineoplastic Potential Against Glioblastoma. Cells. 2020 Mar 3;9(3):599. doi: 10.3390/cells9030599. PMID: 32138190; PMCID: PMC7140435.

15. Moretti, E., Favero, G., Rodella, L. F., & Rezzani, R. (2020). Melatonin's Antineoplastic Potential Against Glioblastoma. *Cells*, *9*(3), 599. https://doi.org/10.3390/cells9030599

16. Jung B, Ahmad N. Melatonin in cancer management: progress and promise. Cancer Res. 2006 Oct 15;66(20):9789-93. doi: 10.1158/0008-5472.CAN-06-1776. PMID: 17047036.

17. Brittney Jung and Nihal Ahmad, Melatonin in Cancer Management: Progress and Promise Cancer Res October 15 2006 (66) (20) 9789-9793; **DOI:** 10.1158/0008-5472.CAN-06-1776

18. Five Year-Survival with High-Dose Melatonin and Other Antitumor Pineal Hormones in Advanced Cancer Patients Eligible for the Only Palliative Therapy (dibellainsieme.org)

19. Five Year-Survival with High-Dose Melatonin and Other Antitumor Pineal Hormones in Advanced Cancer Patients Eligible for the Only Palliative Therapy (dibellainsieme.org)

20. Cohen M, Lippman M, Chabner B. Role of pineal gland in aetiology and treatment of breast cancer. Lancet. 1978 Oct 14;2(8094):814-6. doi: 10.1016/s0140-6736(78)92591-6. PMID: 81365.

21. Cohen M, Lippman M, Chabner B. Role of pineal gland in aetiology and treatment of breast cancer. Lancet. 1978 Oct 14;2(8094):814-6. doi: 10.1016/s0140-6736(78)92591-6. PMID: 81365.

22. JPI_258 360..366 (acesototalhealth.com)

23. Mills E, Wu P, Seely D, Guyatt G. Melatonin in the treatment of cancer: a systematic review of randomized controlled trials and meta-analysis. J Pineal Res. 2005 Nov;39(4):360-6. doi: 10.1111/j.1600-079X.2005.00258.x. PMID: 16207291.

24. Lissoni P, Ardizzoia A, Barni S, Paolorossi F, Tancini G, Meregalli S, Esposti D, Zubelewicz B, Braczowski R. A randomized study of tamoxifen alone versus tamoxifen plus melatonin in estrogen receptor-negative heavily pretreated metastatic breast-cancer patients. Oncol Rep. 1995 Sep;2(5):871-3. doi: 10.3892/or.2.5.871. PMID: 21597833.

25. Lissoni P, Ardizzoia A, Barni S, Paolorossi F, Tancini G, Meregalli S, Esposti D, Zubelewicz B, Braczowski R. A randomized study of tamoxifen alone versus tamoxifen plus melatonin in estrogen receptor-negative heavily pretreated metastatic breast-cancer patients. Oncol Rep. 1995 Sep;2(5):871-3. doi: 10.3892/or.2.5.871. PMID: 21597833.

26. Expression of the MT1 melatonin receptor in ovarian cancer cells. (medscape.com)

27. Koshiyama M, Matsumura N, Konishi I. Recent concepts of ovarian carcinogenesis: type I and type II. Biomed Res Int. 2014;2014:934261. doi: 10.1155/2014/934261. Epub 2014 Apr 23. PMID: 24868556; PMCID: PMC4017729.

28. Janicek MF, Averette HE. Cervical cancer: prevention, diagnosis, and therapeutics. CA Cancer J Clin. 2001 Mar-Apr;51(2):92-114; quiz 115-8. doi: 10.3322/canjclin.51.2.92. PMID: 11577486.

29. Shafabakhsh R, Reiter RJ, Mirzaei H, Teymoordash SN, Asemi Z. Melatonin: A new inhibitor agent for cervical cancer treatment. J Cell Physiol. 2019 Dec;234(12):21670-21682. doi: 10.1002/jcp.28865. Epub 2019 May 27. PMID: 31131897.

30. McAlpine, J.N., Temkin, S.M. and Mackay, H.J. (2016), Endometrial cancer: Not your grand-mother's cancer. Cancer, 122: 2787-2798. https://doi.org/10.1002/cncr.30094

31. Schernhammer, E., Schulmeister, K. Melatonin and cancer risk: does light at night compromise physiologic cancer protection by lowering serum melatonin levels?. *Br J Cancer* **90,** 941–943 (2004). https://doi.org/10.1038/sj.bjc.6601626

32. McAlpine, J.N., Temkin, S.M. and Mackay, H.J. (2016), Endometrial cancer: Not your grand-mother's cancer. Cancer, 122: 2787-2798. https://doi.org/10.1002/cncr.30094

33. Schernhammer, E., Schulmeister, K. Melatonin and cancer risk: does light at night compromise physiologic cancer protection by lowering serum melatonin levels?. *Br J Cancer* 90, 941–943 (2004). https://doi.org/10.1038/sj.bjc.6601626

34. Cabrera J, Negrín G, Estévez F, Loro J, Reiter RJ, Quintana J. Melatonin decreases cell proliferation and induces melanogenesis in human melanoma SK-MEL-1 cells. J Pineal Res. 2010 Aug;49(1):45-54. doi: 10.1111/j.1600-079X.2010.00765.x. Epub 2010 Apr 29. PMID: 20459460.

35. Vijayalaxmi, & Thomas, Charles & Reiter, Russel & Herman, Terence. (2002). Vijayalaxmi, Thomas CRJ, Reiter RJ, Herman TSMelatonin: from basic research to cancer treatment clinics. J Clin Oncol 20: 2575-2601. Journal of clinical oncology : official journal of the American Society of Clinical Oncology. 20. 2575-601. 10.1200/JCO.2002.11.004.

36. Cutando, A., Lopez-Valverde, A., Arias-Santiago, S., De Vicente, J. and De Diego, R.G. (2012) Role of Melatonin in Cancer Treatment. AntiCancer Research, 32, 2747-2753. - References - Scientific Research Publishing (scirp.org)

37. Srinivasan, Venkataramanujam & Spence, D. & Pandi-Perumal, Seithikurippu R. & Trakht, Ilya & Cardinali, Daniel. (2008). Therapeutic Actions of Melatonin in Cancer: Possible Mechanisms. Integrative cancer therapies. 7. 189-203. 10.1177/1534735408322846.

38. Chen, F., Deng, J., Liu, X., Li, W., & Zheng, J. (2015). HCRP-1 regulates cell migration and invasion via EGFR-ERK mediated up-regulation of MMP-2 with prognostic significance in human renal cell carcinoma. *Scientific reports*, *5*, 13470. https://doi.org/10.1038/srep13470

39. Um, Hee & Park, Jong-Wook & Kwon, Taeg Kyu. (2011). Melatonin sensitizes Caki renal cancer cells to kahweol-induced apoptosis through CHOP-mediated up-regulation of PUMA. Journal of pineal research. 50. 359-66. 10.1111/j.1600-079X.2010.00851.x.

40. Costa, G.J., Thuler, L.C., & Ferreira, C.G. (2016). Epidemiological changes in the histological subtypes of 35,018 non-small-cell lung cancer cases in Brazil. *Lung cancer, 97*, 66-72 .

41. Lu JJ, Fu L, Tang Z, Zhang C, Qin L, Wang J, Yu Z, Shi D, Xiao X, Xie F, Huang W, Deng W. Melatonin inhibits AP-2β/hTERT, NF-κB/COX-2 and Akt/ERK and activates caspase/Cyto C signaling to enhance the antitumor activity of berberine in lung cancer cells. Oncotarget. 2016 Jan 19;7(3):2985-3001. doi: 10.18632/oncotarget.6407. PMID: 26672764; PMCID: PMC4823085.

42. Ma Z, Yang Y, Fan C, Han J, Wang D, Di S, Hu W, Liu D, Li X, Reiter RJ, Yan X. Melatonin as a potential anticarcinogen for non-small-cell lung cancer. Oncotarget. 2016

Jul 19;7(29):46768-46784. doi: 10.18632/oncotarget.8776. PMID: 27102150; PMCID: PMC5216835.

43. Peng PL, Kuo WH, Tseng HC, Chou FP. Synergistic tumor-killing effect of radiation and berberine combined treatment in lung cancer: the contribution of autophagic cell death. Int J Radiat Oncol Biol Phys. 2008 Feb 1;70(2):529-42. doi: 10.1016/j.ijrobp.2007.08.034. PMID: 18207031.

44. Peng PL, Kuo WH, Tseng HC, Chou FP. Synergistic tumor-killing effect of radiation and berberine combined treatment in lung cancer: the contribution of autophagic cell death. Int J Radiat Oncol Biol Phys. 2008 Feb 1;70(2):529-42. doi: 10.1016/j.ijrobp.2007.08.034. PMID: 18207031.

45. Crew, Katherine & Neugut, Alfred. (2006). Crew KD, Neugut AIEpideiology of gastric cancer. World J Gastroenterol 12: 354-362. World journal of gastroenterology : WJG. 12. 354-62.

46. Wang, R., Liu, H., Xu, L., Zhang, H., & Zhou, R. (2015). Involvement of nuclear receptor RZR/RORγ in melatonin-induced HIF-1α inactivation in SGC-7901 human gastric cancer cells. Oncology Reports, 34, 2541-2546. https://doi.org/10.3892/or.2015.4238

47. S Zhang, Y Qi, H Zhang, W He, Q Zhou, S Gui & Y Wang (2013) Melatonin inhibits cell growth and migration, but promotes apoptosis in gastric cancer cell line, SGC7901, Biotechnic & Histochemistry, 88:6, 281-289, DOI: 10.3109/10520295.2013.769633

48. Zhang, S., Zuo, L., Gui, S. *et al.* Induction of cell differentiation and promotion of endocan gene expression in stomach cancer by melatonin. *Mol Biol Rep* **39,** 2843–2849 (2012). https://doi.org/10.1007/s11033-011-1043-4

49. Leja-Szpak, A., Jaworek, J., Pierzchalski, P. and Reiter, R.J. (2010), Melatonin induces pro-apoptotic signaling pathway in human pancreatic carcinoma cells (PANC-1). Journal of Pineal Research, 49: 248-255. https://doi.org/10.1111/j.1600-079X.2010.00789.x

50. Han, Sung-Sik MD*; Jang, Jin-Young MD*; Kim, Sun-Whe MD, FACS*; Kim, Woo-Ho MD†; Lee, Kuhn Uk MD*; Park, Yong-Hyun MD, FACS* Analysis of Long-term Survivors After Surgical Resection for Pancreatic Cancer, Pancreas: April 2006 - Volume 32 - Issue 3 - p 271-275 doi: 10.1097/01.mpa.0000202953.87740.93

51. Talar-Wojnarowska R, Malecka-Panas E. Molecular pathogenesis of pancreatic adenocarcinoma: potential clinical implications. Med Sci Monit. 2006 Sep;12(9):RA186-93. PMID: 16940943.

52. Lv, Dong, Cui, Pei-Lin, Yao, Shi-Wei, Xu, You-Qing, AND Yang, Zhao-Xu. "Melatonin inhibits the expression of vascular endothelial growth factor in pancreatic cancer cells" *Chinese Journal of Cancer Research* [Online], Volume 24 Number 4 (15 October 2012)

53. Gonzalez, Antonio & Castillo-Vaquero, Angel & Miro-Moran, Alvaro & Tapia, Jose & Salido, Gines M.. (2010). Melatonin reduces pancreatic tumor cell viability by altering mitochondrial physiology. Journal of pineal research. 50. 250-60. 10.1111/j.1600-079X.2010.00834.x.

54. Xu C, Wu A, Zhu H, Fang H, Xu L, Ye J, Shen J. Melatonin is involved in the apoptosis and necrosis of pancreatic cancer cell line SW-1990 via modulating of Bcl-2/Bax balance. Biomed

Pharmacother. 2013 Mar;67(2):133-9. doi: 10.1016/j.biopha.2012.10.005. Epub 2012 Nov 15. PMID: 23245210.

55. Uguz AC, Cig B, Espino J, Bejarano I, Naziroglu M, Rodríguez AB, Pariente JA. Melatonin potentiates chemotherapy-induced cytotoxicity and apoptosis in rat pancreatic tumor cells. J Pineal Res. 2012 Aug;53(1):91-8. doi: 10.1111/j.1600-079X.2012.00974.x. Epub 2012 Jan 31. PMID: 22288984.

56. Ruiz-Rabelo J, Vázquez R, Arjona A, Perea D, Montilla P, Túnez I, Muntané J, Padillo J. Improvement of capecitabine antitumoral activity by melatonin in pancreatic cancer. Pancreas. 2011 Apr;40(3):410-4. doi: 10.1097/MPA.0b013e318201ca4f. PMID: 21178648.

57. Bułdak RJ, Pilc-Gumuła K, Bułdak Ł, Witkowska D, Kukla M, Polaniak R, Zwirska-Korczala K. Effects of ghrelin, leptin and melatonin on the levels of reactive oxygen species, antioxidant enzyme activity and viability of the HCT 116 human colorectal carcinoma cell line. Mol Med Rep. 2015 Aug;12(2):2275-82. doi: 10.3892/mmr.2015.3599. Epub 2015 Apr 7. PMID: 25873273.

58. García-Navarro A, González-Puga C, Escames G, López LC, López A, López-Cantarero M, Camacho E, Espinosa A, Gallo MA, Acuña-Castroviejo D. Cellular mechanisms involved in the melatonin inhibition of HT-29 human colon cancer cell proliferation in culture. J Pineal Res. 2007 Sep;43(2):195-205. doi: 10.1111/j.1600-079X.2007.00463.x. PMID: 17645698.

59. Wei JY, Li WM, Zhou LL, Lu QN, He W. Melatonin induces apoptosis of colorectal cancer cells through HDAC4 nuclear import mediated by CaMKII inactivation. J Pineal Res. 2015 May;58(4):429-38. doi: 10.1111/jpi.12226. Epub 2015 Mar 20. PMID: 25752481.

60. León J, Casado J, Jiménez Ruiz SM, Zurita MS, González-Puga C, Rejón JD, Gila A, Muñoz de Rueda P, Pavón EJ, Reiter RJ, Ruiz-Extremera A, Salmerón J. Melatonin reduces endothelin-1 expression and secretion in colon cancer cells through the inactivation of FoxO-1 and NF-κβ. J Pineal Res. 2014 May;56(4):415-26. doi: 10.1111/jpi.12131. Epub 2014 Apr 15. PMID: 24628039.

61. Hong Y, Won J, Lee Y, Lee S, Park K, Chang KT, Hong Y. Melatonin treatment induces interplay of apoptosis, autophagy, and senescence in human colorectal cancer cells. J Pineal Res. 2014 Apr;56(3):264-74. doi: 10.1111/jpi.12119. Epub 2014 Jan 31. PMID: 24484372.

62. Nemeth C, Humpeler S, Kallay E, Mesteri I, Svoboda M, Rögelsperger O, Klammer N, Thalhammer T, Ekmekcioglu C. Decreased expression of the melatonin receptor 1 in human colorectal adenocarcinomas. J Biol Regul Homeost Agents. 2011 Oct-Dec;25(4):531-42. PMID: 22217986.

63. Wang J, Guo W, Chen W, Yu W, Tian Y, Fu L, Shi D, Tong B, Xiao X, Huang W, Deng W. Melatonin potentiates the antiproliferative and pro-apoptotic effects of ursolic acid in colon cancer cells by modulating multiple signaling pathways. J Pineal Res. 2013 May;54(4):406-16. doi: 10.1111/jpi.12035. Epub 2013 Jan 17. PMID: 23330808.

64. Seely D, Wu P, Fritz H, Kennedy DA, Tsui T, Seely AJ, Mills E. Melatonin as adjuvant cancer care with and without chemotherapy: a systematic review and meta-analysis of randomized trials. Integr Cancer Ther. 2012 Dec;11(4):293-303. doi: 10.1177/1534735411425484. Epub 2011 Oct 21. PMID: 22019490.

65. Wang YM, Jin BZ, Ai F, Duan CH, Lu YZ, Dong TF, Fu QL. The efficacy and safety of melatonin in concurrent chemotherapy or radiotherapy for solid tumors: a meta-analysis of randomized controlled trials. Cancer Chemother Pharmacol. 2012 May;69(5):1213-20. doi: 10.1007/s00280-012-1828-8. Epub 2012 Jan 24. PMID: 22271210.

66. Lissoni P, Barni S, Ardizzoia A, Paolorossi F, Crispino S, Tancini G, Tisi E, Archili C, De Toma D, Pipino G, et al. Randomized study with the pineal hormone melatonin versus supportive care alone in advanced nonsmall cell lung cancer resistant to a first-line chemotherapy containing cisplatin. Oncology. 1992;49(5):336-9. doi: 10.1159/000227068. PMID: 1382256.

67. Barni S, Lissoni P, Cazzaniga M, Ardizzoia A, Meregalli S, Fossati V, Fumagalli L, Brivio F, Tancini G. A randomized study of low-dose subcutaneous interleukin-2 plus melatonin versus supportive care alone in metastatic colorectal cancer patients progressing under 5-fluorouracil and folates. Oncology. 1995 May-Jun;52(3):243-5. doi: 10.1159/000227465. PMID: 7715908.

68. Cerea G, Vaghi M, Ardizzoia A, Villa S, Bucovec R, Mengo S, Gardani G, Tancini G, Lissoni P. Biomodulation of cancer chemotherapy for metastatic colorectal cancer: a randomized study of weekly low-dose irinotecan alone versus irinotecan plus the oncostatic pineal hormone melatonin in metastatic colorectal cancer patients progressing on 5-fluorouracil-containing combinations. Anticancer Res. 2003 Mar-Apr;23(2C):1951-4. PMID: 12820485.

69. Daniyal M, Siddiqui ZA, Akram M, Asif HM, Sultana S, Khan A. Epidemiology, etiology, diagnosis and treatment of prostate cancer. Asian Pac J Cancer Prev. 2014;15(22):9575-8. doi: 10.7314/apjcp.2014.15.22.9575. PMID: 25520069.

70. Rodriguez-Garcia A, Mayo JC, Hevia D, Quiros-Gonzalez I, Navarro M, Sainz RM. Phenotypic changes caused by melatonin increased sensitivity of prostate cancer cells to cytokine-induced apoptosis. J Pineal Res. 2013 Jan;54(1):33-45. doi: 10.1111/j.1600-079X.2012.01017.x. Epub 2012 Jun 28. PMID: 22738066.

71. Jung-Hynes B, Huang W, Reiter RJ, Ahmad N. Melatonin resynchronizes dysregulated circadian rhythm circuitry in human prostate cancer cells. J Pineal Res. 2010 Aug;49(1):60-8. doi: 10.1111/j.1600-079X.2010.00767.x. Epub 2010 May 27. PMID: 20524973; PMCID: PMC3158680.

72. Sainz RM, Mayo JC, Tan DX, León J, Manchester L, Reiter RJ. Melatonin reduces prostate cancer cell growth leading to neuroendocrine differentiation via a receptor and PKA independent mechanism. Prostate. 2005 Apr 1;63(1):29-43. doi: 10.1002/pros.20155. PMID: 15378522.

73. Cheng, J., Yang, H., Gu, C., Liu, Y., Shao, J., Zhu, R. ... Li, M. (2019). Melatonin restricts the viability and angiogenesis of vascular endothelial cells by suppressing HIF-1α/ROS/VEGF. International Journal of Molecular Medicine, 43, 945-955. https://doi.org/10.3892/ijmm.2018.4021

74. Shiu, S.Y.W., Leung, W.Y., Tam, C.W., Liu, V.W.S. and Yao, K.-M. (2013), Melatonin MT$_1$ receptor-induced transcriptional up-regulation of p27^{Kip1} in prostate cancer antiproliferation is mediated via inhibition of constitutively active nuclear factor kappa B (NF-κB): potential implications on prostate cancer chemoprevention and therapy. J. Pineal Res., 54: 69-79. https://doi.org/10.1111/j.1600-079X.2012.01026.x

75. Gurunathan, S., Qasim, M., Kang, M. H., & Kim, J. H. (2021). Role and Therapeutic Potential of Melatonin in Various Type of Cancers. *OncoTargets and therapy*, *14*, 2019–2052. https://doi.org/10.2147/OTT.S298512

76. Cho SY, Lee HJ, Jeong SJ, Lee HJ, Kim HS, Chen CY, Lee EO, Kim SH. Sphingosine kinase 1 pathway is involved in melatonin-induced HIF-1α inactivation in hypoxic PC-3 prostate cancer cells. J Pineal Res. 2011 Aug;51(1):87-93. doi: 10.1111/j.1600-079X.2011.00865.x. Epub 2011 Mar 11. PMID: 21392092.

77. Jung-Hynes B, Schmit TL, Reagan-Shaw SR, Siddiqui IA, Mukhtar H, Ahmad N. Melatonin, a novel Sirt1 inhibitor, imparts antiproliferative effects against prostate cancer in vitro in culture and in vivo in TRAMP model. J Pineal Res. 2011 Mar;50(2):140-9. doi: 10.1111/j.1600-079X.2010.00823.x. Epub 2010 Nov 9. PMID: 21062352; PMCID: PMC3052633.

78. Jung-Hynes B, Schmit TL, Reagan-Shaw SR, Siddiqui IA, Mukhtar H, Ahmad N. Melatonin, a novel Sirt1 inhibitor, imparts antiproliferative effects against prostate cancer in vitro in culture and in vivo in TRAMP model. J Pineal Res. 2011 Mar;50(2):140-9. doi: 10.1111/j.1600-079X.2010.00823.x. Epub 2010 Nov 9. PMID: 21062352; PMCID: PMC3052633.

79. Dauchy RT, Hoffman AE, Wren-Dail MA, Hanifin JP, Warfield B, Brainard GC, Xiang S, Yuan L, Hill SM, Belancio VP, Dauchy EM, Smith K, Blask DE. Daytime Blue Light Enhances the Nighttime Circadian Melatonin Inhibition of Human Prostate Cancer Growth. Comp Med. 2015 Dec;65(6):473-85. PMID: 26678364; PMCID: PMC4681241.

80. Li Y, Li S, Zhou Y, et al. Melatonin for the prevention and treatment of cancer. Oncotarget. 2017 Jun;8(24):39896-39921. DOI: 10.18632/oncotarget.16379. PMID: 28415828; PMCID: PMC5503661.

81. Shiu SY, Law IC, Lau KW, Tam PC, Yip AW, Ng WT. Melatonin slowed the early biochemical progression of hormone-refractory prostate cancer in a patient whose prostate tumor tissue expressed MT1 receptor subtype. J Pineal Res. 2003 Oct;35(3):177-82. doi: 10.1034/j.1600-079x.2003.00074.x. PMID: 12932201.

82. Chen, L., Deng, H., Cui, H., Fang, J., Zuo, Z., Deng, J., Li, Y., Wang, X., & Zhao, L. (2017). Inflammatory responses and inflammation-associated diseases in organs. *Oncotarget*, *9*(6), 7204–7218. https://doi.org/10.18632/oncotarget.23208

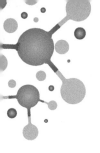

20

PINEAL GLAND

The seat of melatonin production & much more

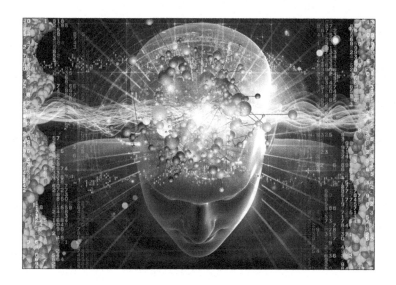

Your pineal gland functions at its highest between 1 and 4 am each night. Melatonin is produced in the enigmatic pineal gland, usually in response to darkness and that's why it's famously coined the hormone of darkness.

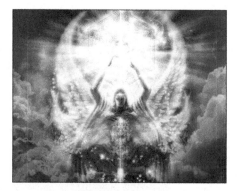

Shaped like a pinecone, the pineal gland is deeply seated within the brain. This small gland has ignited the imagination of philosophers, scholars as well as spiritual leaders from different cultures and religions.

The pineal gland is dubbed as "the seat of the soul" or the "third eye" and conceptualized as the 'tranquilizing organ'.[1] [2] [3]

Interestingly, researchers have suggested that the pineal gland and its hormonal product, melatonin, are possibly associated with improved longevity. Moreover, the pineal gland dysfunctions or failure is what is believed to initiate or accelerate the aging process.

This small gland is extremely vital for our health and lifespan. The pineal also releases DMT which is associated with feelings of love and connection to others. A paper published in 2018 by researchers in the U.K. purported that DMT simulates the near-death experience, wherein people report the sensation of transcending their bodies and entering another realm. It's no wonder the pineal is considered so important, as these 2 hormones are crucial when it comes to health.

I was an expert guest on a film called Psychedelics Revealed and although I don't advocate using DMT recreationally, I am a proponent of using psychedelic medicines in the right setting to work through emotional trauma and to become more spiritually aware through a profound experience that some of these medicines can provide. Many of which work through the DMT pathways and the pineal gland![4] [5] [6] [7]

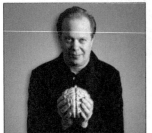

Dr. Joe Dispenza teaches his students to use a particular breath to improve the pressures around the pineal gland. I've taken his advanced course and it is something enormously powerful that creates a similar experience to being on psychedelics. There is a feeling of universal connection, love, and gratitude for being alive. This connection with the "divine source" is the experience I assume all religions speak about.

Becoming more aware of this energy or "doorway" can allow you to be connected to something that many religions speak of that unite us all in an energy that is not yet detectable with modern science. That's the best I can do to explain, as I know some might read this and think it's a bit "woo-woo" but there is no denying the events taking place at these events and the studies soon to be published through Dispenza's meditation practices.

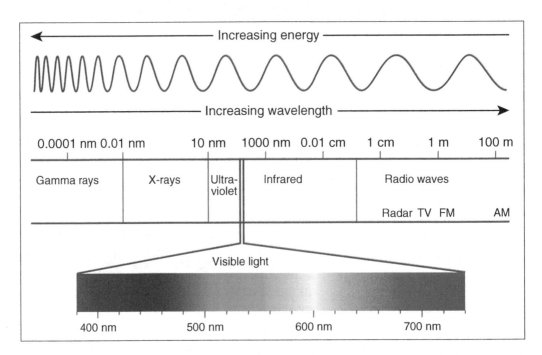

NASA scientists are seeing changes in the blood of these meditators. Tiny vesicles called exosomes found in the plasma of the meditator's were mixed with epithelial cells. They then introduced the COVID-19 virus and compared these cells to a control group without the meditator's exosomes. The COVID-19 virus was unable to enter the epithelial cells mixed with the meditator plasma. In contrast, the control group cells that were not from meditators were infected severely. They found tiny vesicles in much higher amounts in the blood of these meditators which are called exosomes.

Exosomes are packets of RNA which carry information to other cells and parts of the body. Scientists are attributing these exosomes to explain some of the remarkable changes within these meditators. Changes that range from virtually every disease known.

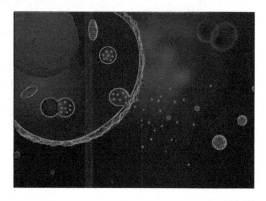

What I'm speaking of is spontaneous healing that occurs due to this heightened connection through the pineal and the other energy centers that run through the body. We use exosomes in my practice to heal various injuries and degenerative conditions that occur in the body. Such as osteoarthritis or even stroke. These exosomes are taken from the placentas of healthy mothers.

These exosomes can be injected just like stem cells, as exosomes are the healing substances delivered by stem cells regardless. Therefore, by bypassing the need for the stem cells to deliver the exosomes they can simply be isolated and injected with great results in many applications.

So, is it possible when we connect with your pineal with certain intentionality's, such as to heal a foot or your brain that the body responds by releasing exosomes that will carry the information you intend?

I believe this is what's happening. If you look at the graph showing the energy spectrum and what a small part of it is the "visible light" you can appreciate there are so many frequencies and wavelengths we are not aware of.

Is it possible the pineal is more of a radio receiver? Do the crystals becoming activated through the CSF creating an energy field that allows us to tap into a source that can allow for powerful changes in our health?

Pineal & CSF Flow

This image of the flow of CSF shows how the circulation goes through what's called ventricles in the brain. These ventricles are like canals carrying the life-giving nutrients the CSF delivers to the brain and spinal cord. The pineal sits right at the end of the 3rd ventricle and CSF has most of its pressure around it and the pituitary.

Take a look at this MRI showing the red areas as the most active.

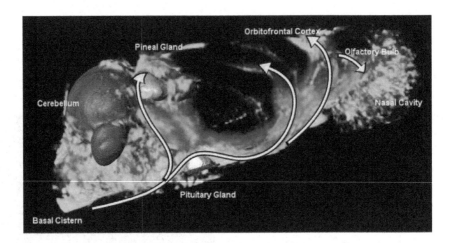

What Dr. Dispenza teaches is a breath that directs your CSF into the pineal by locking down your muscles from the base of your pelvis or perineum up the spine and throat toward the pineal. There is a pumping action upon a full inhale with intentionality to the pineal gland. This is creating hydrostatic pressure to the pineal, which Dr. Dispenza has been discovered in the literature to be involved in an activation to the crystalline structure inside the pineal.

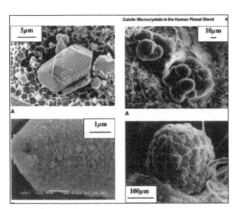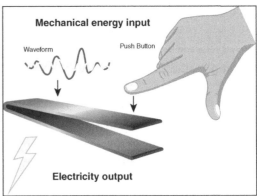

There seems to be a piezoelectric effect from the hydrostatic pressure of CSF as it interacts with the crystalline structures within the pineal.

Piezoelectric is defined as the ability of certain materials to generate an electric charge in response to applied mechanical stress. I always say you're either a swamp or a river and this means better circulation, better health, and the pineal can become a victim or a victor due to good or poor circulation.

Doing things like this pineal breath Dr. Dispenza teaches might hold some promise to improving pineal health, as well as detoxing many of the chemicals that interfere with pineal gland function such as fluoride, which has been proven to create calcifications.

DMT The Spirit Molecule

DMT or N, N-Dimethyltryptamine is so powerful that it was dubbed the "spirit molecule" for its spiritual awakening–type trips. It's defined as a chemical substance that occurs in many plants and animals and is a derivative and a structural analog of tryptamine. DMT is used as a recreational psychedelic drug and prepared by various

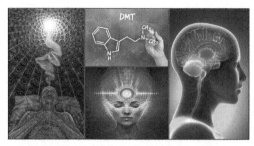

cultures for ritual purposes as an entheogen such as with Ayahuasca. Ayahuasca is traditionally prepared using two plants called *Banisteriopsis caapi* and *Psychotria Viridis*. The latter contains DMT while the former contains MAOIs, which prevent certain enzymes in your body from breaking down DMT.

DMT may also be released when we dream. It's also believed to be released during birth and death. This release of DMT at death may be responsible for those mystical experiences seen with Dispenza's work and psychedelic drugs such as psilocybin and LSD. Trace amounts of DMT have been shown in rat pineal glands.[8]

The pineal gland in humans produces a small amount and it's uncertain if the pineal is a large enough source of DMT to be psychoactive. My personal belief is that DMT can be released by a healthy pineal. Keep in mind 80% of us have calcified pineals and therefore, a healthy pineal is rare, thus meaning that studies on typical pineal glands might not reflect the potential in certain individuals.

In fact, it's quite possible that the pineal can produce more DMT than what scientists have seen thus far given the right circumstance.

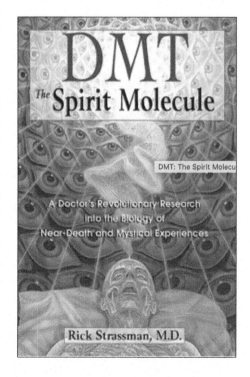

Dr. Dispenza's work as well as other anecdotal methods to activate your "third eye" such as: breathing methods, yoga, meditation, taking certain supplements, doing a detox or cleanse, using crystals and various vibrations tuned to certain frequencies might hold the answers.

Dr. Rick Strassman wrote a book on DMT called "The Spirit Molecule: A Doctor's Revolutionary Research into the Biology of Near-Death and Mystical Experiences". In this amazing book, Strassman sees DMT consistently producing near-death and mystical experiences with his volunteers. Many reported encounters with intelligent nonhuman presences, aliens, angels, and spirits. Nearly all felt that the sessions were among the most profound experiences of their lives.

The pineal gland commonly becomes non-functional and calcified as we age

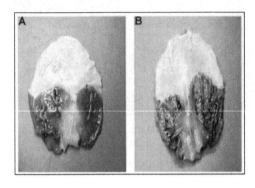

In 80% of adult humans, the pineal gland contains calcifications defined as "corpora arenacea" or "brain sand".[9]

One of the defense mechanisms protecting the body against the effects of fluoride toxicity seems to be its deposition in calcified tissues. The symptoms of excessive fluoride accumulation in bones and teeth are known and well documented, classified as skeletal fluorosis and dental fluorosis, respectively.

Calcium deposition into the pineal gland is like that found in bones. The process of calcium accumulation in the pineal gland is initiated in childhood and even in newborns.

Calcification is accompanied by a reduction in melatonin synthesis. Hence, the conclusion that pineal gland calcification has an indirect effect on the production and secretion of this hormone. The image here shows the severe calcification of the pineal.

In light of this science, it may make sense to limit fluoride intake by avoiding drinking most municipal water sources, which have been fortified with fluoride, as well as many conventional toothpastes. Furthermore, fluoride is also used in pesticides and some chemicals used to create non-stick compounds for pots and pans. Eating organic foods and avoiding processed foods can also reduce fluoride consumption.

This study might support avoiding fluoride fluoride 'Fluoride-Free Diet Stimulates Pineal Growth in Aged Male Rats'.[10]

How to detox your pineal gland

Besides melatonin, there are a few supplements that can be helpful. Here are the ones I found to be most relevant:

- *Iodine* is a mineral found in sea vegetables, like seaweed or kelp. This vital mineral assists the thyroid gland in regulating hormones and is one of the most efficient removers (chelators) of heavy metals from the body. Iodine chelates heavy metals such as mercury, lead, cadmium, and aluminum, as well as fluoride.

- *Shilajit* is plant material produced over millions of years from plants preserved in dark crevices of the Himalayan Mountains. Shilajit forms a thick resin that's packed with 85 different trace minerals including fulvic acid. Fulvic acid helps eliminate toxins and heavy metals, supporting the decalcification process.

- *Turmeric* is another excellent supplement for your pineal gland detox. This study in Pharmacon Magazine shows that curcumin, the active ingredient in turmeric, can prevent and potentially reverse the damage from fluoride exposure.[11]

- *Chaga Mushrooms:* The Chinese call it the "King of Plants." In Siberia, it's the "Gift from God." And for the Japanese, it's the "Diamond of the Forest." Not bad for wood-rotting fungus! Hundreds of scientific studies have demonstrated the potent effects of the Chaga mushroom on the immune, hormonal, and central nervous systems. Studies in Finland and Russia found that Chaga is an efficient anti-tumor agent as well as antiviral. Chaga provides us with phytochemicals, nutrients, and melanin. The pineal gland uses melanin to help shield us from UV light. From my research, the Siberian Chaga appears to be the most potent with the highest recorded levels of antioxidants according to the ORAC Scale. [12] [13] [14] [15]

- *K2 or factor X:* Intestinal microflora in animal tissues produces vitamin K1 & 2. You can find it in organ meats, fermented dairy products, like cheese or butter (grass-fed butter), sauerkraut, and marine oils.

  In 1945, the "Isaac Newton of Nutrition," a former dentist named Weston Price, described a vitamin-like compound that plays a major role in:

  - Growth

  - Reproduction

  - Brain function

  - Tooth decay prevention

  - Protection against calcification of the arteries

- *Tamarind:* One study and a follow-up study from the early 2000s demonstrated that tamarind increased the excretion of fluoride in urine compared to the control group. The researchers believe tamarind may even be able to reverse the effects of skeletal fluorosis caused by ingesting fluoride.[16] [17]

- *Green Superfoods:* Finally, eating raw, green foods that are rich in chlorophyll will also help chelate heavy metals from your blood while nourishing it. Chlorophyll-dense foods like chlorella, spirulina, and wheatgrass also increase oxygen levels, repair damaged tissue, and boost the immune system.

Conclusion

The pineal is an important gland and might play many roles beyond melatonin production. It may also serve as a connection to a "source" or a divine higher power.

It is now being proven in science that the pineal via its piezoelectric effect through the pressures CSF imposed on the gland may be like a radio receiver. Moreover, the pineal may allow us to have the ability to access information in the form of extremely high frequencies.

In other words, the pineal gland may serve as a connection with a force we might classify as mystical, holy, divine, God or the creator. However, one chooses to call this force or energy; it's difficult to deny its existence.

Information may be at the root of this connection and this might explain the dramatic changes in blood with the healing exosomes being discovered with meditators which are connecting and activating the pineal gland through Dr. Joe Dispenza's work.

Cranial work can be very helpful for pineal health. I have been using a technique called FCR or Functional Cranial Release for 26 years with interesting effect. I have a book coming out next called "Its All In Your Head: Endo-Nasal Cranial Therapy" I discuss some of the amazing healing effects using this treatment to restore the normal wider structure of the cranium and something called cranial rhythm that allows cerebral spinal fluid not only to be formed but to circulate and increased the piezoelectric affect to the pineal which as you can see in this chapter may have some benefit. Keep an eye out for this book to be released sometime in the summer of 2022.

Reference

1.   Scripps Study Finds Higher Death Risk With Sleeping Pills (prnewswire.com)

2.   Evans T. Drug error at Eskenazi Hospital killed prominent cancer researcher. Here's how it happened. *Indianapolis Star*. Updated October 31, 2020. 2021. www.indystar.com/story/news/investigations/2020/10/30/drug-error-cancer-researcher-eskenazi-hospital-killed/5979448002/

3.   Andersen, L. P., Werner, M. U., Rosenkilde, M. M., Harpsøe, N. G., Fuglsang, H., Rosenberg, J., & Gögenur, I. (2016). Pharmacokinetics of oral and intravenous melatonin in healthy volunteers. *BMC pharmacology & toxicology*, *17*, 8. https://doi.org/10.1186/s40360-016-0052-2

4.   Sinha, R., Sinha, I., Calcagnotto, A., Trushin, N., Haley, J. S., Schell, T. D., & Richie, J. P., Jr (2018). Oral supplementation with liposomal glutathione elevates body stores of glutathione and markers of immune function. *European journal of clinical nutrition*, *72*(1), 105–111. https://doi.org/10.1038/ejcn.2017.132

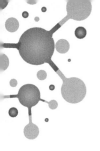

21

SUPRA-PHYSIOLOGICAL DOSING

Dosing Ideas, Conclusion & Final Words on Melatonin

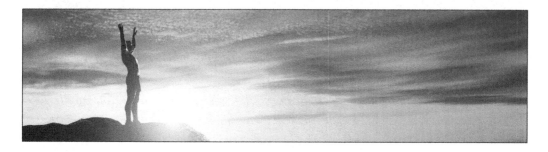

The Silver Bullet & Why Melatonin Is So Important Today

Is Melatonin the Silver Bullet?

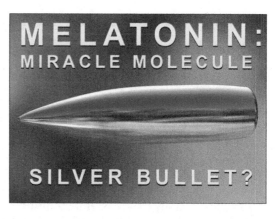

We have all heard the term "Silver Bullet". From Wikipedia: "folklore, a bullet cast from silver is often one of the few weapons that are effective against a werewolf or witch. The term is also a metaphor for a simple, seemingly magical, solution to a difficult problem: for example, penicillin was a silver bullet that allowed doctors to treat and successfully cure many bacterial infections." With all the powerful aspects melatonin is involved with inside your body and how it works to protect you especially during stress it seems that melatonin should absolutely carry this badge of honor as being a Silver Bullet against stress and diseases caused by stress. We discussed stresses as mental-emotional, chemical, physical or structural, microbial, and electromagnetic stress. These stressors are worse now than 10 years ago and especially when compared to how our parents grew up. Moreover, they will only get worse over time due to the reckless advance of technology and the ability for tech to allow us to be even more productive and "busy" 24/7.

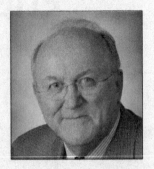

"Taking melatonin may extend your healthy, productive life span. I personally take 100mg every night! As we age, our body produces less and less melatonin, depriving you of this sleep-enhancing, free radical scavenging, heart calming, immune-stimulating, cancer-fighting hormone- in short depriving you of one of your body's best defenses against aging. Replenishing your supply of this vital hormone may allow you to live longer, and allow you to avoid crippling diseases such as arthritis, diabetes, heart disease, cancer, Alzheimer's, and Parkinson's. The possibility of this is more than wishful thinking. Laboratory studies show that giving melatonin to aging animals has extended their lifespan by as much as 20%"

Russel Reiter, MD, PhD

Why Melatonin isn't more well known?

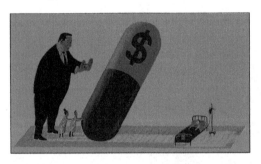

Our healthcare system being sold out to Big Pharma and the revolving door in Washington allowing drugs and drug companies to destroy the true intentions of what a health care system is supposed to stand for versus an FDA that has a design based on keeping the population in a constant state of consumption of Big Pharma's products. Cures are not popular molecules for these companies to study as the ROI or return on investment is not great enough. Yes, that's right, your health is not the most important goal for this, a behemoth of a system called Big Pharma. It is a group of executives that sit around and strategize how to best capitalize. Keeping you in a disease state taking their drug day after day month after month and year after year, making sure their shareholders are happy and their stock price elevated.

Look at our current situation with COVID-19 and how censorship has not allowed anything except vaccines to be heard over social media as well as news channels. I personally know friends and businesses that have been shut down for speaking up about natural solutions to raising the immune system, as well as natural antivirals.

A good example is colloidal silver which has a tremendous antiviral effect and is completely safe to consume. Companies and people who were trying to educate the public about this are either being thrown in jail or silenced another way. Ozone is another therapy.

I had Dr. Frank Shallenberger on my YouTube channel called CellularReset and the interview was taken down due to not conforming to the community standards and or violating spreading misinformation on COVID-19. And of course, melatonin has not gotten its deserving recognition. It's been covered on a couple of small news outlets and various papers here and there but wouldn't you think that Dr. Fauci or other prominent voices would be encouraging the public to consume such a safe and effective hormone?

Dangers of using Sleeping Pills?

Sleeping pills are the 3rd leading cause of death in the United States. In fact, I'd go as far as saying that sleeping pills are criminal in my mind. According to ScienceDaily, based on an article published in the British Medical Journal, *"Feb. 27, 2012 — People are relying on sleeping pills more than ever to get a good night's rest, but a new study by Scripps Clinic researchers links the medications to a 4.6 times higher risk of death and a significant increase in cancer cases among regular pill users."*[1]

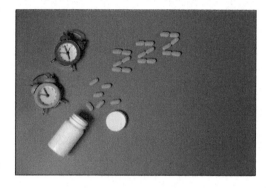

This is just speaking to the overall health risk and danger medications for sleep have in general.

The Pharmacy Times printed a story stating, "Sleeping pill users in the middle third (of sleeping pill consumption) had a 20% increased risk of developing cancer, whereas, those in the top third of users had a 35% increased risk. Zolpidem users in the top third had a 28% increased risk of major cancer. Temazepam users in the middle third had a 44% increased risk of major cancer, and users in the top third had a 99% increased risk. The study's results indicated that the increased risk of death and developing cancer associated with sleeping pill use was not attributable to pre-existing diseases."[2]

That means these medications **CAUSED CANCER** in these cases. By extrapolating their findings to the entire US population, the researchers estimate that sleeping pills may have been associated with 320,000 to 507,000 excess deaths in 2010. Did you read that? 3-500,000 deaths! That makes sleeping pills the **THIRD LEADING CAUSE OF DEATH** in the United States, just 13% behind cancer.

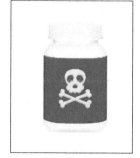

But wait, here's the real kicker! If sleeping pills are associated with these numbers and cancer is a clear side effect, how many cases of the 600,000 cancer deaths a year are due to sleeping pills? The numbers start to blur, but it is clear these medications are causing much more harm than potential good.

Don't support them by using them, someone's life, if not your own may be on the line.

To see the bigger picture and the tremendous danger these drugs represent we have to consider that according to the U.S. Center for Disease Control (CDC), 2,468,435 people died in the U.S. alone in 2010. If this estimate is accurate it means that 13% to 20.5% of those deaths may have been associated with sleeping pills.

Again, a 460% higher risk of death, potentially contributing to 20.5% of all the deaths each year, and a 99% potential increase in cancer for a non-life-threatening condition is insane.

It is time for melatonin and other natural sleep-promoting options to shine. Sleep is like a symphony and it has a flow of changes from light sleep, deep sleep, and REM. If someone were to be knocked out by Mike Tyson then placed next to a person sleeping soundly, they might look the same. However, when each person got up they would feel quite different. The person waking up after an Ambien or any of the other conventional sleeping pills will not have experienced the same level of restful sleep when compared to an individual who'd slept naturally.

In fact, many sleeping pills actually suppress melatonin, and when one considers the powerful effects of melatonin as a cancer inhibitor it makes sense that suppressing natural melatonin production will increase cancer risks. Also, we have discussed many diseases and negative aspects of health caused by poor sleep. Low melatonin leads to poor sleep and many acute and chronic diseases.

Supra physiological dose Melatonin – Safe and Effective

Studies show that melatonin is often beneficial at high therapeutic doses to achieve the desired effect. Also, many studies have proved that melatonin use at these high doses say higher than 100mg per day, is safe for humans. '**The Therapeutic Potential of Melatonin: A Review of Science'**[3] Melatonin toxicity in both animal and human studies is extremely rare. However, minor side effects such as headache, rash, stomach upset, and nightmare are noticed on rare occasions. As high as 800mg per kg body weight was not lethal[4]. That's 56,000mg for a 160 lb person! Studies were also carried out on human subjects who were given varying doses of melatonin ranging from 1 g to 6.6 g per day for 30 to 45 days (1,000mg – 6,600mg), after which comprehensive tests were done on them to detect potential toxicity. Findings showed that apart from drowsiness, all findings were normal at the end of the test period.

Melatonin use as a form of contraceptive for women has been proposed, giving rise to the question of if melatonin damages the female reproductive system. However, no adverse effects were reported in a phase 2 clinical trial done on 1400 women who were given 75mg of melatonin every night for four consecutive years[5]. That's a nice stretch that would tell me its plausible melatonin at very high doses are safe for long term use. 1400 people enrolled in this study is a large study and these results should not be ignored! Another study showed that melatonin at high doses has no significant toxicity, aside from some rare exceptions. This study showed melatonin is safe for 100 mg per day. Another study using a high dose of melatonin – 1g per day for one month in humans, shows no adverse effect on the individuals. In a study, 80mg of melatonin were given to healthy men every hour for 4 hours with no adverse effects other than drowsiness. Also, in healthy women, 300 mg of melatonin per day were used for 4 months with no adverse effects . Another study in children with muscular dystrophy using 70 mg per day of melatonin revealed reduced cytokines and lipid peroxidation. A randomized, controlled, double-blind clinical trial done recently on 50 patients referred for liver surgery demonstrated a single preoperative oral dose of 50 mg per kg of melatonin which is up to 3g for an adult, was both safe and well-tolerated[6].

When looking over the available research on supra physiological melatonin dosing with some of the research even going as high as 3000 mg it's evident that melatonin is extremely safe. Although

Although I've not ever tried a full 3000 mg of melatonin in an evening, I have taken 1000mg and besides tolerating it, it felt beneficial. I am certainly not suggesting anybody reading this take these high of doses especially outside of medical supervision.

The most common dosage I prescribed to a lot of my patients in my clinic is 100 to 200 mg about 30 minutes before bedtime. I recommend folks that are interested in super physiological melatonin dosing should start low and work their way up to allow for adaptation and cellular detoxification.

Contraindications to melatonin supplementation

People that are taking steroids such as cortisone or dexamethasone may consider that melatonin may counter some of the effects of these medications. Due to the unknown risks with pregnancy it is recommend not to take melatonin. Women that are wanting to conceive may not want to take more than 10 mg per day as it might prevent ovulation.[7] A small subset of individuals may have insulin, diabetic reactions to high dose melatonin due to the MTNR1B Gene. Currently there is no known strategies that allow these individuals to continue melatonin without those side effects?

I have noticed there has been a subset of individuals who experience more pronounced grogginess or drowsiness the day after taking larger or even small doses of melatonin. There is a polymorphisms of a gene called CYP1A2 which slows the breakdown of

"Caution for individuals with MTNR1B a gene mutation is warranted. In all my years I have not come across even one case of this. I am aware of a dietetic friend who take as much as 1 gram (yes, gram) daily without consequence. I am not diabetic, but if I was melatonin would even be of greater interest to me, because it is usually very beneficial in these cases."

Russell Reiter, MD, PhD

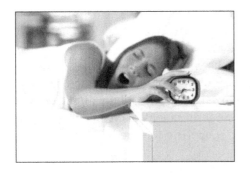

melatonin.[8] It also relates to caffeine and for those who are Especially sensitive to caffeine wise the effects seem to be much longer lasting this might be a window that you have this gene variant. What that means is that you will also break down melatonin slowly. This could cause melatonin to continue to be in the bloodstream much longer than normal. With cases like this I have had success dosing people hours earlier than their bedtime. Keep in mind that melatonin with light exposure should not cause drowsiness so taking melatonin in the late afternoon or dinner time might work better for some so that by the time they wake up the melatonin has been fully metabolized and cleared out of the blood. Since melatonin also asked to chelate heavy metals out of the central nervous system as well as could create a detox reaction in the body it could be possible that there might be temporary side effects for a few days when one first starts dosing higher amounts of melatonin. I have found in my own clinic that many people that might have side effects initially seem to be able to adapt to the melatonin after a few days on that higher dose. I consider this the same as if you we're experiencing fatigue for many days or weeks leaving you with very little energy to keep your home clean and organized. Imagine that all the sudden you got lots of energy and motivation came with it because your brain started working better such as is the case with melatonin. You would then likely begin fixing things that are broken in your home, cleaning and throwing things away that you no longer need. This is exactly what happens at the cellular level when there is poor mitochondrial function and the cells can

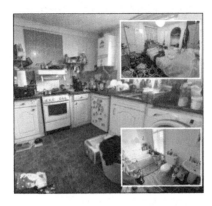

no longer adequately maintained themselves, which involves maintaining all of the functional components within the cell as well as clearing toxins that normally develop when we make energy. The world we live in has so many different toxins that that is an additional stressor that each cell needs to deal with as well resulting in even more energy are requirements to clear these toxins. Although it would be best to talk to your doctor or healthcare practitioner about any side effects resulting from melatonin supplementation this phenomenon should be considered an adaptation phase can be normal.

Naturally Improve Melatonin through Sauna or Hot Baths.

Doing saunas, hot baths preferably with Epson salts, hot showers and Jacuzzis could all be a way to naturally boost melatonin levels. The effect of increasing melatonin levels through heat might be one reason that hot therapies improve health and life span.

A study in April 2015 in JAMA showing that regular use of saunas can decrease all cause mortality, improve and extend life. Association Between Sauna Bathing and Fatal Cardiovascular and All-Cause Mortality Events.[9]

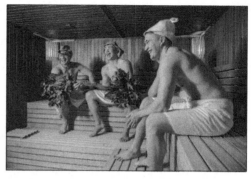

Another paper in 2001 published in the Journal of American College of Cardiology 'Repeated thermal therapy improves impaired vascular endothelial function in patients with coronary risk factors'.[10] It has long been known that taking a hot bath before bed can sometimes improve sleep onset or help you fall asleep faster. Melatonin works to drop your temperature and this is why sleeping in a cold room supports sleep throughout the night. Perhaps melatonin is working to normalize your temperature after the heat then Sandman comes along to take you into a beautiful night sleep.

Route of Delivery: Melatonin Supplementation

One major consideration regarding supplementing with melatonin is the different routes of delivery or administration. Of course, the most common is oral supplementation. Like with all oral routes of delivery melatonin must have indoor gastric acid and pancreatic enzymes before it is then metabolized through the liver. This is the reason in this study that oral administration of melatonin only demonstrated a 2.5 % absorption rate.[11]

By contrast, an intravenous or subcutaneous injection may bypass hepatic metabolism for what's called "first pass" through the liver.

When I was first introduced to the term *peak plasma* it was when I was considering beginning using glutathione suppositories during my personal journey with chronic Lyme disease and mold illness. At the time I didn't know what was wrong with me and I just knew that I had massive inflammation in my body. After looking at the role of glutathione in the body I knew this would be a helpful nutrient, however, I wasn't interested in regular visits to a doctor's office to receive these intravenously It was then that I discovered suppositories.

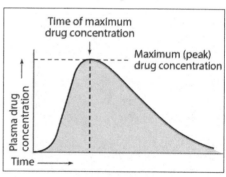

Suppository Delivery

I began using glutathione suppositories and noticing the drastic improvement in my condition I decided to try intravenous administration. What I found was I actually had a better response with the suppositories than I did with the procedure that can cost $150 and

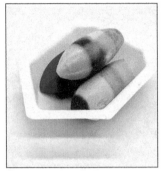

two hours of my day to go to the doctor's office. This got my attention and wanted to understand why the suppositories seem to work better. This is where the concept of peak plasma had the answers to my question.

The term peak plasma is simply referring to maximal blood levels of a certain nutrient after it is administered. This is where one can look at various routes of administration and judge the most effective in order to promote the most absorption into the body.

With this in mind let's look at a study by Kennaway and Seamark which showed that subcutaneous injection of melatonin quickly leads to high peak plasma levels, but it *declines rapidly*. By contrast, oral administration leads to a *lower* but *longer-lasting and constant* peak plasma melatonin level.[12]

DeMuro demonstrated that intravenous injection of melatonin can reach a much higher serum peak plasma levels of melatonin concentration when compared to oral administration. However, the half-life of melatonin in the serum showed no significant difference between these two different routes of administration. What this means is that the routes of melatonin administration will influence the peak plasma level of melatonin but not the half-life of melatonin. This means melatonin will last just as long-circulating in the blood no matter what route of delivery of administration you use.[13]

What about liposomal delivery?

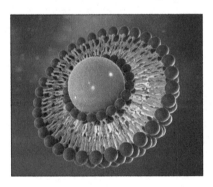

Liposomal delivery systems, with their advanced nutrient bioavailability, are becoming more popular. There are over 65,000 peer reviewed published studies on liposomal delivery. They are utilized in medicine for the delivery of vaccines, hormones, enzymes, vitamins and botanicals.

Liposomes are tiny lipid bubbles about the width of a single human hair. They are made out of the same type of fat as our own cell membranes called phospholipids. Liposomes are stable, and can carry both water and fat-soluble nutrients. When formulated correctly, they can facilitate absorption as soon as they land on the tongue, and can help protect breakdown by digestive acids, enzymes and first pass through the liver. Because they are made of the same lipids that compose our own cell membranes, they may assist nutrients to gain access into the cell membrane and optimize cellular support.

Liposomal technology like suppository has been said to provide the power of intravenous therapy. Because of enhanced delivery and absorption, nutrients delivered in liposomal form at lower doses may offer equal or greater efficacy than higher doses provided in forms that are less bioavailable.[14],[15]

Their potency is impressive. In liposomal form, the absorption of melatonin or glutathione can compare to that of intravenous formulations, and appears to help maintain intracellular storage.[16],[17] Even better, the phospholipids in liposomes are therapeutic. They help nourish every cell membrane by providing the lipids needed to function optimally and flush out toxins that accumulate there.

With all of the documentation, many have concluded that a very high pharmacological dose of melatonin under the supervision of a physician or healthcare provider in the therapy of various conditions should be safe and acceptable. Melatonin protects us under stress therefore it might make sense to supplement melatonin under times of stress or when our body is dealing with various disease conditions.

The aging process seems to be slowed through the supplementation of melatonin and for those looking to simply be healthier and live longer than the use of melatonin supplementation may make sense in this situation as well.

Being the author of this book, I've made it evident and stated it before that I take 100 mg to 200 mg of melatonin each night personally. I either take it in a suppository or in a liposomal delivery forum which is much more absorbable than the 2.5 % oral absorption. I have done this for nearly 2 years now and have never felt better. This may not be for everyone and it is certainly important that this is discussed with your healthcare provider before you start something like a super physiological melatonin dosing schedule.

For the vast majority of people reading this book these high doses would be safe and very effective in supporting the body and brain in a wide range of natural stress and disease states.

Recap of all the ways Melatonin can Support your Health

- *Degenerative Neurological Disease*
- *Memory and Cognitive Problems*
- *Immune System Weakness; Susceptibility to Infections: both acute and chronic*
- *Autoimmune Diseases*
- *Digestive Diseases*
- *Skin Conditions*
- *Premature Aging*
- *Mood, Mental/Emotional Conditions*
- *Cancer*
- *Liver Disease*
- *Cardiovascular Disease*
- *Sexual Decline and Infertility*
- *Low-Stress Resistance, Poor Mitochondrial Function*
- *Autism & Childhood Development Issues*
- *Metabolic diseases like Diabetes*

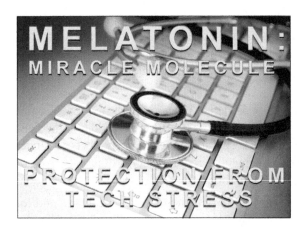

I think it's important to consider at this point that we are no longer really living in a natural environment. In the past, we did not have to deal with this unnatural green and blue light emitting from our cell phones, computers, televisions, and the lighting in our homes. We did not have to deal with the melatonin-destroying medications that some of us are on. We did not have to deal with the electromagnetic stress that lowered our melatonin levels, and hopefully, after reading this book you've chosen to turn your Wi-Fi router off at night. Moreover, we also have not evolved to have to deal with all of the chemical toxins in our environment.

Technology has created a situation for us to be ultra productive with our mobile devices, being able to run a business through a handheld device creates a situation where there is never really downtime and unless we make it so. I am just as guilty of this as anybody, as it becomes an addiction to be more and more productive and to share your life with others on social media instead of taking time to enjoy quiet and peace.

Lastly, there is the lack of sunshine on our skin and into our eyes which allow us to store melatonin only to be dumped when we are in complete darkness. Avoiding the sun and wearing sunglasses is a massive headwind to us producing and releasing the maximum amount of melatonin each night.

Indeed we are living in a much more stressful time in many regards than we have been evolutionarily able to evolve to handle with regards to the production of melatonin allowing us to buffer these stressors. I for one would not be without my melatonin after taking into account all of the facts presented in the research we've discussed throughout this book.

Conclusion

I've been working on this book for nearly a year and a half and it has been a labor of love, and there has been a tremendous feeling of purpose to deliver this information to the world. Although there have been a couple of other very well-written books on melatonin

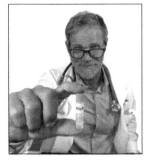

there has been new research since those were published and I felt that a holistic and naturopathic viewpoint on integrating melatonin to support various health concerns was needed.

I honestly can't think of one condition that wouldn't benefit from supplementing with melatonin as it has such a wide range and diverse and positive effect on so many aspects of health through the stress responses. Just think of all the changes that have occurred over the years with the invention of light bulbs and artificial light, harmful EMFs, drugs, toxins in our water supply, chemicals from plastics in our food and water, poor air quality, aluminum, mercury-laden fish and other heavy metals, GMO's, pesticide and chemical-laden food, microbiome destroying antibiotics, technologies that adrenalize us throughout the day and superbugs like COVID-19.

In our current state of a global pandemic, we also have concerns with the safety and efficacy of the experimental vaccines that are being forced on us. With the isolation, social distancing, and fear-based media it is no wonder people are suffering from many mental and emotional afflictions.

There has never been a more appropriate time for the widespread use of melatonin. Of course, it is my opinion that high-dose supraphysiological dosing in many cases might be the most effective use of the miracle molecule. Through my own biohacking experiences using supraphysiological melatonin dosing I have literally done months at 800 mg and I've had nothing but positive effects in my resilience to stress. I have also not found any challenges when abruptly discontinuing the use, which supports the research showing that it doesn't shut down our own production, but also on a personal level I find this to be true.

I'm certainly not advocating everybody go out and start supplementing that much melatonin right away, and as always my advice would be to find a doctor that understands melatonin who can help guide you with an appropriate dosing schedule and protocol created for your unique case.

Unfortunately, there are not enough doctors that know of the incredibly long list of benefits melatonin has to offer. Yet, other prominent physicians like Dr. Joe Mercola, Dr. Russell Reiter, and Dr. Frank Shallenberger share my viewpoint after digging into the research, as I have.

Indeed it is a time for melatonin's miracle story to be told and this was my intention with this book. Now that you have the knowledge regarding melatonin, the miracle molecule, it is your responsibility to share this with the people that you love and care about.

Thank you for reading my book and I hope that the information you have acquired from this book helps you to be healthier, live longer, and be more resilient to stress.

When we are healthier we're happier and when we're happier we treat ourselves better. When we treat ourselves better we treat other people better. When we treat other people better, other people are happier and the world is a better place for it. Let us use melatonin to become healthier and happier and start the cascade into creating a better world for us all.

References

1. Kripke, D. F., Langer, R. D., & Kline, L. E. (2012). Hypnotics' association with mortality or cancer: a matched cohort study. *BMJ open*, *2*(1), e000850. https://doi.org/10.1136/bmjopen-2012-000850

2. Sleeping Pills May Dramatically Increase Death Rate (pharmacytimes.com)

3. Malhotra, S., Sawhney, G., & Pandhi, P. (2004). The therapeutic potential of melatonin: a review of the science. *MedGenMed : Medscape general medicine*, *6*(2), 46.

4. Savage RA, Zafar N, Yohannan S, et al. Melatonin. [Updated 2021 Aug 15]. In: StatPearls [Internet]. Treasure Island (FL): StatPearls Publishing; 2021 Jan-. Available from: https://www.ncbi.nlm.nih.gov/books/NBK534823/

5. Silman RE. Melatonin: a contraceptive for the nineties. Eur J Obstet Gynecol Reprod Biol. 1993 Apr;49(1-2):3-9. doi: 10.1016/0028-2243(93)90099-x. PMID: 8365512.

6. Tordjman, S., Chokron, S., Delorme, R., Charrier, A., Bellissant, E., Jaafari, N., & Fougerou, C. (2017). Melatonin: Pharmacology, Functions and Therapeutic Benefits. *Current neuropharmacology*, *15*(3), 434–443. https://doi.org/10.2174/1570159X14666161228122115

7. Massion AO, Teas J, Hebert JR, Wertheimer MD, Kabat-Zinn J. Meditation, melatonin and breast/prostate cancer: hypothesis and preliminary data. Med Hypotheses. 1995 Jan;44(1):39-46. doi: 10.1016/0306-9877(95)90299-6. PMID: 7776900.

8. Härtter, S., Nordmark, A., Rose, D.-M., Bertilsson, L., Tybring, G. and Laine, K. (2003), Effects of caffeine intake on the pharmacokinetics of melatonin, a probe drug for CYP1A2 activity. British Journal of Clinical Pharmacology, 56: 679-682. https://doi.org/10.1046/j.1365-2125.2003.01933.x

9. Laukkanen T, Khan H, Zaccardi F, Laukkanen JA. Association between sauna bathing and fatal cardiovascular and all-cause mortality events. JAMA Intern Med. 2015 Apr;175(4):542-8. doi: 10.1001/jamainternmed.2014.8187. PMID: 25705824.

10. Imamura M, Biro S, Kihara T, Yoshifuku S, Takasaki K, Otsuji Y, Minagoe S, Toyama Y, Tei C. Repeated thermal therapy improves impaired vascular endothelial function in patients with coronary risk factors. J Am Coll Cardiol. 2001 Oct;38(4):1083-8. doi: 10.1016/s0735-1097(01)01467-x. PMID: 11583886.

11. Andersen, L. P., Werner, M. U., Rosenkilde, M. M., Harpsøe, N. G., Fuglsang, H., Rosenberg, J., & Gögenur, I. (2016). Pharmacokinetics of oral and intravenous melatonin in healthy volunteers. *BMC pharmacology & toxicology*, *17*, 8. https://doi.org/10.1186/s40360-016-0052-2

12. Kennaway DJ, Seamark RF. Circulating levels of melatonin following its oral administration or subcutaneous injection in sheep and goats. Aust J Biol Sci. 1980 Jun;33(3):349-53. doi: 10.1071/bi9800349. PMID: 7425968.

13. DeMuro RL, Nafziger AN, Blask DE, Menhinick AM, Bertino Jr JS. The absolute bioavailability of oral melatonin. J Clin Pharmacol. 2000;40:781–4.

14. Silva AC, Santos D, et al. Lipid-based nanocarriers as an alternative for oral delivery of poorly water-soluble drugs: Peroral and mucosal routes. Curr Med Chem. 2012;19(26):4495-4510. View Abstract

15. Rogers JA, Anderson KE. The potential of liposomes in oral drug delivery. Crit Rev Ther Drug Carrier Syst. 1998;15(5):421-480. View Abstract

16. Levitskaia TG, Morris JE. Aminothiol receptors for decorporation of intravenously administered (60)Co in the rat. Health Phys. 2010 Jan;98(1):53-60. View Full Paper

17. Zeevalk GD, Bernard LP Liposomal-glutathione provides maintenance of intracellular glutathione and neuroprotection in mesencephalic neuronal cells. Neurochem Res. 2010 Oct;35(10):1575-87. View Abstract